OAT™

Fourth Edition

OAT™

Fourth Edition

The Staff of Kaplan Test Prep and Admissions

KAPLAN
PUBLISHING
New York

Published by Kaplan Publishing, a division of Kaplan, Inc.
1 Liberty Plaza, 24th Floor
New York, NY 10006

Printed in the United States of America

10 9 8 7 6 5 4 3 2 1

ISBN 13: 978-1-4195-5035-5

Table of Contents

How to Use This Book

Congratulations on buying the best Optometry Admissions Test (OAT) test-prep book available. Kaplan's *OAT* provides you with key test strategies, practice sets for each of the four OAT sections, and two full-length OAT practice tests. All the questions in this book are followed by thorough, detailed explanations.

This book will test your understanding of college-level biology, general chemistry, organic chemistry, and physics, as well as your reading comprehension ability. In addition, you will become familiar with the format and style of the OAT. Here's how to use the various components of Kaplan's *OAT.*

STEP ONE: READ THE OAT STRATEGIES SECTION

In this section, we've distilled the main techniques and approaches from our popular live OAT course in a clear, easy-to-grasp format. We'll introduce you to the idiosyncrasies of the OAT and show you how to take control of the test-taking experience on all levels, including:

- Test strategies
- Specific methods and strategies for tackling OAT passages and questions
- Test expertise
- Test mentality

You'll review item-specific techniques, and get advice on how to pace yourself on each section and how to decide when to answer questions and when to guess. We'll teach you how the peculiarities of a standardized test can be used to your advantage. Plus, you'll learn the winning attitude for executing all you've learned and for facing the OAT with confidence.

STEP TWO: COMPLETE THE PRACTICE SETS

The practice tests in Section Two are shorter than the related sections on an actual OAT examination. These problem sets will help you warm up for the more grueling experience of a full-length OAT. They contain simulated OAT passages and questions that are followed by detailed explanations, including rationales for why the right answers are right and why each of the other choices is incorrect. By working through these problems, you'll familiarize yourself with the design of OAT questions. By analyzing the explanations, you'll appreciate how solid OAT-style thinking can get you to the correct answers quickly. In short, you'll learn to think like the test makers. As you work through these problems, try to identify your strengths and weaknesses. After completing these tests, you'll be ready tackle the two full-length practice OATs at the end of the book.

STEP THREE: TAKE KAPLAN'S FULL-LENGTH PRACTICE OATs

After you've learned valuable test strategies and completed the practice sets, take the full-length practice tests—two timed, simulated OATs—as a test run for the real thing. The explanations for every question on the test are included in this book so you can understand your mistakes. Try not to confine your review to the explanations for the questions you've gotten wrong. Instead, read all the explanations to reinforce key concepts and sharpen your skills.

STEP FOUR: REVIEW TO SHORE UP WEAK POINTS

If you find your performance was weak in any area, go back to the section in which that material was tested and review the explanations.

After you're finished, relax! You've prepared with the best and are ready for Test Day!

kaptest.com/publishing

The material in this book is up-to-date at the time of publication. However, the American Association of Schools and Colleges of Optometry may have instituted changes in the test after this book was published. Be sure to carefully read the materials you receive when you register for the test. For any important late-breaking developments—or changes or corrections to the Kaplan test preparation materials in this book—we will post that information online at **kaptest.com/publishing.** Check to see if there is any information posted there regarding this book.

kaplansurveys.com/books

What did you think of this book? We'd like to hear your comments and suggestions. We invite you to fill out our online survey form at **kaplansurveys.com/books**. Your feedback is extremely helpful as we continue to develop high-quality resources to meet your needs.

| SECTION ONE |

OAT Strategies

Chapter 1: **Introduction to the OAT**

- **The Computer-Based OAT**
- **Registration**
- **Anatomy of the OAT**
- **Scoring**
- **Take Control: The OAT Mindset**

The Optometry Admission Test, affectionately known as the OAT, is different from any other test you've encountered in your academic career. It's not like the knowledge-based exams from high school and college, whose emphasis was on memorizing and regurgitating information. Optometry schools can assess your academic prowess by looking at your transcript. The OAT isn't even like other standardized tests you may have taken, where the focus was on proving your general skills.

The Optometry Admission Test (OAT) was developed by the American Optometry Association and is sponsored by the Association of Schools and Colleges of Optometry. All schools and colleges of optometry require candidates to submit OAT scores for admission. The OAT is designed to predict general academic ability and measure the two skills needed by future optometrists: scientific knowledge and analytical ability. It does this by testing your knowledge of physics, chemistry, and biology; your reading comprehension ability; and your quantitative reasoning skills.

Optometry schools use OAT scores to assess whether you possess the foundation upon which to build a successful career in optometry. Though you certainly need to know the content to do well, the stress is on thought process, because the OAT is above all else a thinking test. That's why it emphasizes reasoning, critical and analytical thinking, reading comprehension, data analysis, and problem-solving skills.

The OAT's power comes from its use as an indicator of your abilities. Good scores can open doors. Your power comes from preparation and mindset, because the key to OAT success is knowing what you're up against. And that's where this section of this book comes in. We'll explain the philosophy behind the test, review the sections one by one, share some of Kaplan's proven methods, and clue you in to what the test makers are really after. You'll get a handle on the process, find a confident new perspective, and achieve your highest possible scores.

THE COMPUTER-BASED OAT

Now that a computer-based version of the Optometry Admission Test is available, the paper-based OAT has been phased out. Now instead of being restricted to two testing dates a year, testing is available year round and an examinee can select the date, time, and place.

A summary of the test changes is as follows:

- Students must wait 90 days between test administrations.
- The computer-based test (CBT) will be offered year round.
- Students may take the test an unlimited number of times, but only scores from the four most recent attempts will be reported.
- OAT CBT test-takers will get their scores on the day of their test. Schools will have a three-week period after the test to receive the scores.
- Once students begin any section of the test, they cannot void or cancel it.
- An extra 10 minutes have been added to the computer OAT Reading Comprehension section, to provide time for scrolling the passages on the computer.
- The fee for the OAT CBT will be $195.

REGISTRATION

The OAT is offered in a computer-based format. The CBT is offered year round. It is offered by Prometric at testing centers in the U.S. and its territories and in Canada. Most students take the exam after completing several years of college, including courses in advanced sciences like biology, chemistry, and physics. You can contact the OAT Program Office at the following address and ask for a registration packet:

Optometry Admission Testing Program
211 East Chicago Avenue, Suite 600
Chicago, IL 60611-2678
(800) 232-2159

Note that there is no longer any overseas testing.

ANATOMY OF THE OAT

Before mastering strategies, you need to know exactly what you're dealing with on the OAT. Let's start with the basics: The OAT is, among other things, an endurance test. It consists of close to four hours of stand-alone multiple-choice questions. Add in the administrative details at both ends of the testing experience, plus breaks (including lunch), and you can count on being in the test room for well over five hours. It's a grueling experience, to say the least. If you can't approach it with confidence and stamina, you'll quickly lose your composure. That's why it's so important that you take control of the test.

The OAT consists of four timed sections: Survey of the Natural Sciences, Reading Comprehension, Physics, and Quantitative Reasoning. Later in this book you will have an opportunity to attempt individual practice sets in all four sections plus two full-length practice tests. For now, you'll find a general overview in the table below.

Section	Time	Number of Questions	Topics Tested
1. Survey of Natural Sciences	90 minutes	100 questions	Biology Inorganic Chemistry Organic Chemistry
2. Reading Comprehension	60 minutes	50 questions	Ability to find main idea Ability to process information Ability to read and understand dense passages
3. Physics	50 minutes	40 questions	Vectors Energy and Momentum Thermodynamics Magnetism Optics
4. Quantitative Reasoning	45 minutes	50 questions	Arithmetic Algebra Geometry Trigonometry

The sections of the test always appear in the same order as above. There is a 15-minute introductory tutorial and a 10-minute post-test survey. Examinees may request scratch paper from the administrator. All scratch paper must be returned to the administrator before leaving the testing center. You won't be allowed to use a calculator.

SCORING

The OAT is given a scaled score of 200–400, 300 being the median representing the 40th–52nd percentile. Separate subscores are reported for biology, general chemistry, organic chemistry, reading comprehension, and quantitative reasoning.

Each question within a section is worth the same amount, and *there's no penalty for guessing*. That means that *you should always answer every question whether you get to that question or not!* This is an important piece of advice, so pay it heed. Never let time run out on any section without filling in an answer for every question.

Your score report will tell you (and optometry schools) not only your scaled scores but also your percentile ranking. Students often ask: what's a good score? Much depends on the strength of the rest of your application (if your transcript is first-rate, the pressure to strut your stuff on the OAT isn't as intense) and on where you want to go to school (different schools have different score expectations). Recent statistics show that the average score on the OAT is a 300.

TAKE CONTROL: THE OAT MINDSET

In addition to being a thinking test, as we've stressed, the OAT is a standardized test. As such, it has its own consistent patterns and idiosyncrasies that can actually work in your favor. This is the key to why test preparation works. You have the opportunity to familiarize yourself with those consistent peculiarities, to adopt the proper test-taking mindset.

The OAT Mindset is something you want to bring to every question and section you encounter. Being in the OAT Mindset means reshaping the test-taking experience so that you are in the driver's seat:

- Answer questions when you want to—feel free to skip tough but doable passages and questions, coming back to them only after you've racked up points on easy ones.
- Answer questions how you want to—use our shortcuts and methods to get points quickly and confidently, even if those methods aren't exactly what the test makers had in mind when they wrote the test.

The following are some overriding principles of the OAT Mindset that are covered in depth in the chapters to come:

- Read actively and critically.
- Translate prose into your own words.
- Save the toughest questions for last.
- Know the test and its components inside and out.
- Do OAT-style problems in each topic area after you've reviewed it.
- Allow your confidence to build on itself.
- Take full-length practice tests a week or two before the test to break down the mystique of the real experience.
- Learn from your mistakes—get the most out of your practice tests.
- Look at the OAT as a challenge, the first step in your optometry career, rather than as an arbitrary obstacle.

And that's what the OAT Mindset boils down to: taking control, being proactive, being on top of the testing experience so that you can get as many points as you can as quickly and as easily as possible. Keep this in mind as you read and work through the material in this book and, of course, as you face the challenge on Test Day.

Chapter 2: **Test Expertise**

- **Kaplan's Five Basic Principles of Test Expertise**
- **OAT Section-Specific Pacing**
- **Computer-Based OAT Strategies**

The first year of optometry school is a frenzied experience for most students. In order to meet the requirements of a rigorous work schedule, they either learn to prioritize and budget their time or else fall hopelessly behind. It's no surprise, then, that the OAT, the test specifically designed to predict success in the first year of optometry school, is a high-speed, time-intensive test.

It's one thing to answer a Reading Comprehension question correctly; it's quite another to answer 60 of them correctly in 50 minutes (60 on the computer test). And the same goes for Natural Sciences, Physics, and Quantitative Reasoning. It's a whole new ball game once you move from doing an individual passage at your leisure to handling a full section under actual timed conditions. When it comes to the multiple-choice sections, time pressure is a factor that affects virtually every test taker.

So when you are comfortable with the content of the test, your next challenge will be to take it to the next level, test expertise, which will enable you to manage the all-important time element of the test.

KAPLAN'S FIVE BASIC PRINCIPLES OF TEST EXPERTISE

On some tests, if a question seems particularly difficult, you spend significantly more time on it, since you'll probably be given more points for correctly answering a hard question. Not so on the OAT. Remember, every OAT question, no matter how hard, is worth a single point. There's no partial credit or "A" for effort. And since there are so many questions to do in so little time, it wouldn't make sense to spend ten minutes getting a point for a hard question and then not have time to get a couple of quick points from three easy questions later in the section.

Given this combination—limited time, all questions equal in weight—you have to develop a way of handling the test sections to make sure you get as many points as you can as quickly and easily as you can. Here are the principles that will help you do that:

1. Feel Free to Skip Around

One of the most valuable strategies to help you finish the sections in time is to learn to recognize and deal first with the questions that are easier and more familiar to you. That means temporarily skipping those that promise to be difficult and time-consuming, if you feel comfortable doing so. You can always come back to these at the end, and if you run out of time, you're much better off not getting to questions you may have had difficulty with, rather than missing out on potentially score-raising material. Of course, since there's no guessing penalty, always fill in an answer to every question on the test, whether you get to it or not.

This strategy is difficult for most test takers; we're conditioned to do things in order. But give it a try when you practice. Remember, if you do the test in the exact order given, you're letting the test makers control you. But *you* control how you take this test. On the other hand, if skipping around goes against your moral fiber and makes you a nervous wreck—don't do it. Just be mindful of the clock and don't get bogged down with the tough questions.

2. Learn to Recognize and Seek Out Questions You Can Do

Another thing to remember about managing the test sections is that OAT questions and passages, unlike items on the SAT and other standardized tests, are not presented in order of difficulty. There's no rule that says you have to work through the sections in any particular order; in fact, the test makers scatter the easy and difficult questions throughout the section, in effect rewarding those who actually get to the end. Don't lose sight of what you're being tested for along with your reading and thinking skills: efficiency and cleverness. If organic chemistry questions are your thing, head straight for them when you first turn to the Natural Sciences section.

Don't waste time on questions you can't do. We know that skipping a possibly tough question is easier said than done; we all have the natural instinct to plow through test sections in their given order. But it just doesn't pay off on the OAT. The computer won't be impressed if you get the toughest question right. If you dig in your heels on a tough question, refusing to move on until you've cracked it, well, you're letting your ego get in the way of your test score. A test section (not to mention life itself) is too short to waste on lost causes.

3. Use a Process of Answer Elimination

Using a process of elimination is another way to answer questions both quickly and effectively. There are two ways to get all the answers right on the OAT. You either know all the right answers, or you know all the wrong answers. Since there are three times as many wrong answer choices, you should be able to eliminate some if not all of them. By doing so, you either get to the correct response or increase your chances of guessing the correct response. You start out with a 25 percent chance of picking the right answer, and with each eliminated answer, your odds go up. Eliminate one, and you'll have a 33 1/3 percent chance of picking the right one; eliminate two, and you'll have a 50 percent chance; and, of course, eliminate three, and you'll have a 100 percent chance. Increase your efficiency by actually crossing out the wrong choices in your test booklet. Remember to look for wrong-answer traps when you're eliminating. Some answers are designed to seduce you by distorting the correct answer.

4. Remain Calm

It's imperative that you remain calm and composed while working through a section. You can't allow yourself to become so rattled by one hard reading passage that it throws off your performance on the rest of the section. Expect to find at least a few killer questions in every section, but remember, you won't be the only one to have trouble with it. The test is curved to take the tough material into account. Having trouble with a difficult question isn't going to ruin your score—but getting upset about it and letting it throw you off track will. When you understand that part of the test-maker's goal is to reward those who keep their composure, you'll recognize the importance of not panicking when you run into challenging material.

5. Keep Track of Time

Of course, the last thing you want to happen is to have time called on a particular section before you've gotten to half the questions. Therefore, it's essential that you pace yourself, keeping in mind the general guidelines for how long to spend on any individual question. Have a sense of how long you have to do each question, so you know when you're exceeding the limit and should start to move faster.

When working on a section, always remember to keep track of time. Don't spend a wildly disproportionate amount of time on any one question or group of questions. Also, give yourself 30 seconds or so at the end of each section to fill in answers for any questions you haven't gotten to.

OAT SECTION-SPECIFIC PACING

Natural Sciences

You have 90 minutes to answer 40 questions on Biology, 30 questions on General Chemistry, and 30 questions on Organic Chemistry for a total of 100 stand-alone multiple-choice questions. Essentially, you have a little under a minute per question (52 seconds, to be exact). The key to remember is that some questions require more time whereas others don't take as much time. Begin with your strengths and answer all questions that you are comfortable with. Mark the tough questions and come back to them at the end.

Reading Comprehension

You have 60 minutes to do three passages, each of which has 16–17 questions for a total of 50 questions. Allow yourself approximately 17–20 minutes per passage. It may seem like a lot of time, but it goes by quickly. Do the easiest passages first. Within a section, if you're deciding which passage to do based on time alone, do the one with the most questions. That way you maximize your reading efficiency. However, keep in mind that some passages are longer than others. On average, give yourself about 7 or 8 minutes to read and then 9 or 10 minutes for the questions.

Physics and Quantitative Reasoning

You have 50 minutes to answer 40 stand-alone multiple-choice questions in Physics (a little over a minute per question) and 45 minutes to answer 50 stand-alone multiple-choice questions in Quantitative Reasoning (a little under a minute per question). The same strategy that is useful in Natural Sciences applies here. Go with your strengths and answer the questions that are easiest for you. Mark the tough questions so you can come back to them at the end.

COMPUTER-BASED OAT STRATEGIES

Since the OAT is only given in the CBT format, it is important to keep the following strategies in mind:

Tutorial

Don't ignore this section of your test experience. Even if you are a computer whiz, this is a source of important information. Be as prepared and comfortable with your test station as possible.

Marking Function

On the computer-based OAT, it is a bit less easy to jump around the testing sections and go back and forth between questions than it was on the paper-and-pencil test. You can go back and forth within a section, but this takes time. However, you have a function available to you called "Mark" that you can use to mark the tough questions with. You can get back to these after you've answered all the easy questions. At the end of the section, the screen will prompt you to review marked questions, and you can go back to answer these then. There is no penalty for guessing, so answer them all.

Chapter 3: **Test Mentality**

- **Kaplan's Four Basic Principles of Good Test Mentality**
- **Quick Tips for the Days Just Before the Exam**
- **Handling Stress During the Test**
- **Kaplan's Top Ten OAT Tips**

In this section, we first glanced at the content that makes up each specific section of the OAT, focusing on the strategies and techniques you'll need to tackle individual questions and passages. Then we discussed the test expertise involved in moving from individual items to working through full-length sections. Now we're ready to turn our attention to the often-overlooked attitudinal aspects of the test, to put the finishing touches on your comprehensive OAT approach.

KAPLAN'S FOUR BASIC PRINCIPLES OF GOOD TEST MENTALITY

Knowing the test content arms you with the weapons you need to do well on the OAT. But you must wield those weapons with the right frame of mind and in the right spirit. Otherwise, you could end up shooting yourself in the foot. This involves taking a certain stance toward the entire test. Here's what's involved:

1. Test Awareness

To do your best on the OAT, you must always keep in mind that the test is like no other test you've taken before, both in terms of content and in terms of the scoring system. If you took a test in high school or college and got a number of the questions wrong, you wouldn't receive a perfect grade. But on the OAT, you can get a handful of questions wrong and still get a "perfect" score. The test is geared so that only the very best test takers are able to finish every section. But even these people rarely get every question right.

What does this mean for you? Well, just as you shouldn't let one bad question ruin an entire section, you shouldn't let what you consider to be a subpar performance on one section ruin your performance on the entire test. If you allow that subpar performance to rattle you, it can have a cumulative negative effect, setting in motion a downward spiral. It's that kind of thing that could potentially do serious damage to your score. Losing a few extra points won't do you in, but losing your cool will.

Remember, if you feel you've done poorly on a section, don't sweat it. Chances are it's just a difficult section, and that factor will already be figured into the scoring curve. The point is, remain calm and collected. Simply do your best on each section, and once a section is over, forget about it and move on.

2. Stamina

You must work on your test-taking stamina. Overall, the OAT is a fairly grueling experience, and some test takers simply run out of gas on the last section. To avoid this, you must prepare by taking a few full-length Practice Tests in the weeks before the test, so that on Test Day, all four sections will seem like a breeze. (Well, maybe not a breeze, but at least not a hurricane.)

Take the full-length practice tests included in this book. You'll be able to review answer explanations and assess your performance. You should, of course, keep in mind that every OAT administration differs; you can't assume that your actual score will be predicted by your score on a Practice Test. The score you'll get on any Practice Test is less important than the practice itself.

For those students who want more intensive preparation, Kaplan offers a wide range of OAT prep options, including classroom-based courses, private tutoring, and online courses. Visit **kaptest.com** for more information or to enroll in these courses. Your best option, if you have time, would be to take the live Kaplan course. We'll give you access to all the released material plus loads of additional material, so you can really build up your OAT stamina. You'll also have the benefit of our expert live instruction on every aspect of the OAT. To go this route, call 800-KAP-TEST or visit **kaptest.com** for a Kaplan center location near you.

Reading this chapter is a great start in your preparation for the test, but it won't get you your best score. That can happen only after lots of practice and skill-building. You've got to train your brain to be test-smart! Kaplan has been helping people do that for over 60 years, so giving us a call would be a great way to move your test prep into high gear!

3. Confidence

Confidence feeds on itself, and unfortunately, so does the opposite of confidence—self-doubt. Confidence in your ability leads to quick, sure answers and a sense of well-being that translates into more points. If you lack confidence, you end up reading the sentences and answer choices two, three, or four times, until you confuse yourself and get off track. This leads to timing difficulties, which only perpetuate the downward spiral, causing anxiety and a tendency to rush in order to finish sections.

If you subscribe to the OAT Mindset we've described, however, you'll gear all of your practice toward the major goal of taking control of the test. When you've achieved that goal—armed with the principles, techniques, strategies, and approaches set forth in this book—you'll be ready to face the OAT with supreme confidence. And that's the one sure way to score your best on Test Day.

4. The Right Attitude

Those who approach the OAT as an obstacle, who rail against the necessity of taking it, who make light of its importance, who spend more time making fun of the OAT than studying for the test, usually don't fare as well as those who see the OAT as an opportunity to show off the reading and reasoning skills that the optometry schools are looking for. Don't waste time making value judgments about the OAT. It is not going to go away, so deal with it. Those who look forward to doing battle with the OAT—or, at least, who enjoy the opportunity to distinguish themselves from the rest of the applicant pack—tend to score better than do those who resent or dread it.

It may sound a little dubious, but take our word for it: attitude adjustment is a proven test-taking technique. Here are a few steps you can take to make sure you develop the right OAT attitude:

- Look at the OAT as a challenge, but try not to obsess over it; you certainly don't want to psyche yourself out of the game.
- Remember that, yes, the OAT is obviously important, but contrary to what some students think, this one test will not single-handedly determine the outcome of your life.
- Try to have fun with the test. Learning how to match your wits against the test makers can be a very satisfying experience, and the reading and thinking skills you'll acquire will benefit you in optometry school as well as in your future optometry career.
- Remember that you're more prepared than most people. You've trained with Kaplan. You have the tools you need, plus the know-how to use those tools.

QUICK TIPS FOR THE DAYS JUST BEFORE THE EXAM

- The best test takers do less and less as the test approaches. Taper off your study schedule and take it easy on yourself. Give yourself time off, especially the evening before the exam. By that time, if you've studied well, everything you need to know is firmly stored in your memory bank.
- Positive self-talk can be extremely liberating and invigorating, especially as the test looms closer. Tell yourself things such as "I will do well," rather than "I hope things go well"; "I can," rather than "I cannot." Replace any negative thoughts with affirming statements that boost your self-esteem.
- Get your act together sooner rather than later. Have everything (including choice of clothing) laid out in advance. Most important, make sure you know where the test will be held and the easiest, quickest way to get there. You'll have great peace of mind by knowing that all the little details—gas in the car, directions, etc.—are set before the day of the test.
- Go to the test site a few days in advance, particularly if you are especially anxious. Better yet, bring some practice material and do at least a section or two.
- Forego any practice on the day before the test. It's in your best interest to marshal your physical and psychological resources for 24 hours or so. Even horses are kept in the paddock and treated like princes the day before a race. Keep the upcoming test out of your consciousness; go to a movie, take a pleasant hike, or just relax. Don't eat junk food or

tons of sugar. And, of course, get plenty of rest the night before—just don't go to bed too early. It's hard to fall asleep earlier than you're used to, and you don't want to lie there worrying about the test.

HANDLING STRESS DURING THE TEST

The biggest stress monster will be the test itself. Fear not; there are methods of quelling your stress during the test.

- Keep moving forward instead of getting bogged down in a difficult question. You don't have to get everything right to achieve a fine score. So don't linger out of desperation on a question that is going nowhere even after you've spent considerable time on it. The best test takers skip difficult material temporarily in search of the easier stuff. They mark and return to the questions that require extra time and thought.
- Don't be thrown if other test takers seem to be working more busily and furiously than you are. Don't mistake the other people's sheer activity as signs of progress and higher scores.
- Keep breathing! Weak test takers tend to share one major trait: they don't breathe properly as the test proceeds. They might hold their breath without realizing it or breathe erratically or arrhythmically. Improper breathing hurts confidence and accuracy. Just as importantly, it interferes with clear thinking.
- Some quick isometrics during the test—especially if concentration is wandering or energy is waning—can help. Try this: Put your palms together and press intensely for a few seconds. Concentrate on the tension you feel through your palms, wrists, forearms, and up into your biceps and shoulders. Then quickly release the pressure. Feel the difference as you let go. Focus on the warm relaxation that floods through the muscles. Now you're ready to return to the task.
- Here's another isometric that will relieve tension in both your neck and eye muscles. Slowly rotate your head from side to side, turning your head and eyes to look as far back over each shoulder as you can. Feel the muscles stretch on one side of your neck as they contract on the other. Repeat five times in each direction.

With what you've just learned here, you're armed and ready to do battle with the test. This book and your studies have given you the information you'll need to answer the questions. It's all firmly planted in your mind. You also know how to deal with any excess tension that might come along, both when you're studying for and taking the exam. You've experienced everything you need to tame your test anxiety and stress. You're going to get a great score.

KAPLAN'S TOP TEN OAT TIPS

1. Relax!
2. Remember: It's primarily a thinking test. Never forget the purpose of the OAT: it's designed to test your powers of analytical reasoning. You need to know the content, as each section has its own particular "language," but the underlying OAT intention is consistent throughout the test.
3. Feel free to skip around within each section. Attack each section confidently. You're in charge. Move around if you feel comfortable doing so. Work your best areas first to maximize your opportunity for OAT points. Choose the order in which to complete questions. Don't be a passive victim of the test structure!
4. Avoid wrong-answer traps. Try to anticipate answers before you read the answer choices. This helps boost your confidence and protects you from persuasive or tricky incorrect choices. Most wrong answer choices are logical twists on the correct choice.
5. Think, think, think! We said it before, but it's important enough to say again: think. Don't compute.
6. Don't look back. Don't spend time worrying about questions you had to guess on. Keep moving forward. Don't let your spirit start to flag, or your attitude will slow you down. You can recheck answers within a section if you have time left, but don't worry about a section after time has been called.
7. Be sure to take the computer tutorial. Learn how to mark questions so you can return to review them at the end of each section. There is no penalty for wrong answers, so be sure to answer every question.
8. Don't leave any questions unanswered. There are no points taken off for wrong answers, so if you're unsure of an answer, guess.
9. Take advantage of the "Mark" feature on the computer for questions you may want to revisit. At the end, you can review all your marked answers before you submit them as final.
10. Call us! We're here to help! 800-KAP-TEST. Or visit us on the Web at **kaptest.com**.

| SECTION TWO |

OAT Practice Sets

PERIODIC TABLE OF THE ELEMENTS

1 **H** 1.0																	2 **He** 4.0
3 **Li** 6.9	4 **Be** 9.0											5 **B** 10.8	6 **C** 12.0	7 **N** 14.0	8 **O** 16.0	9 **F** 19.0	10 **Ne** 20.2
11 **Na** 23.0	12 **Mg** 24.3											13 **Al** 27.0	14 **Si** 28.1	15 **P** 31.0	16 **S** 32.1	17 **Cl** 35.5	18 **Ar** 39.9
19 **K** 39.1	20 **Ca** 40.1	21 **Sc** 45.0	22 **Ti** 47.9	23 **V** 50.9	24 **Cr** 52.0	25 **Mn** 54.9	26 **Fe** 55.8	27 **Co** 58.9	28 **Ni** 58.7	29 **Cu** 63.5	30 **Zn** 65.4	31 **Ga** 69.7	32 **Ge** 72.6	33 **As** 74.9	34 **Se** 79.0	35 **Br** 79.9	36 **Kr** 83.8
37 **Rb** 85.5	38 **Sr** 87.6	39 **Y** 88.9	40 **Zr** 91.2	41 **Nb** 92.9	42 **Mo** 95.9	43 **Tc** (98)	44 **Ru** 101.1	45 **Rh** 102.9	46 **Pd** 106.4	47 **Ag** 107.9	48 **Cd** 112.4	49 **In** 114.8	50 **Sn** 118.7	51 **Sb** 121.8	52 **Te** 127.6	53 **I** 126.9	54 **Xe** 131.3
55 **Cs** 132.9	56 **Ba** 137.3	57 **La** * 138.9	72 **Hf** 178.5	73 **Ta** 180.9	74 **W** 183.9	75 **Re** 186.2	76 **Os** 190.2	77 **Ir** 192.2	78 **Pt** 195.1	79 **Au** 197.0	80 **Hg** 200.6	81 **Tl** 204.4	82 **Pb** 207.2	83 **Bi** 209.0	84 **Po** (209)	85 **At** (210)	86 **Rn** (222)
87 **Fr** (223)	88 **Ra** 226.0	89 **Ac** † 227.0	104 **Rf** (261)	105 **Db** (262)	106 **Sg** (263)	107 **Bh** (264)	108 **Hs** (269)	109 **Mt** (268)	110 **Ds** (269)	111 **Rg** (272)	112 **Uub** (277)	113 **Uut** (284)	114 **Uug** (289)	115 **Uup** (288)	116 **Uuh** (292)	117 **Uus** (291)	118 **Uuo** (293)

*	58 **Ce** 140.1	59 **Pr** 140.9	60 **Nd** 144.2	61 **Pm** (145)	62 **Sm** 150.4	63 **Eu** 152.0	64 **Gd** 157.3	65 **Tb** 158.9	66 **Dy** 162.5	67 **Ho** 164.9	68 **Er** 167.3	69 **Tm** 168.9	70 **Yb** 173.0	71 **Lu** 175.0
†	90 **Th** 232.0	91 **Pa** (231)	92 **U** 238.0	93 **Np** (237)	94 **Pu** (244)	95 **Am** (243)	96 **Cm** (247)	97 **Bk** (247)	98 **Cf** (251)	99 **Es** (252)	100 **Fm** (257)	101 **Md** (258)	102 **No** (259)	103 **Lr** (260)

Survey of the Natural Sciences: **Practice Set 1**

40 questions—36 minutes

Directions: Choose the best answer for each question from the five choices provided.

1. Mushroom is to Basidiomycota as moss is to
   (A) Myxomycophyta.
   (B) Bryophyta.
   (C) Rhodophyta.
   (D) angiosperm.
   (E) gymnosperm.

2. The red color of blood is produced by a pigment that requires
   (A) copper.
   (B) zinc.
   (C) iron.
   (D) sodium.
   (E) phosphorous.

3. A movement of muscle that tends to bend one part of the body upon the other is termed
   (A) flexion.
   (B) insertion.
   (C) tonus.
   (D) diastole.
   (E) extension.

4. Components of blood include
   (A) plasma.
   (B) red blood cells.
   (C) white blood cells.
   (D) cell fragments known as platelets.
   (E) All of the above

5. Which enzyme breaks down starch to disaccharides?
   (A) Amylase
   (B) Gastrin
   (C) Secretin
   (D) Pepsin
   (E) Maltase

6. Homeostasis
   (A) is the secretion of enzymes by the digestive glands.
   (B) is demonstrated by the action of the endocrine glands.
   (C) is shown by a cross of two homozygous traits.
   (D) is the capacity of living things to change internal conditions to meet environmental changes.
   (E) results in the death of living tissue.

GO ON TO THE NEXT PAGE

7. All of the following are essential for blood clotting EXCEPT
   (A) Na^+ ions.
   (B) Ca^{2+} ions.
   (C) prothrombin.
   (D) vitamin K.
   (E) platelets.

8. Which of the following is NOT a function of bone?
   (A) Formation of blood cells
   (B) Protection of vital organs
   (C) Maturation of T lymphocytes
   (D) Framework for movement
   (E) All of the above

9. Nematocysts are characteristic of
   (A) Porifera.
   (B) Protozoa.
   (C) Coelenterata.
   (D) Annelida.
   (E) Echinodermata.

10. A factor that tends to keep the gene pool constant is
    (A) nonrandom mating.
    (B) freedom to migrate.
    (C) mutations.
    (D) large populations.
    (E) None of the above

11. Bicarbonate ion in the blood
    (A) keeps the pH of the blood from fluctuating.
    (B) promotes phagocytosis by leukocytes.
    (C) carries O_2 to the lungs.
    (D) functions in the blood-clotting mechanism.
    (E) None of the above

12. Which of the following acts as the primary pacemaker of the heart?
    (A) Foramen ovale
    (B) Sino-atrial node
    (C) Ductus arteriosus
    (D) Bundle of His
    (E) Vagus nerve

13. The breathing center, which is located in the medulla oblongata, will cause an increase in the rate of breathing when the blood concentration of
    (A) O_2 decreases.
    (B) CO_2 decreases.
    (C) O_2 increases.
    (D) CO_2 increases.
    (E) N_2 decreases.

14. The glomerular filtrate in Bowman's capsule contains all of the following EXCEPT
    (A) glucose.
    (B) amino acids.
    (C) plasma proteins.
    (D) urea.
    (E) Na^+.

15. The lymphatic system
    (A) filters the capillary ultrafiltrate.
    (B) has its fluid propelled by muscular contraction.
    (C) returns lymph to the circulatory system via the thoracic duct.
    (D) Two of the above
    (E) All of the above

GO ON TO THE NEXT PAGE

16. In the pituitary gland

(A) the anterior pituitary directs pancreatic endocrine function.
(B) the anterior pituitary directs thyroid gland production.
(C) the posterior pituitary secretes progesterone.
(D) synthesis of steroid hormones takes place.
(E) the anterior pituitary secretes estrogen.

17. Which of the following will NOT affect the frequency of a gene in an ideal population?

(A) Environmental selective pressure
(B) Mutation
(C) Random breeding
(D) Nonrandom matings
(E) Selective emigration

18. The epiphyseal plate

(A) is a bone located in the skull.
(B) is part of the neuromuscular junction.
(C) is observed during mitosis.
(D) is the region of growth in a long bone.
(E) None of the above

19. Which of the following statements about systemic respiration is FALSE?

(A) O_2 and CO_2 exchange by passive diffusion.
(B) Oxyhemoglobin transports O_2 to the tissues.
(C) Hemoglobin is incapable of binding CO_2.
(D) Cellular respiration is a source of serum CO_2.
(E) O_2 and CO_2 are exchanged across the alveolar capillary membrane.

20. The anterior pituitary gland is able to affect all of the following directly EXCEPT

(A) adrenal gland function.
(B) concentration of the urine.
(C) thyroid gland function.
(D) egg follicle growth.
(E) lactation.

Questions 21–22 refer to the table below:

Half Reaction	E°
$Mg \rightarrow Mg^{2+} + 2e-$	2.37 V
$Mn \rightarrow Mn^{2+} + 2e-$	1.03 V
$H_2 \rightarrow 2H^+ + 2e-$	0.00 V
$Cu \rightarrow Cu^{2+} + 2e-$	−0.16 V

21. Which of the following reactions is spontaneous?

(A) $Mn^{2+} + H_2 \rightarrow$
(B) $Mg + Mn^{2+} \rightarrow$
(C) $Mg^{2+} + Mn \rightarrow$
(D) $Cu + 2H^+ \rightarrow$
(E) $Mg^{2+} + Cu \rightarrow$

22. What will be the maximum cell potential for the reaction in the answer to question 21?

(A) −0.16 V
(B) −1.34 V
(C) +1.03 V
(D) +1.34 V
(E) +2.21 V

23. If 3.0 liters of 0.50 M NaCl(*aq*) is mixed with 9.0 liters of 0.2777 M NaCl(*aq*), what is the final concentration of the resulting solution?

(A) 0.33 M
(B) 0.39 M
(C) 0.44 M
(D) 0.58 M
(E) 5.33 M

GO ON TO THE NEXT PAGE

24. How many grams of H_3PO_4 are needed to make 50 mL of a 2.5 N H_3PO_4 solution? (Atomic weights: H = 1, P = 31, O = 16)

(A) 12.36 g
(B) 4.08 g
(C) 12.36×10^3 g
(D) 4.08×10^3 g
(E) 98 g

25. What happens to the entropy of a solid when it is dissolved in a solvent?

(A) It increases.
(B) It decreases.
(C) It remains the same.
(D) It decreases, then increases.
(E) It increases, then decreases.

26. At 760 torr, Solution X boils at 100.26°C and Solution Y boils at 101.04°C. If both aqueous solutions contain the same nonvolatile solute, which of the following is a correct conclusion?

(A) The freezing point of solution X is lower than that of Solution Y.
(B) Solution Y is saturated.
(C) The vapor pressure of Solution X is higher than that of Solution Y at 25°C.
(D) Solution X is hypertonic to Solution Y.
(E) The vapor pressure of Solution X at boiling is greater than the vapor pressure of Solution Y at boiling.

27. The half-life of the radioactive element Weissonium is 6 days. How much of an original sample of 30 grams will have decayed after 24 days?

(A) $1\frac{7}{8}$ g
(B) 7.5 g
(C) 22.5 g
(D) 25 g
(E) $28\frac{1}{8}$ g

28. The normality of a potassium permanganate solution is 2.10. What is the molarity of the product of the reaction of postassium permanganate to manganese dioxide?

(A) 0.30 M
(B) 0.70 M
(C) 2.10 M
(D) 6.30 M
(E) 10.50 M

29. How many grams of $Al_2(SO_4)_3$ are needed to make 87.5 g of 0.3 *m* $Al_2(SO_4)_3$ solution? (Atomic weights: Al = 27, S = 32, O = 16)

(A) $102.6/(87.5 \times 1{,}000)$
(B) $(87.5 \times 102.6)/1{,}000$
(C) $87.5/1{,}102.6$
(D) $102.6/(87.5 \times 1{,}102.6)$
(E) $(87.5 \times 102.6)/1{,}102.6$

30. Which of the following describes a possible synthesis of *m*-nitrobenzoic acid from toluene?

(A) Reaction with alkaline $KMnO_4$, followed by HNO_3 and H_2SO_4
(B) Reaction with HNO_3 and H_2SO_4, followed by acidic $K_2Cr_2O_7$
(C) Reaction with alkaline $KMnO_4$, followed by $NaNO_2$ and HCl
(D) Reaction with $NaNO_2$ and HCl, followed by acidic $K_2Cr_2O_7$
(E) Reaction with alkaline $KMnO_4$, followed by $NaNO_2$ and NaOH

GO ON TO THE NEXT PAGE

31. Which of the following most properly depicts a pair of tautomers?

(A) 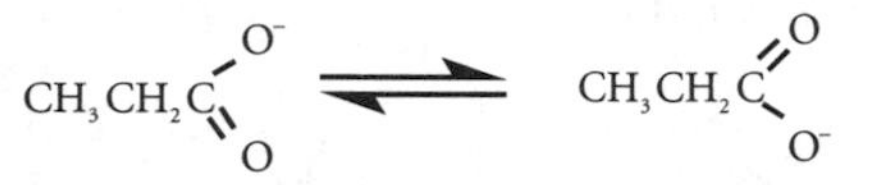

(B) $H_2C{=}CHCH_2^+ \rightleftharpoons {}^+H_2CCH{=}CH_2$

(C) 

(D) 

(E) 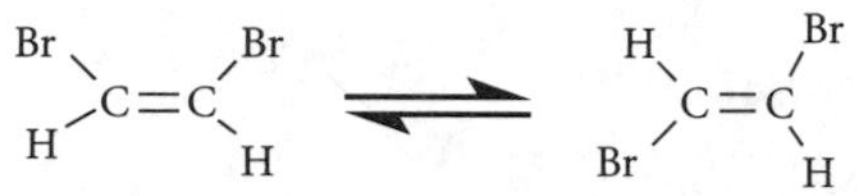

32. Which of the following substituents has the greatest electron-withdrawing effect?

(A) Br
(B) Cl
(C) F
(D) CH_3
(E) NH_2

33. Which of the following alkenes would react MOST rapidly with HCl?

(A) Chloroethene
(B) *Cis*-1,2-dichloroethene
(C) *Trans*-2-butene
(D) Propene
(E) 2-methylpropene

34. When pure Compound X is subjected to ozonolysis, the only organic product formed is butanal. Compound X can be

(A) *trans*-2-butene.
(B) *cis*-2-pentene.
(C) *cis*-3-hexene.
(D) *trans*-3-heptene.
(E) *cis*-4-octene.

35. Which hydrogen is most acidic?

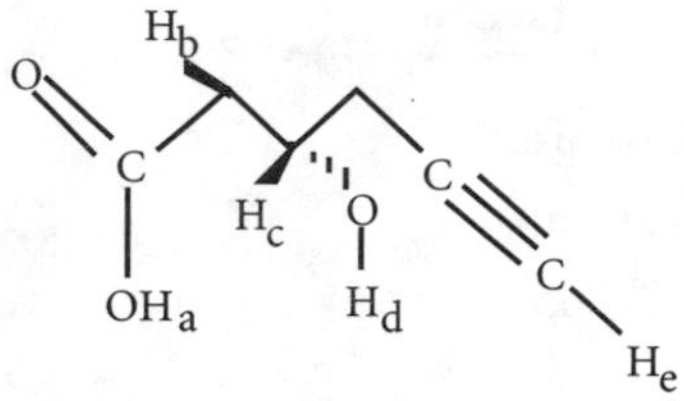

(A) H_a
(B) H_b
(C) H_c
(D) H_d
(E) H_e

36. In the reaction below, which of the following would be made?

$$CH_4 \xrightarrow[h\upsilon]{Cl_2} ?$$

(A) CH_3Cl
(B) CH_2Cl_2
(C) $CHCl_3$
(D) CCl_4
(E) All of the above

37. The NMR spectrum for a compound shows a signal at 8.5 ppm. Based on this evidence alone, it can be inferred that the compound most likely has at least one

    (A) isolated double bond.
    (B) nonterminal triple bond.
    (C) aromatic ring.
    (D) localized negative charge.
    (E) localized positive charge.

38. What is the product of the following reaction?
    n-propyl chloride $\xrightarrow{\text{KOH(alc)}}$?

    (A) Isopropyl chloride
    (B) Isopropyl alcohol
    (C) *n*-propyl alcohol
    (D) Propylene
    (E) 2-chloro-1-propanol

39. Rank the following compounds in order of decreasing reactivity for electrophilic aromatic substitution.

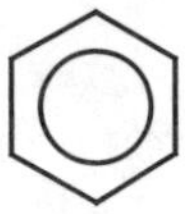

I

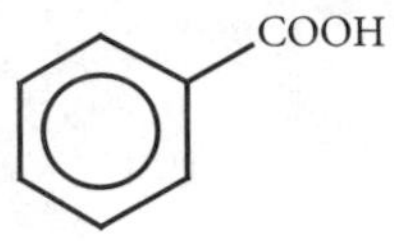

II

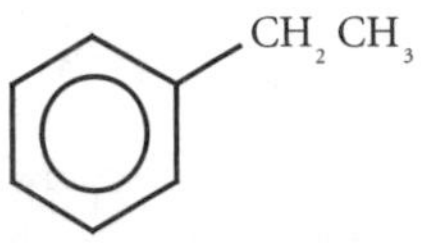

III

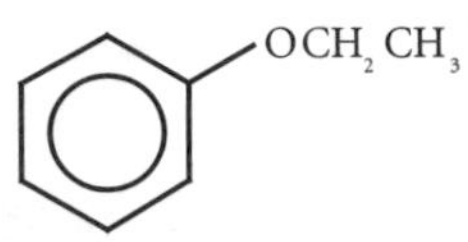

IV

    (A) II, IV, III, I
    (B) III, IV, II, I
    (C) IV, III, I, II
    (D) IV, III, II, I
    (E) III, IV, I, II

40. What is the missing reagent in the following reaction?

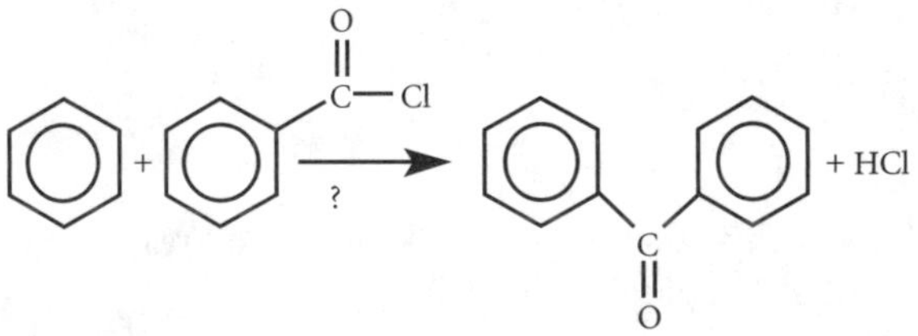

    (A) $AlCl_3$
    (B) MgBr
    (C) MgCl
    (D) PCl_3
    (E) NaOH(*aq*)

IF YOU FINISH BEFORE TIME IS CALLED, YOU MAY CHECK YOUR WORK ON THIS SECTION ONLY. DO NOT TURN TO ANY OTHER SECTION IN THE TEST. **STOP**

THE ANSWER KEY APPEARS ON THE FOLLOWING PAGE.

ANSWERS AND EXPLANATIONS

1. B	11. A	21. B	31. D
2. C	12. B	22. D	32. C
3. A	13. D	23. A	33. E
4. E	14. C	24. B	34. E
5. A	15. E	25. A	35. A
6. D	16. B	26. C	36. E
7. A	17. C	27. E	37. C
8. C	18. D	28. B	38. D
9. C	19. C	29. E	39. C
10. D	20. B	30. A	40. A

1. B

Basidiomycota is the division of the plant kingdom that includes mushrooms. A division is a major category on the same level as a phylum in the animal kingdom. The question is asking for the division of the plant kingdom that includes moss. Mosses are members of the division Bryophyta, which is characterized by simple plants with few specialized organs and tissues. They lack water-conducting woody material (xylem), which functions as support in higher plants; and retain flagellated sperm cells, which must swim to the eggs. Thus, they have never become successful terrestrial plants. Mosses are primitive bryophytes in which the gametophyte has a filamentous protonema (young moss plant) from which grows a vertical "stem" with radial leaves and a short sporophyte consisting of a foot, stalk, and a capsule filled with spores. (A) is incorrect because Myxomycophyta are slime molds. (C) is incorrect because Rhodophyta contains the red algae. (D) and (E) are incorrect because angiosperms and gymnosperms are members of the division Tracheophyta (higher plants) and are differentiated from each other by their seeds. Angiosperms such as maple and banana trees have covered seeds whereas gymnosperms such as pines and firs have naked seeds.

2. C

The oxidized form of iron present in hemoglobin causes the blood to appear red. (A) is incorrect because oxidized copper would cause the blood to have a bluish appearance, and (B), (D), and (E) would not affect the color of the blood.

3. A

Flexion is the bending of a joint to an acute angle. (B) is incorrect because insertion is the portion of the muscle attached to the bone that moves during contraction. (C) is incorrect because tonus is the continuous state of muscle contraction. (D) is incorrect because diastole is a period of relaxation of cardiac muscles when the AV valves open and the ventricles fill with blood. (E) is incorrect because extension is the straightening of the bones at a joint.

4. E

Blood is made up of answer choices (A), (B), (C), and (D). Plasma is the liquid part of blood containing dissolved nutrients, wastes, proteins, hormones, and fibrinogen. Red blood cells are the anucleated, biconcave discs filled with hemoglobin, which unites with oxygen to form oxyhemoglobin. White blood cells are cells of the body's defense system. These large cells include phagocytes, which engulf bacteria, and lymphocytes, which are involved in the specific immune responses.

5. A

Amylase (pancreatic or salivary) breaks down complex carbohydrates into disaccharides (pancreatic or salivary). (B) is incorrect because gastrin is a hormone secreted by the stomach wall of mammals when food makes contact with the wall; it stimulates other parts of the wall to secrete gastric juice. (C) is incorrect because secretin is secreted by the small intestine and stimulates the pancreas to secrete pancreatic juice containing bicarbonate ions to buffer the chyme. (D) is incorrect because pepsin breaks down proteins into amino acids, and (E) is incorrect because maltase breaks down maltose into glucose.

6. D

Homeostasis is the maintenance of a stable internal physiological environment in an organism. Answer choices (A), (B), (C), and (E) are incorrect as they are not part of this process.

7. A

Clotting occurs when platelets in an open wound release thromboplastin, which initiates a series of reactions ultimately leading to the formation of a fibrin plug. Thromboplastin, with calcium and vitamin K as cofactors, leads to the conversion of inactive plasma prothrombin to the active form thrombin. Thrombin converts fibrinogen into the fibrinous protein, fibrin. Threads of fibrin trap red blood cells to form clots.

8. C

The bony skeleton serves as a framework within all vertebrate organisms. Muscles are attached to the bones, permitting movement. The skeleton also provides protection for vital organs. For example, the rib cage protects the heart and the lungs whereas the skull and vertebral column protect the brain and the spinal cord. The hollow cavity formed within each bone is subsequently filled with bone marrow, which is the site of formation of blood cells. Although all hematopoietic cells are formed in the bone marrow, T lymphocytes are educated and matured in the thymus.

9. C

Nematocysts are stinging cells found in coelenterates and are used to immobilize prey. Coelenterates are organisms such as hydra and jellyfish, which are radially symmetrical and have one opening to their digestive tract that acts as both a mouth and an anus. (A) is incorrect because Porifera are organisms (i.e., sponges) that have no defined tissue or organs. (B) is incorrect because protozoa are one-celled organisms such as paramecia and amoebae. (D) is incorrect because annelids are segmented invertebrates such as earthworms with a true body cavity (coelom) having two openings in their digestive tract. (E) is incorrect because echinoderms are organisms such as starfish and sea cucumbers thought to be a primitive predecessor to vertebrates. They are radially symmetrical as adults and bilaterally symmetrical as larvae, have a circulatory system made up of a water vascular system, and move via tube feet.

10. D

The Hardy-Weinberg Law states that gene ratios and allelic frequencies remain constant through the generations in a nonevolving population. Four criteria must be met for this to occur: (1) random mating, (2) a large population, (3) no migration into or out of the population, and (4) a lack of mutation. If all four of these are met, the gene frequencies will remain constant. Anytime all four of these are not met, the gene frequencies will change and evolution may occur.

11. A

Bicarbonate ion acts as a buffer to maintain the pH of the blood. For example, alkalosis will cause hyperventilation, which will effectively increase the concentration of CO_2 in the blood, which will then lead to the production of more carbonic acid, decreasing the pH of the blood. (C) is incorrect because while bicarbonate transports CO_2 from the tissues to the lungs for exhalation, bicarbonate cannot carry O_2 to the lungs. (B) and (D) are not affected by levels of bicarbonate in the blood. (E) is untrue because (A) is true.

12. B

The heartbeat begins in the sino-atrial (SA) node located in the wall of the right atrium approximately where the vena cava enters and travels through the atria. It is then picked up by the AV nodes and carried to the AV bundle (also known as the bundle of His) and transported through the ventricles through the Purkinje fibers. (A) and (C) are structures in the fetal heart that ensure that blood is shunted away from the fetus's developing lungs. (E) is incorrect because the vagus nerve is a cranial nerve that regulates the heartbeat due to signals from the parasympathetic nervous system although it does not determine the heartbeat. The SA node is able to maintain the heartbeat without any stimulation from the nervous system.

13. D

The breathing center in the medulla oblongata monitors the increase in serum CO_2 through its sensory cells. It also will detect a decrease in pH in the blood, which is also indicative of an increase of CO_2 levels in the blood. (A) is incorrect because a decrease in O_2 is monitored peripherally by chemoreceptors in the carotid bodies in the carotid arteries and aortic bodies in the aorta. (B) and (C) would not lead to an increase in breathing, and (E) is not pertinent to the rate of breathing.

14. C

The glomerulus is a capillary ball in the nephron where glucose, water, amino acids, ions, and urea enter, whereas plasma proteins and cells remain behind. (A) and (B) are filtered and completely reabsorbed, and (D) is incorrect because urea is filtered and excreted. (E) is incorrect because Na^+ is filtered and partially reabsorbed. Plasma proteins are never filtered in a normal, healthy kidney, therefore (C) is the correct answer.

15. E

The lymphatic system collects the plasma from the interstitial spaces and filters out cellular debris, foreign material, and bacteria in the lymph nodes and the spleen. Fluid is propelled through the system of lymphatic vessels through the contraction of surrounding muscles. The lymphatic system joins the circulatory system at the thoracic duct located in the superior vena cava immediately before it enters the heart.

16. B

In the pituitary gland, the anterior pituitary gland secretes TSH (thyroid-stimulating hormone), GH (growth hormone), ACTH (adrenocorticotropic hormone), FSH (follicle-stimulating hormone), and LH (luteinizing hormone). TSH stimulates the thyroid gland to produce thyroxin, which affects the basal metabolic rate. The posterior pituitary gland releases ADH (antidiuretic hormone, also known as vasopressin) and oxytocin. The secretions of the pituitary gland are all protein hormones, so (D) is incorrect. (A) is incorrect because the pancreas is not under the influence of any of these hormones. (C) is incorrect because progesterone is secreted by the corpus luteum in response to LH. (E) is incorrect because estrogen is secreted by the ovary in response to FSH.

17. C

The Hardy-Weinberg law states that for a population to have stability in its gene frequencies, it must be a large, randomly mating population with no migration and no mutation. Only if these criteria are met will gene frequencies not change. Only (C) is one of these criteria. The other answer choices will all affect the gene frequency.

18. D

At the ends of long bones, there are regions of cartilage and bone cells that specialize, calcify, and leave deposits of bone tissue between them as they extend the length of the bones. These areas are called the epiphyseal plates.

19. C

Hemoglobin binds CO_2, O_2, and CO. (A) is true; the gas exchange travels from an area of high concentration to an area of low concentration via passive transport. (B) is true because hemoglobin in red blood cells bound to oxygen is known as oxyhemoglobin. (D) is true because serum CO_2 is released by both aerobic and anaerobic respiration, and (E) is true because exchange does occur at the alveolar capillary membrane.

20. B

The anterior pituitary gland releases trophic hormones that affect other glands such as TSH (thyroid gland function); ACTH (adrenal gland function); GH, FSH, and LH (egg follicle growth); and prolactin (lactation). The posterior pituitary gland releases vasopression (ADH), which increases the permeability of the tubules and causes an increase in the concentration of urine.

21. B

Before checking each choice against the table of oxidation potentials given, it would be most efficient, logically, to notice that (B) and (C) are two sides of the same redox reaction:

$$Mg + Mn^{2+} \rightarrow Mg^{2+} + Mn$$

If we apply the fundamental concept that if the forward reaction is not spontaneous, then the reverse reaction must be (and vice versa), we can eliminate the other three choices. We then only need to determine which of these two, (B) or (C), is spontaneous as written. According to the tabulated values, the oxidation of magnesium, Mg, has a larger E^0 value, at 2.37 V, than does manganese, Mn, at 1.03 V. Larger, more positive values of E^0 correspond to more favorable processes. The magnesium is the more likely candidate for oxidation. (B) is therefore correct.

22. D

We need to determine the numerical value of the cell potential for the reaction just selected. This is most conveniently accomplished by subtracting the oxidation potential of the reduction product, Mn, from that of the oxidized species, Mg:

$$E^0(Mg) - E^0(Mn) = 2.37 - 1.03 = 1.34 \text{ V}$$

That makes (D) the correct response.

Note that (A) and (B) could have been eliminated immediately: spontaneous reactions have positive cell potentials.

23. A

You are probably already familiar with the equation $V_1C_1 = V_2C_2$ for dilutions. This equation comes from the conservation of matter, more precisely that of the solute: volume × concentration is the number of moles of solute, which is constant under dilution. We can apply this same general principle to mixing, where the equation can be written as:

$$V_1C_1 + V_2C_2 = V_fC_f$$

The total amount of solute is the sum of the amount of solute in Solution 1 and the amount of solute in Solution 2. Rearranging and plugging in the given values:

$$Cf = [(3.0)(0.50) + (9.0)(0.2777)]/(3.0 + 9.0)$$
$$= (1.5 + 2.5)/12 = 4/12 = 0.33 \text{ M}$$

The calculation above utilized the conversion: $0.2777 = 5/18$, which you may not be familiar with. A convenient approximation might have been: $0.2777 > 0.25$. Either approach leads to the credited choice.

24. B

Because H_3PO_4 has three acidic hydrogens per formula, its normality, N, will be three times its molarity, M. Thus the molarity of the solution is 2.5/3 M. We can calculate the formula weight as 98 g/mol, convert the volume, 50 mL, to 0.050 L, and then set up the final calculation as:

$$0.050 \text{ L} \times \frac{2.5 \text{ mol}}{3 \text{ L}} \times \frac{98\text{g}}{1 \text{ mol}} = 4.08 \text{ g}$$

Notice that the choices are numerically far apart, which can allow you to determine an approximate answer. For example, we could round the 98 up to an even 100, convert 0.05 to a fraction (1/20), and approximate 2.5/3 as 2.4/3 without loss of accuracy:

$$\frac{1}{20} \times \frac{2.4}{3} \times 100 = \frac{240}{3 \times 20} = \frac{24}{6} = 4$$

25. A

Entropy increases when a system becomes more random. When a solid dissolves, the highly ordered crystal structure is replaced by the relatively disordered solution phase. As an example, take $MgCl_2$: in the solid state, the magnesium and chloride ions alternate in the lattice because of their opposing charges. The ions are fixed rather rigidly in place throughout the solid and vibrate about some relatively small equilibrium distance from each other. The fixed nature of their relative positions and distances from one another results in a high level of three-dimensional order throughout the crystal. Additionally, the relatively high density of the solid implies that the mass of solid will occupy a relatively small volume of space. When the $MgCl_2$ is dissolved in water, the ions separate and are now free to move about the entire solution. The particles experience an increased freedom of motion in an increased volume of space. This results in more possibilities for location, speed, and direction. There is a net increase in the randomness of their motion, and entropy is thus increased as well.

26. C

Of the solutions named, Solution Y has a higher boiling point than Solution X at the given pressure. Because both solutions are aqueous and contain the same nonvolatile solute, it follows that Solution Y is more concentrated ($\Delta T_b = K_b m$, where m is for molality) and thereby experiences a more significant boiling point elevation. Vapor pressure is decreased by increasing solute concentration ($PA = X_A P_{total}$, where X_A is the mole fraction of *solvent* in the mixture and thus decreases with increasing mole fraction of *solute*), so the vapor pressure above the less concentrated solution, Solution X, will be greater than that above Solution Y at the same temperature. (A) is incorrect because freezing point decreases with increasing concentration ($\Delta T_f = K_f m$, where m is for molality), so the more concentrated solution, Solution Y, would be predicted to have a lower freezing point. (B) is an unwarranted assumption: Solution Y can be more concentrated without necessarily being saturated. (D) is false because "hypertonic to" means "more concentrated than." Solution X is actually *hypotonic* to Solution Y. Finally, (E) is incorrect because at the boiling point, the vapor pressure above either solution will be equal to the atmospheric pressure. The vapor pressures above the two solutions, at their respective boiling points, will thus be the same.

27. E

This question requires an understanding of the meaning of the term *half-life* and a careful reading of the question stem. Because the half-life is given as 6 days, 50% of the sample will decay (and therefore the other 50% will remain) every 6 days; after 24 days, or 4 half-lives, $\left(\frac{1}{2}\right)^4$, or $\frac{1}{16}$, will remain. One-sixteenth of 30 g would give us (A), but the question asks how much will have decayed rather than how much would be left. The correct answer is $\frac{15}{16}$ of the original 30 g, or (E).

$$30\text{g} \xrightarrow{\text{6 days}} 15\text{g} \xrightarrow{\text{6 days}} 7\tfrac{1}{2}\text{g} \xrightarrow{\text{6 days}} 3\tfrac{3}{4}\text{g} \xrightarrow{\text{6 days}} 1\tfrac{7}{8}\text{g}$$

$$30\text{g} - 1\tfrac{7}{8}\text{g} = 28\tfrac{1}{8}\text{g}.$$

28. B

This question requires knowledge of the definition of normality as well as some skill at balancing redox equations, including the determination of oxidation numbers. Normality is defined as the molarity of the "reactive species"; in the case of electrochemistry, the reactive species are the electrons involved in the redox reaction. Because we are told that potassium permanganate is converted to manganese dioxide, we can set up and solve the manganese half-reaction to determine the number of electrons transferred:

$$KMnO_4 \rightarrow MnO_2 \Rightarrow Mn^{7+} \xrightarrow{3e-} Mn^{4+}$$

From this result, we can see that three electrons are absorbed for each formula of permanganate ion; the relationship between normality and molarity is therefore N = 3 M, and a 2.10 N solution is thus 0.70 M. (D) and (E) could have been easily eliminated if we remembered that normality is always greater than or equal to molarity. (C) is wrong, but it is tempting if one forgets that normality and molarity are only equal in a 1:1 reaction or if you had incorrectly balanced the redox half-reaction.

29. E

This rather tricky question on concentration units and solution stoichiometry requires that you apply the definition of *molality*, or moles of solute per kg solvent, although a glance at the answer choices indicates that full calculation is unnecessary. We can calculate the formula weight of aluminum sulfate as 342 g/mol ($2 \times 27 + 3 \times 32 + 12 \times 16$, or $54 + 3 \times 96$) and thus deduce that 102.6 g are required per kg of solvent ($0.3 \times 342 = 102.6$). The total mass of a solution produced by dissolving 102.6 g of aluminum sulfate in 1 kg (i.e., 1,000 g) of solvent will then be 1,102.6 g. We can set up and rearrange a ratio now to find the quantity of $Al_2(SO_4)_3$ required for the 87.5 g of solution given in the question:

$$\frac{102.6\,g_{solute}}{1{,}102.6\,g_{solution}} = \frac{X\,g_{solute}}{87.5\,g_{solution}} =$$

$$\Rightarrow X = \frac{87.5 \times 102.6}{1{,}102.6}$$

30. A

The methyl group in toluene is *ortho/para*-directing, and thus the first step in synthesizing a *meta*-substituted product would be to turn it into a *meta*-directing substituent. This can be done by oxidation with hot alkaline potassium permanganate, which upon subsequent acidification would yield benzoic acid. The carboxylic acid functional group is *meta*-directing and will therefore lead to the addition of the nitro group in the position we want in the second step. Nitration of benzene is accomplished by heating it with a mixture of concentrated nitric and sulfuric acids (the latter is needed to generate the electrophilic nitronium ion).

31. D

Tautomerization in organic chemistry is the keto-enol tautomers, which is the interconversion of a ketone to an alkene with an alcohol group next to the double bond. Tautomers are constitutional isomers (notice that a hydrogen atom needs to be shifted) but nonetheless interconvert readily in the presence of traces of acids or bases. (A), (B), and (C) are all resonant forms, which are actually identical compounds that differ only in the electron density distribution. (E) depicts *cis-trans* isomerism, which are diastereomers. (D) is a textbook example of keto-enol tautomers.

32. C

Fluorine is the most electronegative of all species, so it should be obvious that it will exert the strongest electron-withdrawing effect.

33. E

Addition of HX to alkenes proceeds through a carbocation intermediate. As with all such reactions, the intermediate with the most stable carbocation will react the fastest. The alkenes with halide substitution listed, (A) and (B), are poor choices because the electron-withdrawing effect of the halides will actually destabilize the carbocation. Of the three remaining choices, the one with the most substituted alkene will react the fastest. (C) and (D) would both yield secondary carbocations, whereas (E) would give one that is tertiary. (E) is therefore correct.

34. E

Ozonolysis cleaves double bonds to form two separate carbonyl products:

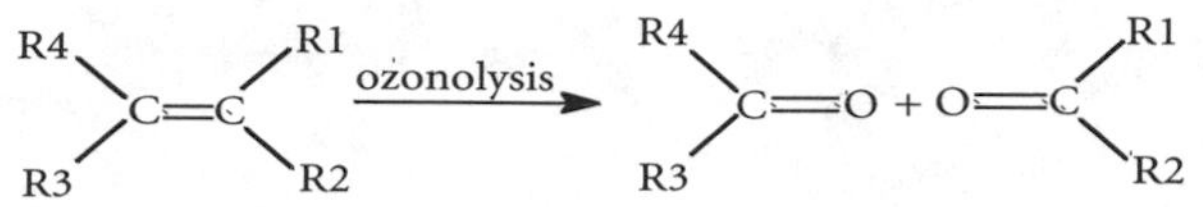

If there is only one product, this must mean that the molecule has the same number of carbons on either side of the double bond. Because butanal, with four carbon atoms, is the product of the reaction, the parent molecule must be the eight-carbon octene, either cis or *trans*. Thus, (E) is the correct choice.

35. A

The most acidic hydrogen is on the carboxylic acid. The most acidic hydrogen is the one that would leave behind the most stable anion. (A) is correct because the anion is stabilized by resonance between two electronegative oxygen atoms, characteristic of the conjugate base of carboxylic acids. It has a pK_a of about 5. All the other four protons can only be removed by much stronger bases: H_b is an α-hydrogen and has a pK_a of 19–20, much lower than that of hydrogens attached to normal saturated carbons because the enolate ion formed upon its extraction is stabilized by resonance. H_c and H_d are also slightly more acidic than expected because of their proximity to the electronegative oxygen atom. H_e is an acetylenic hydrogen and has a pK_a of about 25, compared with a pK_a of 50 for the hydrogen atoms of ethane. None of these, however, is as acidic as H_a.

36. E

The chlorine-chlorine bond is cleaved homolytically by UV photons, forming reactive radicals. Free radical chlorination is quite rapid and unselective, leading to multiple substitution products. (It is therefore not a useful synthetic pathway.) (A), (B), (C), and (D) will all be produced, in that order, to some extent, so (E) is correct.

37. C

It pays for the student to memorize a few facts about NMR and other spectrographic values for certain compounds. Aromatic hydrogens are found in the 6–8.5 ppm range. Hydrogen atoms near double bonds (A) run at 4.6–6 ppm, and those near triple bonds (B) at 2–3 ppm. (A) and (B) are incorrect. NMR does not identify charges, so (D) and (E) are also incorrect.

38. D

Alkyl halides are subject to elimination reactions in the presence of strong bases, such as alcoholic KOH. None of the other four choices is a very realistic product for this reaction. (A) would be the result of a rearrangement reaction, which would not occur spontaneously under the listed conditions. (B) would be indicative of an S_N1 type reaction, but an S_N1 reaction would be difficult to achieve here because it would involve a very unstable primary carbocation intermediate. (C) is perhaps the most likely of the incorrect answers. *n*-Propyl chloride might react in an S_N2-like manner (sterically unhindered target for a nucleophile), but the strength of the base makes elimination much more likely. (E) is also incorrect because it would involve the migration of the chloride ion and the displacement of a hydride ion, which is a highly unlikely reaction scheme.

39. C

Electrophilic additions to benzene rings have as a rate-determining step the formation of a positively charged arenium ion. Electron-donating groups increase the rate by stabilizing this intermediate, whereas electron-withdrawing groups decrease the reactivity. Benzene with no substituents is somewhere in the middle. –OR groups are moderately activating because the lone pairs on oxygen can stabilize the carbocation by resonance. Alkyl groups are electron donating as well. The carboxylic acid is electron withdrawing and thus deactivating. Therefore, the order in decreasing order of electrophilic addition activity is $–OCH_2CH_3$, $–CH_2CH_3$, unsubstituted, and –COOH, or (C).

40. A

Aluminum chloride is an essential requirement for the Friedel-Crafts acylation reaction. (B) and (C), superficially resembling Grignard reagents, are not even stable molecules that could be added to a reaction! (D) is used to generate acyl chlorides from carboxylic acids (we may, for example, have used it to make the second reactant from benzoic acid). (E) is incorrect because any aqueous solution, regardless of acidic or basic quality, will quickly degrade the acyl chloride and will not assist in the electrophilic addition.

Reading Comprehension: Practice Set 1

20 minutes—17 questions

Directions: The following practice set consists of a reading passage and questions that test your comprehension of the passage. Choose the best answer for each question from the five choices provided.

The growth and development of mammalian teeth is the result of a complex series of tissue interactions that occurs during the embryonic and postnatal periods. The permanent tooth and its associated structures are composed of a wide variety of tissue types including bone, epithelium, connective tissue, nerves, and blood vessels. Its anatomic structure is based upon a central pulp cavity containing the neural and vascular supply. This is surrounded by a layer of dentin, a yellowish material that is somewhat harder than bone. Finally, the dentin is covered by a layer of mineralized enamel, the hardest substance in the body. The dentin and enamel are each produced by highly specialized cells known as odontoblasts and ameloblasts, respectively.

The nerves responsible for pain sensation in the teeth are the superior and inferior alveolar nerves, which are derived from the fifth cranial (trigeminal) nerve. These are the sole sensory nerves for the teeth. The autonomic nervous system also innervates the teeth, through the parasympathetic vasodilator fibers of the otic ganglion of the ninth cranial (glossopharyngeal) nerve and the fibers of the cervical sympathetic chain.

The blood supply to the upper jaw is provided by the superior alveolar arteries, which arise from the infraorbital and maxillary arteries. Blood to the lower jaw is carried by the inferior alveolar artery, another branch of the maxillary artery. These arteries are controlled by the vasoconstrictor fibers of the cervical sympathetic system, which stimulates contraction of the arterial smooth-muscle fibers. All of the blood to the teeth comes originally from the right and left common carotid arteries, which supply the entire head and face.

The rate of tooth eruption in mammals has been studied for over 150 years. Early observations in 1823 led Oudet to conclude that rat incisors were capable of persistent growth, even in mature animals. Although it was long suspected that innervation might be responsible for control of this growth, it was not until 1919 that Moral and Hosemann were the first to measure tooth growth after cutting the inferior alveolar nerve. In 1927, Leist reported increased growth of guinea pig incisors after cutting the inferior alveolar nerve and the cervical sympathetic chain. However, he believed that the observed increase may have been due to secondary hyperemia of the pulp following the cervical sympathectomy.

This belief shifted attention, at least temporarily, away from the nervous system and toward the circulatory system. Despite the wide range of possible explanations for the control of tooth growth, the most commonly accepted theory was that first proposed by Leist—that blood supply was the important regulatory influence. It was not until the work of Butcher and Taylor in 1951 that any significant change in thought evolved.

GO ON TO THE NEXT PAGE

The two investigators, working at New York University, studied five factors—blood supply, innervation, the shape of the tooth, physical stress and the consistency of the diet—and their influence upon tooth growth rates. They explained that rat incisors were capable of two processes, eruption and attrition. The former refers to extrusion of a tooth into the oral cavity, while the latter results in a shortening of the tooth due to breakage or grinding, usually the result of normal feeding activity. Changes in tooth length were measured by initially cutting a notch in the tooth at the gingival crest. Eruption was quantified by measuring the distance between the notch and the gingival crest after a period of a few days during which the tooth was allowed to grow. Attrition was measured as the decrease in distance from the notch to the incisal edge after breaking or grinding had occurred.

Studying the blood supply, Butcher and Taylor found that unilateral ligation of the common carotid artery decreased blood supply to teeth on the corresponding side, but also produced bilateral fluctuation in eruption rate, although there was no clear decrease in tooth growth. Further, they showed that ligation of the inferior alveolar artery, while decreasing blood flow considerably, had no effect on rate of eruption. However, when all blood flow to a tooth was stopped by applying retroactive tension to the tooth, eruption ceased. Thus, the demonstration that only complete ischemia, or total lack of blood, would drastically reduce tooth growth led Butcher and Taylor to conclude that circulation was not the most important regulatory factor.

Considering innervation, they discovered that cutting the inferior alveolar nerve resulted in an average increase in growth rate of 26 to 30 percent. Teeth so denervated appeared microscopically normal, except for a decrease in nerve fibers in the periodontal tissue and pulp cavity. Sympathetic denervation in the rats had no effect on tooth growth, despite contrary results observed in guinea pigs. Likewise, removal of the rat's otic ganglion had no effect upon the rate of growth. Thus, Butcher and Taylor surmised that the role of the inferior alveolar nerve was due to its sensory fibers, since the autonomic system had no apparent influence. They hypothesized that the phenomenon was due to sensory impulses conducted from the tooth by the inferior alveolar nerve whenever the tooth met its antagonist in occlusion. This suggested the presence of a feedback system where lack of sensory impulse served as a stimulus to additional growth and presence of sensory impulse served to inhibit additional growth. A loss of the sensory nerve, then, would render the animal unable to detect normal occlusion of the tooth or injury to the tooth.

This hypothesis was tested by artificially altering the physical stress upon a tooth by adjusting its shape. When all occlusal stress was relieved by repeated fracture of the incisor, eruption rate was accelerated. Extrusion rate was increased in every case of relieved functional pressure, and the increase reached a maximum of 200 percent above normal with prolonged repeated fracture. This was considered to be the maximum growth potential of the tooth. When the tooth was allowed to resume normal contact with its antagonist, there was an immediate return of growth rate to the normal levels. Rapidly erupting teeth were found to be abnormal in cross-sectional appearance, with decreased content of dentin and enamel and a widely dilated pulp cavity. Individual odontoblasts and ameloblasts, however, were found to be normal.

Finally, the consistency of the diet and its relation to functional stress were considered, and the results further supported the sensory feedback hypothesis. The standard-consistency diet of all experiments was Purina Dog Chow™. To prevent fracture and grinding, a soft-consistency diet of cornmeal was used; to promote fracture and grinding, a hard-consistency diet of whole-kernel corn was used. When animals were placed on the soft-consistency diet, eruption rate decreased 20 percent from the normal value of 0.5 mm/day. The rate gradually returned to normal when the animals were returned to the dog chow. Similarly, eruption rate increased when the rats were fed whole-kernel corn, a food which caused increased fracture and grinding. The overall difference in

GO ON TO THE NEXT PAGE

eruption rate from the hard to soft-consistency diets was 35 percent.

Thus, the work of Butcher and Taylor shifted the focus of attention from the circulatory system to the nervous system and was largely responsible for the direction and emphasis of future research. To date, no major evidence in opposition to the theory of Butcher and Taylor has been found.

1. Vasodilator nerve fibers that innervate teeth in mammals are found in

    (A) the trigeminal nerve.
    (B) the otic ganglion.
    (C) the cervical sympathetic chain.
    (D) the inferior alveolar nerve.
    (E) the superior alveolar nerve.

2. Since the work of Butcher and Taylor, the accepted theory for control of tooth eruption rate has been based upon

    (A) sensory nerve feedback.
    (B) blood supply.
    (C) the role of odontoblasts.
    (D) the role of ameloblasts.
    (E) None of the above

3. In the experiment described in the passage, when a rat on a soft diet was returned to the standard consistency diet, its tooth growth rate

    (A) remained depressed.
    (B) immediately returned to normal.
    (C) gradually returned to normal.
    (D) remained elevated.
    (E) decreased even further.

4. Which of the following statements correctly summarizes the sensory feedback hypothesis of Butcher and Taylor?

    (A) Lack of sensory impulse causes increased blood flow to the tooth.
    (B) Lack of sensory impulse causes decreased tooth growth rate.
    (C) Lack of sensory impulse causes gradual pulp ischemia.
    (D) Lack of sensory impulse causes increased tooth growth rate.
    (E) The absence of a feedback system allows for an increased tooth growth rate.

5. Teeth that are denervated by cutting the inferior alveolar nerve show

    (A) an average decrease in growth rate of 30 percent.
    (B) no change in normal growth rate.
    (C) an average increase in growth rate of 45 percent.
    (D) no change in microscopic appearance except for a proliferation of capillaries.
    (E) no change in microscopic appearance except for a decrease in nerve fibers.

6. Removal of the otic ganglion in rats

    (A) caused an immediate increase in growth rate.
    (B) caused an immediate decrease in growth rate.
    (C) caused a delayed decrease in growth rate.
    (D) caused a delayed increase in growth rate.
    (E) had no effect on growth rate.

7. Before 1951, tooth growth was commonly thought to be regulated by

    (A) diet.
    (B) physical stress.
    (C) blood supply.
    (D) innervation.
    (E) both (C) and (D).

GO ON TO THE NEXT PAGE

8. Which of the following would be MOST likely to cause the greatest increase in blood supply to the teeth in mammals?
   (A) A cervical sympathectomy
   (B) Ligation of the common carotid artery
   (C) Cutting the inferior alveolar nerve
   (D) Removal of the otic ganglion
   (E) Ligation of the inferior alveolar nerve

9. Based on information in the passage, which of the following statements BEST defines the term "antagonistic teeth"?
   (A) Two adjacent teeth on the upper jaw
   (B) Two adjacent teeth on the lower jaw
   (C) Two teeth with opposite functional properties
   (D) One tooth on the upper jaw, one on the lower
   (E) Upper and lower teeth that meet in normal biting

10. According to the author, odontoblasts are responsible for the production of
   (A) enamel.
   (B) dentin.
   (C) pulp.
   (D) gingival tissue.
   (E) dentin and enamel.

11. In the experiments on normal adult rats, significant incisor growth could be measured within
   (A) 24 hours.
   (B) 48 hours.
   (C) 72 hours.
   (D) 1 week.
   (E) 2 weeks.

12. The greatest increase in eruption rate was achieved by
   (A) altering the consistency of the diet.
   (B) relieving the tooth of all functional stress.
   (C) ligating the common carotid artery.
   (D) removing the otic ganglion.
   (E) returning the tooth to normal contact with its antagonist.

13. The central structure of the adult tooth is composed of
   (A) epithelium.
   (B) mineralized enamel.
   (C) cementum.
   (D) nerves and blood vessels.
   (E) bone.

14. To destroy pain sensation in the teeth, which of the following nerves must be cut?
   (A) The ninth cranial nerve
   (B) The cervical sympathetic fibers
   (C) The otic ganglion
   (D) The glossopharyngeal nerve
   (E) The inferior alveolar nerve

15. What observation was made about rat teeth that were permitted to grow at their maximum potential rate?
   (A) They were more prone to fracture.
   (B) They were lacking in nerve fibers.
   (C) They had decreased amounts of dentin and enamel.
   (D) They had unusually small pulp cavities.
   (E) They appeared normal at the microscopic level.

GO ON TO THE NEXT PAGE

16. Which of the following may be concluded from the observation of Butcher and Taylor?

    (A) Teeth are more likely to fracture in older mammals.
    (B) Occlusal stress may account for suppression of the maximum tooth growth rate.
    (C) Mammals fed a "soft" diet will exhibit an increased number of ameloblasts.
    (D) Occlusion involves only antagonistic teeth.
    (E) Circulation plays a critical role in the regulation of tooth growth.

17. Butcher and Taylor's findings on the effects of dietary consistency upon tooth growth rate

    (A) are inconsistent with the hypothesis of a sensory feedback system.
    (B) show that consistency of the diet has little effect on rate of tooth eruption in rats, even if the diet consists solely of Purina Dog Chow™.
    (C) suggest that a mechanism other than sensory feedback affects tooth growth rate.
    (D) are irrelevant, since rats would never duplicate the experimental diet under normal circumstances.
    (E) indicate that tooth growth rate is affected by more than one factor.

IF YOU FINISH BEFORE TIME IS CALLED, YOU MAY CHECK YOUR WORK ON THIS SECTION ONLY. DO NOT TURN TO ANY OTHER SECTION IN THE TEST. STOP

ANSWERS AND EXPLANATIONS

1. B	6. E	11. C	16. B
2. A	7. C	12. B	17. E
3. C	8. A	13. D	
4. D	9. E	14. E	
5. E	10. B	15. C	

1. B

The passage states that the vasodilator nerve fibers are parasympathetic fibers found in the otic ganglion of the glossopharyngeal nerve, making choice (B) correct. They are not found in the inferior alveolar nerve, the superior alveolar nerve, a branch of the trigeminal nerve, or the cervical sympathetic chain. Thus, answer choices (A), (C), (D), and (E) are all incorrect.

2. A

Each of the five factors (blood supply, innervation, shape of the tooth, physical stress, and the consistency of the diet) that Butcher and Taylor examined pointed to sensory nerve feedback, choice (A), as the predominant controller of the rate of tooth growth. While the blood supply was thought at one point in time to be important in tooth eruption, Taylor and Butcher concluded that it was not the most important regulatory factor. In addition, the accepted theory for control of tooth eruption rate since Butcher and Taylor has not been based in the roles of odontoblasts or of ameloblasts.

3. C

Although animals who were placed on a soft consistency diet experienced decreases of tooth eruption rate of up to 20 percent from the normal value of 0.5 mm/day, the passage states that the animals' eruption rates gradually returned to normal when the animals returned to the dog chow (the standard consistency diet).

4. D

The passage states that Butcher and Taylor surmised that the sensory fibers of the inferior alveolar nerve would provide a feedback system where a lack of sensory impulse would serve as a stimulus for a tooth to grow—choice (D)—and, conversely, the presence of a sensory impulse would serve to inhibit a tooth's growth. The sensory feedback hypothesis did not address the lack of sensory impulses and their relation to blood flow or ischemia.

5. E

After cutting the inferior alveolar nerve, Butcher and Taylor discovered that teeth demonstrated an average increase in growth rate of 26-30 percent, not 45 percent as in choice (C). When examined microscopically, these teeth were normal except for a decrease in nerve fibers. Therefore, choice (D) is incorrect.

6. E

In contrast to the question above, denervation of the otic ganglion had no effect on growth rate. Butcher and Taylor surmised that this was due to the presence of sensory fibers in the inferior alveolar nerve that were not present in the autonomic nerves.

7. C

The passage states that prior to 1951 and subsequent to 1927, the most commonly accepted theory of tooth growth was the one proposed by Leist—that blood supply was the important regulatory influence. Although innervation was considered at one time, it is not the optimal answer because in the years pursuant to 1951, blood supply was more highly considered. Physical stress and diet were never thought to be extremely important regulators of tooth growth.

8. A

The passage states that following cervical sympathectomy, a secondary hyperemia (increase in blood flow to the site of innervation) occurs. Therefore, choice (A) would be most correct. Ligation of the common carotid artery would decrease the amount of blood flow to teeth, and the denervation of the inferior alveolar nerve would have little to do with blood supply. Finally, the removal of the otic ganglion may actually decrease the amount of blood to the teeth due to the presence of parasympathetic autonomic nerve fibers.

9. E

The use of the word *antagonists* in the passage refers to a tooth that makes normal contact with another. Therefore, answer choice (E) is most correct. While the word *antagonist* might conjure up images of teeth with opposite functional properties, choice (C), it was not used in this context in the passage. Clearly, answer choices (A) and (B) are incorrect; they are not mentioned as valid choices in the passage. Finally, answer choice (D) is too vague—choice (E) is far more accurate.

10. B

The author states that odontoblasts are responsible for the production of dentin and that ameloblasts are responsible for the production of enamel. The pulp is littered with neural and vascular supply, and the author does not mention the origin of gingival tissue.

11. C

The passage states that eruption (the extrusion of a tooth into the oral cavity) was measured by examining the distance between the notch (cut initially at the gingival crest) and the gingival crest after a period of a few days (during which time the tooth was allowed to grow). Three days, or 72 hours, is the best choice.

12. B

The passage states that ligating the common carotid artery or removing the otic ganglion did nothing to affect the eruption rate. Altering the consistency of the diet, while affecting the eruption rate slightly, could not compare to relieving the tooth of all functional stress (which was shown to increase eruption to 200 percent). Finally, returning the tooth to normal contact with its antagonist reinstituted normal growth rates.

13. D

(D) is the correct answer choice, as the passage specifically states that the central pulp cavity of a tooth contains the neural and vascular supply. The mineralized enamel is a layer that covers the dentin, which in turn surrounds the central pulp cavity. No mention is made of cementum or bone in the composition of the central structure of the adult tooth.

14. E

The inferior alveolar nerve carries sensory nerve fibers that the cervical sympathetic fibers and the otic ganglion do not. While the glossopharyngeal nerve does have sensory fibers, this nerve does not innervate the teeth. Therefore, the inferior alveolar nerve is the most correct answer.

15. C

The passage states that Butcher and Taylor found that rapidly erupting teeth were abnormal in cross-sectional appearance (thus, answer choice (E) is not correct). They possessed decreased contents of dentin and enamel—choice (C)—and a widely dilated pulp cavity. Therefore, choice (D) is not correct. No mention was made of their propensity for fracture or their abundance of nerve fibers; therefore, these answers—choices (A) and (B)—are incorrect.

16. B

According to the sensory feedback hypothesis proposed by Butcher and Taylor, it is the absence of sensory influences that causes an increase in the growth rate of teeth. No mention is made of tooth fracture and older mammals or of the occlusive ability of nonantagonistic teeth. Mammals fed on a "soft" diet exhibit a decrease in the eruption rate, indicating—if anything—a decrease in the number of ameloblasts.

17. E

Butcher and Taylor's experiments revealed that both occlusal stress and diet consistency affected tooth eruption. This corresponds to many other findings in science, namely, that they are multifactorial. The fact that dietary consistency affected tooth growth rate does not obviate the hypothesis of a sensory feedback system, nor does it suggest that a sole mechanism other than sensory feedback affects tooth growth rate. These diet consistency experiment results are relevant and should be examined from a multifactorial perspective.

Physics: **Practice Set 1**

20 questions – 25 minutes

Directions: Choose the best answer for each question from the five choices provided.

The values for the physical constants below are to be used as needed:

Gravitational acceleration at the surface of the Earth: $g = 10 m/s^2$

Speed of light in a vacuum: $c = 3 \times 10^8$ m/s

Charge of an electron: $e = 2.0 \times 10^{-19}$ Coulomb

1. When a spring is compressed to its minimum length and not permitted to expand

   (A) potential energy is at its maximum, and kinetic energy is at its minimum.

   (B) kinetic energy is at its maximum, and potential energy is at its minimum.

   (C) the sum of the potential and kinetic energies is zero.

   (D) potential energy and kinetic energy are at their maximum.

   (E) potential energy and kinetic energy are at their minimum.

2. A block starts with a certain speed at the top of a frictionless inclined plane with an unknown angle to the horizontal. To calculate the time required for the block to reach the bottom of the plane, all of the following are required EXCEPT

   (A) the height of the plane.

   (B) the length of the plane.

   (C) the speed of the block at the top of the plane.

   (D) the weight of the block.

   (E) the acceleration due to gravity.

GO ON TO THE NEXT PAGE

Questions 3–5 refer to following scenario:

A 6-ft man lifts a 100-lb weight from the floor to a height 1 ft above his head.

3. How much work is done in lifting the weight?

(A) 0 ft·lb

(B) 6 ft·lb

(C) 14 ft·lb

(D) 600 ft·lb

(E) 700 ft·lb

4. What force must be exerted by the man to sustain the object above his head?

(A) 0 lb

(B) 50 lb

(C) 100 lb

(D) 150 lb

(E) 200 lb

5. How much work does the man perform in sustaining the object above his head?

(A) 0 ft·lb

(B) 50 ft·lb

(C) 100 ft·lb

(D) 150 ft·lb

(E) 200 ft·lb

6. A billiard ball of mass m and velocity v undergoes an elastic, head-on collision with another billiard ball, also of mass m, which is initially at rest. What is the velocity of the first ball after the collision?

(A) 0

(B) $\frac{1}{3}v$

(C) $\frac{2}{3}v$

(D) v

(E) Cannot be determined from the information given.

7. A car is parked on a ramp inclined at an angle θ. What is the minimum value of the coefficient of static friction between the tires and the road such that the car does not slip down the ramp?

(A) $\cos\theta$

(B) $\cos^{-1}\theta$

(C) $\tan\theta$

(D) $\tan^{-1}\theta$

(E) Cannot be determined from the information given.

8. A passenger stands on a scale that is inside an elevator. If the scale reads 110 lb when the elevator is at rest, what would it read when the elevator begins to accelerate upward at 3 ft/s^2?

(A) 105 lb

(B) 115 lb

(C) 120 lb

(D) 130 lb

(E) 135 lb

9. Three weights are suspended from a beam by a rope of negligible weight, as shown in the diagram below. What is the tension T in the middle rope?

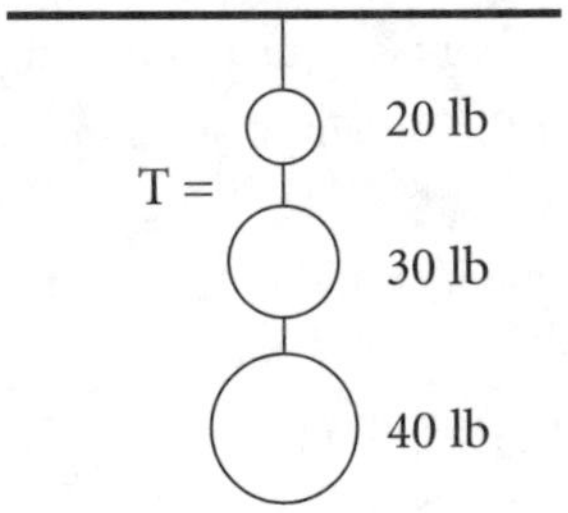

(A) 0 lb

(B) 20 lb

(C) 70 lb

(D) 90 lb

(E) Cannot be determined from the information given.

GO ON TO THE NEXT PAGE

10. Forces F_1 and F_2 support the 60-lb weight of a uniform beam as shown below. What is the magnitude of force F_2?

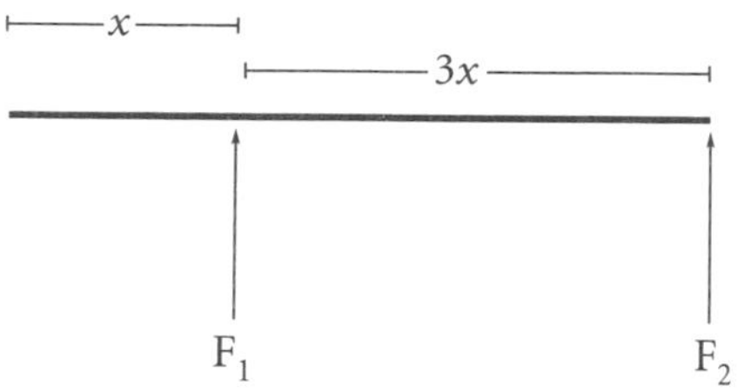

(A) 15 lb
(B) 20 lb
(C) 25 lb
(D) 30 lb
(E) 40 lb

11. For most liquids, viscosity

(A) varies directly with temperature.
(B) is measured in dynes.
(C) varies indirectly with the force necessary to turn a rotor in the fluid.
(D) increases as temperature decreases.
(E) varies directly with flow.

12. It requires 5×10^{-5} J of work to carry a 10-μC point charge from A to B. What is the potential difference between the two points?

(A) 5×10^{-10} V
(B) 5×10^{-5} V
(C) 0.2 V
(D) 5 V
(E) 2×10^{5} V

13. During an adiabatic expansion

(A) the system is at the same temperature after the expansion as it was before the expansion.
(B) the internal energy of the system decreases.
(C) heat is put into the system.
(D) work equal to PΔV is put into the system.
(E) the internal energy of the system remains the same; the system did work, but the heat content remained the same.

14. If an object is placed between a concave mirror and its focal point, what is the nature of the image formed?

(A) Real, inverted, reduced
(B) Real, inverted, enlarged
(C) Virtual, erect, same size
(D) Real, inverted, same size
(E) Virtual, erect, enlarged

15. Q_1, Q_2, Q_3 are all charges of equal magnitude and sign. If the sign of Q_3 is reversed, what happens to the net force vector of charge Q_1?

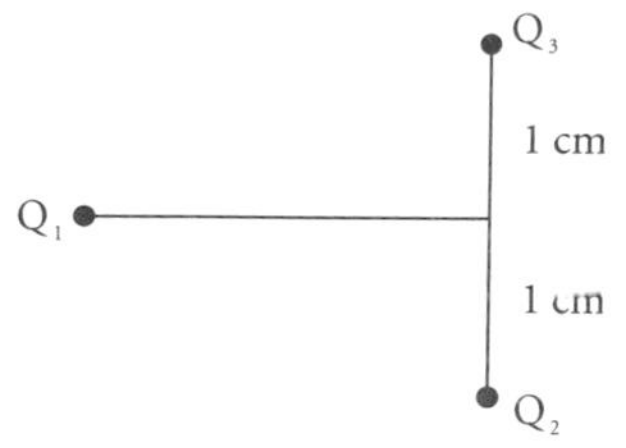

(A) The net force vector will be 0.
(B) The net force vector will rotate 90° clockwise.
(C) The net force vector will rotate 90° counterclockwise.
(D) The net force vector will rotate 180°.
(E) The net force vector will rotate 45° clockwise.

ANSWERS AND EXPLANATIONS

1. A	6. A	11. D	16. D
2. D	7. C	12. D	17. E
3. E	8. C	13. B	18. B
4. C	9. C	14. E	19. B
5. A	10. B	15. B	20. A

1. A

Compressing a spring requires work, which is then transformed into potential energy. If the spring is not permitted to expand then it is being held motionless, which means it has zero kinetic energy. Because total energy (kinetic plus potential) is conserved, we can say that the point of minimum kinetic energy is also the point of maximum potential energy. (A) is therefore correct.

For completeness, (B) says that the potential energy is a minimum. We know this to be false because the spring has been compressed. (C) says that the sum of the kinetic and potential energies is zero, which means that the total energy is zero. Again this is false, because the spring has a nonzero potential energy due to its compression. (D) and (E) can be ruled out because of conservation of energy. You can't have both kinetic and potential energies either minimum or maximum at the same time. If kinetic energy is a maximum, then potential energy is a minimum, and vice versa.

2. D

To determine the amount of time required for the block to reach the bottom of the plane, we would have to develop an equation to describe the block's motion. The equation $x = v_o t + \left(\frac{1}{2}\right)at^2$ will suffice if x is the distance measured along the plane, v_o is the speed at the top of the plane, and a is the acceleration down the plane. We'd then be able to determine the time if we knew the distance down the plane (i.e., the length of the plane). So far, we know we'll need the initial speed at the top of the plane and the length of the plane. Thus, we can eliminate (B) and (C). Let's consider how to determine the acceleration down the plane. We find acceleration by applying Newton's second law, $F = ma$. To find the acceleration down the plane, we'll need the force down the plane, which is the component of the object's weight along the plane. The object's weight along the plane is $mg\sin q$, where q is the angle of the incline. Putting all this together, we have that $mg\sin q = ma$, or $a = g\sin q$. Notice how the mass of the object canceled out. We see that computing the acceleration requires knowing the acceleration of gravity and the sine of the angle of incline of the plane. We can then directly rule out (E). Because $\sin q$ = (height of plane)/(length of plane), we know that we'll need the height of the plane. We can thus rule out (A), which leaves only (D), the correct answer.

3. E

Work done is determined from the equation $W = Fd\cos\theta$. In this case, the direction of the force and the direction of the displacement are the same, so $\theta = 0$ means that $\cos\theta = 1$. So $W = Fd$. Now we note that the force required to lift an object is simply the weight of the object. So we have $W = (100\text{ lb})(7\text{ ft}) = 700$ ft·lb.

4. C

If the 100-lb weight is sustained above the man's head, then it is motionless and remains so. This can be true only if the net force on the weight = 0. The two forces on the weight are the force of gravity downward and the upward force supplied by the man. For the net force to be zero, we must have (weight of object) = (upward force exerted by man), which tells us simply that the upward force exerted by the man = 100 lb.

5. A

Recall the equation used to determine work, $W = Fd\cos\theta$, where F is the force, d is the displacement, and θ is the angle between the force and the displacement. In the present case, the man holds the weight stationary above his head. There is no displacement ($d = 0$) and no work done, which is the same as saying $W = 0$ ft·lb. The correct answer is (A). The key point is that work is only done when a displacement occurs. The presence of forces is itself not sufficient to say that work is done.

6. A

An elastic collision means the kinetic energy of the system before the collision equals the kinetic energy after the collision. For all types of collision, both elastic and inelastic, momentum is conserved. Consider the answer choices. (A) says the velocity of the incoming ball is 0 after the collision. The initial momentum is mv, so for momentum to be conserved, we require $mv_2 = mv$, where v_2 is the velocity of the other ball. This means $v_2 = v$. Notice that this will also guarantee conservation of kinetic energy because the initial kinetic energy is $\frac{1}{2}mv^2$ and the final kinetic energy will now be $\frac{1}{2}mv_2{}^2 = \frac{1}{2}mv^2$. Thus, 0 final velocity for the incoming ball results in conservation of momentum and conservation of kinetic energy, which means it's the correct value.

7. C

For a car to remain stationary on an inclined ramp, the maximum static friction force must be at least as great as the component of the gravitational force directed down the ramp. Recall that for an incline with angle of θ relative to the horizontal, the component of the gravitational force down the ramp is $mg\sin\theta$. The static frictional force has a maximum magnitude $f = \mu N$, where N is the normal force, and μ is the coefficient of friction. The normal force, in turn, must equal the component of the gravitational force perpendicular to the incline, which is given by $mg\cos\theta$. Thus, $f = \mu\, mg\cos\theta$. We must have $\mu\, mg\cos\theta = mg\sin\theta$, which implies $\mu = \tan\theta$.

8. C

The value of the normal force of the scale upwards on a person standing on the scale is also the weight read by the scale. By Newton's third law, the downward force on the scale caused by the person is the same magnitude as the normal force of the scale upward on the person.

Now consider the case of an upward acceleration of 3 ft/s^2. The net force on the person is now $N - mg = N - 110 = ma$, where N is the normal force of the scale upward on the person and we've used the fact that their weight is $mg = 110$. So we have a reading on the scale of $N = 110 + ma$. From $mg = 110$, we have $m = 110/g = \frac{110}{32}$ ($g = 32$ ft/s^2). Thus, $N = 110 + 3\left(\frac{110}{32}\right)$, so $N = 120$ lb.

9. C

To solve this problem, notice that the tension in the middle rope is the only force supporting the 30-lb and 40-lb weights. The total force being supported by this middle rope is then 70 lb, which means that the tension in the rope is 70 lb.

10. B

A uniform beam is shown supported by two forces. Because the beam is in static equilibrium, we know that the net force and the net torque on the beam are 0. Our approach will be to write down equations that describe translational and rotational equilibrium and then obtain F_2 from them. Translational equilibrium means no net force, so we have $F_1 + F_2 = 60$ (i.e., the two external forces support the 60-lb weight of the beam).

Now consider rotational equilibrium, which requires that the net torque be zero. When calculating total torque, we need to choose a pivot point (i.e., the point about which the torque is calculated). In fact, we're free to choose this point wherever we like. Recall that torque = $rF\sin\theta$. Notice if we choose the pivot point at the center of the beam, then there will be no torque from the weight of the beam, because the weight acts through the center of the beam and that would mean $r = 0$ in the torque equation. We only need consider the torques from F_1 and F_2. We'll take the convention that counterclockwise torques are positive and clockwise torques are negative. Then the net torque on the beam is $\tau = (2x)F_2 - xF_1$, where we've used the fact that F_1 is a distance x from the pivot point, F_2 is a distance $2x$ from the pivot point, and both forces are perpendicular to their respective lever arms. Rotational equilibrium requires $\tau = 0$, so $(2x)F_2 = xF_1$. Crossing out x on both sides, we get $F_1 = 2F_2$. Substituting for F_1 in the force equation above gives $2F_2 + F_2 = 60$, so $F_2 = 20$ lb.

11. D

First, recall that viscosity is a measure of the internal friction in a liquid and that the greater the internal friction, the more resistance to flow. A good home example of a viscous liquid is honey. At room temperature, it's pretty resistant to flow. If you heat it up, however, you'll find that it flows much more readily. This means that the viscosity has decreased with increased temperature.

12. D

Work, W, and potential difference, ΔV, are related by the equation $W = q\Delta V$, where q is the charge that is moved through the potential difference. Thus, $\Delta V = W/q = \dfrac{5 \times 10^{-5}}{10 \times 10^{-6}} = 5\ V$.

13. B

An adiabatic process is one in which no heat enters or leaves the system. Consider a system undergoing an adiabatic expansion. Because the system is expanding, its volume is increasing. Thus, it is doing an amount of work equal to $P\Delta V$ where P is the pressure and ΔV is the change in volume. According to the first law of thermodynamics, we have $\Delta U = Q - W$, where ΔU is the change in the internal energy, Q is the heat absorbed, and W is the work done by the system. Because the process is adiabatic, $Q = 0$, which leaves $\Delta U = -W$. Be careful with signs here. W is positive when work is done by the system, as is the case here. Thus, $\Delta U < 0$, which says that the internal energy decreases.

For completeness, take a look at the other answer choices. (A) says the temperature remains constant. When a system does work and doesn't absorb heat, its temperature drops because its internal energy drops. (C) says heat is put into the system. This is simply testing whether you know the definition of an adiabatic process and is clearly incorrect. (D) suggests that work is put into the system, whereas exactly the opposite occurs (i.e., the system does work in the expansion). (E) says that the internal energy of the system remains the same, which is simply incorrect, as shown above. During an adiabatic expansion, the internal energy decreases.

14. E

First, recall that a concave mirror has a positive focal length. We then need to employ the equation $\frac{1}{o} + \frac{1}{i} = \frac{1}{f}$, where o is the object distance, i is the image distance, and f is the focal length. We're given that $o < f$. Let's solve for $\frac{1}{i} = \frac{1}{f} - \frac{1}{o}$. Given that $o < f$, we have $\frac{1}{f} - \frac{1}{o} < 0$, which tells us that $\frac{1}{i} < 0$, which says that the image is virtual. At this point, we can eliminate all answer choices but (C) and (E). Notice that now we only have to determine if the image is the same size or enlarged. To do this, we'll employ the magnification $m = -\frac{i}{o}$. The only way the image can be the same size as the object is if $|m| = 1$, and this can only happen if $-i = o$. From the above, we've determined that $\frac{1}{i} = \frac{1}{f} - \frac{1}{o}$, so the only way $-i$ can equal o is if $f =$ infinity. Recall that f is related to the radius of curvature and that f equal to infinity means an infinite radius of curvature, which simply means a plane mirror. We're specifically told, though, that the mirror is concave, so we can rule out the choice f = infinity. Then we have that $-i$ is not equal to o, which means that the magnification differs from 1. By process of elimination, (E) is correct.

For completeness, we'll carry out the analysis and convince ourselves that the image is enlarged. We need to compute $m = -\frac{i}{o}$. From $\frac{1}{i} = \frac{1}{f} - \frac{1}{o}$ we have $\frac{1}{i} = \frac{(o - f)}{of}$, which gives $i = \frac{of}{(o - f)}$. This means that $m = -\frac{f}{(o - f)}$. We can simplify this to $m = \frac{f}{(f - o)}$. Notice that $\frac{f}{(f - o)}$ is greater than 1, which tells us that $m > 1$. Thus, the image is enlarged.

15. B

Before we can decide what happens when we change the sign of Q_3, we have to determine the direction of the force given by the initial charges. The force on Q_1 due to Q_3 is toward the bottom left side of the page, and the force on Q_1 due to Q_2 is toward the top left side of the page. Because Q_2 and Q_3 have equal magnitude and are the same distance from Q_1, we know that the magnitude of the force due to each is the same. When the forces are added vectorially, their vertical components will cancel, and the net force on Q_1 will then be toward the left.

Consider what happens when the sign of Q_3 is reversed. The force due to Q_3 is now toward the top right side of the page. We now have the case that the horizontal components of the forces F_2 and F_3 will cancel, which means that the new force on Q_1 will be in the vertical direction. Relative to the original force, the new force is rotated 90° clockwise.

16. D

The specific gravity of an object is the ratio of the density of the object to the density of water. Because the object is floating, we know that the downward force of gravity is balanced by the upward buoyant force. Recall that the upward buoyant force is given by $\rho_w gV$, where ρ_w is the density of water and V is the volume of the object immersed in the water. We're given that $V = 0.8V_o$ where V_o is the total volume of the object. Thus, the buoyant force is given by $\rho_w g(0.8)V_o$. We know this must equal mg, where m is the mass of the object. Because we're trying to find the ratio of the density of the object to that of water, we'll express m in terms of its density by $m = \rho V_o$. The object's weight is $mg = \rho g V_o$. Setting weight equal to buoyant force, we have $\rho g V_o = \rho_w g(0.8)V_o$, which reduces to $\rho = \rho_w(0.8)$. We then have specific gravity $\rho/\rho_w = 0.8$.

17. E

We're told that water pressure increases by 1 atmosphere for every 33 ft of depth. Given that the pressure at the surface is atmospheric pressure (1 atm), the pressure at a depth of 33 ft will be 2 atm. At 66 ft the pressure is 3 atm, and at 99 ft the pressure is 4 atm. So the approximate pressure at 100 ft is 4 atm. The key here is to include the atmospheric pressure at the surface.

18. B

Wavelength, period, and speed are related by $v = \lambda f$. Frequency and period are related by $T = \frac{1}{f}$. We have $v = \frac{\lambda}{T}$, which means that wavelength is given by $\lambda = vT$. Given that $v = 300$ m/s and $T = 0.1$ s, we have $\lambda = (300)(0.1) = 30$ m.

19. B

We're told that radium, with atomic number 88, decays via alpha decay to radon. An alpha particle is simply a helium nucleus. Helium has atomic number 2, which means it has two protons. Thus, two protons have been ejected from a radium nucleus, resulting in the formation of a radon nucleus. The number of protons (atomic number) of the radon nucleus is $88 - 2 = 86$.

20. A

To answer the question, we'll have to recall that resistance depends on length and cross section through the equation $R = \rho L/A$, where R is the resistivity of asbestos. We're told the length and diameter are reduced by a factor of 2. Note that $A = \pi r^2$ and that reducing the diameter by a factor of 2 means reducing the radius by a factor of 2. The new area is then $A_1 = \pi\left(\frac{r}{2}\right)^2 = \frac{A}{4}$. The new resistance is

$$R_1 = \rho\frac{\left(\frac{L}{2}\right)}{\left(\frac{A}{4}\right)} = 2R.$$

Quantitative Reasoning: **Practice Set 1**

20 questions—18 minutes

Directions: Choose the best answer for each question from the five choices provided.

1. A roulette wheel consists of 38 slots. Thirty-six of these are numbered 1–36 and colored red or black so that there are 9 red even-numbered slots, 9 black odd-numbered slots, etc. These slots occur with equal probability. The 2 slots marked 0 or 00 are each 3 times as likely to occur as any one of the other 36. What is the probability that a red even number, a red 23, or a 00 will occur on one roll of the wheel?

   (A) $\frac{2}{7}$

   (B) $\frac{5}{18}$

   (C) $\frac{13}{38}$

   (D) $\frac{13}{42}$

   (E) $\frac{3}{10}$

2. It takes five painters 12 days to paint a certain office. How long would it take six painters to paint an office with 50% more wall space?

   (A) 10 days

   (B) 14.4 days

   (C) 15 days

   (D) 16 days

   (E) 21.6 days

3. A rectangular fence whose width is one-half its length encloses a field of area 648 square feet. How long is the shorter side?

   (A) 6 feet

   (B) 12 feet

   (C) 18 feet

   (D) $6\sqrt{2}$ feet

   (E) $12\sqrt{2}$ feet

4. If $x \neq 0$ and $xy + 1 = (x + 1)(y + 1)$, then $\frac{y}{x} + 1 =$

   (A) -1

   (B) $\frac{y+1}{x+1}$

   (C) $\frac{x}{y} - 1$

   (D) 0

   (E) 2

GO ON TO THE NEXT PAGE

5. $1\frac{1}{2} - \frac{6}{7} \times 1\frac{2}{5} =$

(A) $\frac{3}{10}$

(B) $\frac{4}{10}$

(C) $\frac{19}{20}$

(D) $\frac{19}{14}$

(E) None of the above

6. What is the average of 40%, $\frac{3}{10}$, and 1.25?

(A) $\frac{8}{5}$

(B) $\frac{13}{20}$

(C) 1

(D) $\frac{8}{15}$

(E) $\frac{277}{20}$

7. Mr. Al leaves City X at 6:00 AM, and drives at an average speed of 50 mph to City Y. Mr. Bob leaves City X at 7:00 AM, and arrives in City Y at 10:00 A.M., 30 min ahead of Mr. Al. Assuming they took the same route, what was Mr. Bob's average speed?

(A) 33.3 mph

(B) 55 mph

(C) 66.7 mph

(D) 67.5 mph

(E) 75 mph

8. A dining room table is selling at a 20% discount, which is $120 more than 50% of the list price. What is the list price of the table?

(A) $240

(B) $400

(C) $200

(D) $360

(E) $300

9. Mr. Albert owns 80% of the stock in Albert Glass Works, Inc., which leaves 10,000 shares owned by others. He decides to put some of these shares up for sale to found a sister company, which will have an initial worth of $200,000. If the market value of Albert Glass Works, Inc. is currently $20 per share, what percentage of his own holdings must Mr. Albert put up for sale?

(A) 20%

(B) 25%

(C) 33.3%

(D) 40%

(E) 150%

10. A certain clothing store marks down any stock that is over 1 month old by 20%, and anything over 2 months old is marked down to 50% of its original price. Of one lot of 100 sweaters, 20 sell during the first month, 35 sell during the second month, and the remainder sell quickly after the final markdown. If the cost of the lot was $1,500 and the store's original markup was 100%, what is the total profit on the lot?

(A) $615.00

(B) $775.00

(C) $720.00

(D) $1,027.50

(E) $1,132.50

11. $4x - 3(x - 1) + 2(x + 4) - (x - 2) = 7; x = ?$

(A) -3

(B) -2

(C) -1

(D) 1

(E) 3.5

GO ON TO THE NEXT PAGE

12. $\frac{2}{7} = \frac{d}{5}; d = ?$

(A) $\frac{2}{35}$

(B) $\frac{10}{35}$

(C) $\frac{7}{10}$

(D) $1\frac{3}{7}$

(E) $1\frac{9}{14}$

13. What is the next term in this sequence?

$\frac{1}{3}, \frac{3}{6}, \frac{5}{12},$ ——

(A) $\frac{5}{24}$

(B) $\frac{5}{18}$

(C) $\frac{7}{24}$

(D) $\frac{11}{24}$

(E) $\frac{11}{18}$

14. At the Atlanta 500 car race, a blue car is traveling at 198 mph. A red car, which is three laps behind, is running at 3.5 miles/min. If each lap is 2.4 miles, how long will it take for the red car to catch up with the blue car?

(A) 12 min

(B) 14.4 min

(C) 36 min

(D) 72 min

(E) The red car will never catch up.

15. The volume of a cone is $\frac{1}{3}$ of the area of its circular base times its height. Approximately what is the volume of a cone with a height of $2\frac{8}{11}$ ft and a base of diameter 7 ft? $\left(\pi = \frac{22}{7}\right)$

(A) $32\frac{2}{3}$ cubic ft

(B) 35 cubic ft

(C) 105 cubic ft

(D) 140 cubic ft

(E) 420 cubic ft

16. The two hands of a clock are 14 cm and 21 cm in length. When the small hand travels 120°, approximately what distance does the tip of the large hand cover? $\left(\pi = \frac{22}{7}\right)$

(A) 66 cm

(B) 132 cm

(C) 264 cm

(D) 528 cm

(E) 792 cm

17. $0.84 \div 0.007 = ?$

(A) 120

(B) 1.2

(C) 0.12

(D) 0.012

(E) 0.00012

18. $\frac{x}{3}$ is $\frac{y}{4}$% of $50z$. In terms of x and z, $y = ?$

(A) $\frac{8x}{3z}$

(B) $\frac{8xz}{3}$

(C) $\frac{2x}{75z}$

(D) $\frac{600z}{x}$

(E) $\frac{8x}{z}$

GO ON TO THE NEXT PAGE

19. $\dfrac{495}{\frac{5}{9}} = ?$

(A) $961\frac{2}{5}$

(B) 891

(C) 275

(D) $291\frac{1}{5}$

(E) $945\frac{4}{9}$

20. $\dfrac{1 \text{ gal } 4 \text{ oz}}{1 \text{ qt } 8 \text{ oz}} = ?$

(A) $\frac{1}{2}$

(B) $\frac{33}{10}$

(C) $\frac{2}{1}$

(D) $\frac{19}{4}$

(E) $\frac{17}{4}$

IF YOU FINISH BEFORE TIME IS CALLED, YOU MAY CHECK YOUR WORK ON THIS SECTION ONLY. DO NOT TURN TO ANY OTHER SECTION IN THE TEST. **STOP**

ANSWERS AND EXPLANATIONS

1. D	6. B	11. A	16. D
2. C	7. E	12. D	17. A
3. C	8. B	13. C	18. A
4. D	9. B	14. C	19. B
5. A	10. A	15. B	20. B

1. D

The first step in solving the problem is to determine the likelihood of each slot's occurrence. Say, then, that the likelihood of each of the 36 regular slots is x. Then the likelihood of each of the two special slots (0 and 00) is $3x$. To solve for x, we note that the sum of the probabilities for all 38 slots is 1, so $36x + (2 \times 3x) = 1$ and $x = \frac{1}{42}$. This means that the probability for each special slot is $\frac{3}{42}$ (or $\frac{1}{14}$, but we won't reduce the fraction here because we're going to add it to another in a moment). The probability that (A), a red even number, will occur is $9 \times \frac{1}{42}$, or $\frac{9}{42}$. The probability that (B), a red 23, will occur is $\frac{1}{42}$. The probability that (C), 00, will occur is $\frac{3}{42}$. So the probability that (A) or (B) or (C) will occur is the sum of these probabilities, $\frac{9}{42} + \frac{1}{42} + \frac{3}{42} = \frac{13}{42}$.

All of the other answers are designed to catch you if you make various simple mistakes. For example, (C) is designed to catch you if you decide that the denominator for each probability is 38. The discussion above shows that this is not the case: there are 38 slots, but because they are differently weighted, none of them has a $\frac{1}{38}$ chance of occurring.

2. C

The implicit hypothesis of this question is that every painter paints a fixed amount of wall space in a day. Thus, "the amount one painter paints in one day" becomes our standard unit of wall space. The explicit hypothesis is that it takes five painters 12 days to paint our office, so our office has 60 times the wall space one painter paints in one day.

An office with 50% more wall space therefore has 1.5×60, or 90 times the wall space one painter paints in one day. The question boils down to "90 days of work for one painter is how many days of work for six painters?" This question is expressed by the equation: $6x = 90$. Obviously $x = 15$. It takes six painters 15 days to paint 1.5 offices.

3. C

This problem is just one of setting up an equation. The area of a rectangle is its length times its width. If the shorter side of the rectangular field in the question is x, then the length of the longer side is $2x$. The equation for the area is then $x \times 2x = 648$ or $x^2 = 324$.

Because this is a multiple-choice set, at this point you could square each possible answer if you did not want to find the square root of 324 explicitly. But just in case, let us use the latter, more general method. First we factor the number, so we divide it first by 2, which yields 162, and then again by 2, which yields 81, so $324 = 2 \times 2 \times 81$. It should be clear then that factored 324 is $2^2 \times 3^4$, and so $x = 2 \times 3^2 = 18$.

4. D

Try to rearrange the equation so that the value of $\frac{y}{x} + 1$ will be solved for.

	$xy + 1 = (x + 1)(y + 1)$
Multiply out the right side using FOIL	$xy + 1 = xy + x + y + 1$
Subtract $xy + 1$ from both sides	$0 = x + y$
Divide both sides by x:	$\frac{0}{x} = \frac{x + y}{x}$
The left side of this last equation is just 0:	$0 = \frac{x + y}{x}$
Rewrite the right side so that $\frac{y}{x}$ appears	$0 = \frac{x}{x} + \frac{y}{x}$
$\frac{x}{x}$ is equal to 1	$0 = 1 + \frac{y}{x}$

Thus, $1 + \frac{y}{x} = 0$, so $\frac{y}{x} + 1 = 0$.

5. A

Here one must remember the order of operations: multiplication is performed before addition or subtraction. So

$$1\frac{1}{2} - \frac{6}{7} \times 1\frac{2}{5} = 1\frac{1}{2} - \left[\frac{6}{7} \times \left(1\frac{2}{5}\right)\right] = \frac{3}{2} - \left(\frac{6}{7} \times \frac{7}{5}\right),$$

and multiplying and canceling,

$$\frac{3}{2} - \left(\frac{6}{7} \times \frac{7}{5}\right) = \frac{3}{2} - \left(\frac{7 \times 6}{7 \times 5}\right) = \frac{3}{2} - \left(\frac{6}{5}\right).$$

The lowest common denominator of 2 and 5 is 2×5, or 10, so $\frac{3}{2} - \frac{6}{5} = \frac{15}{10} - \frac{12}{10} = \frac{3}{10}$. The expression is equal to $\frac{3}{10}$.

6. B

To find the average, we must decide on a common mode for expressing these values. We'll use decimals, because it's easiest with them to add and subtract. So 40% = 0.40, $\frac{3}{10} = 0.30$, and we can leave 1.25 alone. Their sum is $0.40 + 0.30 + 1.25 = 1.95$, so their average is $\frac{1.95}{3} = 0.65$, or $\frac{65}{100}$, which in fully reduced terms is $\frac{13}{20}$.

7. E

Because Mr. Bob arrives in City Y at 10:00 AM, *30 min ahead of* Mr. Al, Mr. Al clearly arrives at 10:30 A.M. Because he left at 6:00 AM, the total time of Mr. Al's trip is 4.5 hours. Mr. Bob's trip, on the other hand, takes 3 hours total, only $\frac{2}{3}$ as long. One might think we need here to derive the actual distance based on Mr. Al's trip time and average speed, but we don't. We only need to recognize that the two distances are equal and then to set up the equation: (3 hours) $\times \left(x \frac{\text{miles}}{\text{hour}}\right)$ = (4.5 hours) $\times \left(50 \frac{\text{miles}}{\text{hour}}\right) \times$ (3x miles) = (4.5 × 50 miles). Dividing both sides by 3 and canceling the units gives $x = 1.5 \times 50 = 75$. Mr. Bob's average speed is 75 mph.

8. B

A 20% discount is 80% of regular price. Half of the list price is the same as 50% of the list price, so if we let the list price of the table in dollars be x, we get the equation $80\% \times x = (50\% \times x) + 120$. Subtracting 50% of x from both sides and reversing the distributive property, we get $30\% \times x = 120$, or $\frac{3}{10} \times x = 120$. Multiplying both sides by 10 and dividing by 3 gives $x = 400$. The list price is $400.

9. B

Because we know the value of each share ($20), we have to figure out how many shares Mr. Albert holds. Because he owns 80% of the company, the rest of the company is 100% – 80% = 20% of the company, or $\frac{1}{5}$, and we're also told that this is 10,000 shares. So the total number of shares in the company is 5 × 10,000 = 50,000, and Mr. Albert owns 50,000 – 10,000 = 40,000 of them. At $20 per share, his holdings are valued at 40,000 × $20 = $800,000, and he wants to sell $200,000 of this to start his new company. $200,000 is $\frac{1}{4}$ of $800,000, so he must sell $\frac{1}{4}$, or 25%, of his stock.

10. A

The cost of the lot was \$1,500 for 100 sweaters, or \$15 per sweater. The original markup was 100%, so the first-month price was \$30 per sweater. The second month price is 80% of this, so the second month price is $80\% \times \$30 = \frac{4}{5} \times \$30 = \$24$ per sweater. The final price is 50% of the original price, or $\frac{1}{2} \times \$30 = \$15$, and $100 - 20 - 35 = 45$ is the number of sweaters sold at this price. So the total cash sales are:

$(20 \times \$30) + (35 \times \$24) + (45 \times \$15) = \$600 + \$840 + \$675 = \$2{,}115$. Profit is equal to sales minus cost, so the profit on the lot is $\$2{,}115 - \$1{,}500 = \$615$.

11. A

We can simplify $4x - 3(x - 1) + 2(x + 4) - (x - 2)$ to the expression $4x - 3x + 3 + 2x + 8 - x + 2$. Combining like terms, this expression is equal to $(4 - 3 + 2 - 1)x + 3 + 8 + 2$, or $2x + 13$. The hypothesis is $2x + 13 = 7$. Subtracting 13 from both sides gives $2x = -6$. Dividing both sides by 2 gives $x = -3$.

12. D

Multiplying both sides of the equation by 5 gives $\frac{5(2)}{7} = d$. That is, $d = \frac{10}{7} = \frac{7}{7} + \frac{3}{7} = 1 + \frac{3}{7} = 1\frac{3}{7}$.

13. C

The key is to find the simplest pattern possible in the sequence of terms that is given. Sometimes it helps to look at the numerators and denominators separately for a while. Inspecting the three terms, we see that the numerators appear to be an *arithmetic* progression. That is, they increase by adding the same amount each step, in this case, by adding 2. Because the first three terms are 1, 3, and 5, according to this pattern, the fourth would be 7. Looking now at the denominators, we see that they appear to be a *geometric* progression—they increase by *multiplying* the same amount each step, again, in this case, 2. According to this interpretation of their pattern, because the first three terms are 3, 6, and12, the fourth would be 24; the pattern is clear: 2 times 3 is 6, 2 times 6 is 12, 2 times 12 is 24. Likewise, the next after 24 would be 2 times 24, or 48, but let's not confuse ourselves. The fourth denominator is 24, and the fourth numerator is 7. So the fourth fraction is $\frac{7}{24}$.

14. C

This is about a car race. We have a blue car traveling 198 mph and a red car traveling 3.5 miles/min. First let's convert the red car's rate, which is miles/min, to mph. There are 60 min in an hour, so the rate of the red car is $3\frac{1}{2} \times 60$ mph, which is 210 mph. The blue car is going 198 mph. The rate at which the red car gains on the blue car is (210 – 198) mph = 12 mph. The red car is three laps behind the blue car. Because each lap is 2.4 miles, the red car is behind the blue car 7.2 miles. Because the red car gains on the blue car at 12 mph, if T is the number of hr it takes the red car to catch up with the blue car, then (12 mph) × (T hr) = 7.2 miles. The units all cancel, and we have $12T = 7.2$. Then $T = \frac{7.2}{12} = 0.6$. It takes the red car 0.6 hr to catch up with the blue car. The first four answer choices are all in minutes (and the fifth choice says that the red car will never catch up), so let's convert 0.6 hr to min. There are 60 min in 1 hr, so in 0.6 hr there are 0.6 × 60 min = 36 min. It takes the red car 36 min to catch up. (C) is correct.

15. B

We are asked to find the approximate volume of a cone with a height of $2\frac{8}{11}$ ft and a base diameter of 7 ft. The volume of a cone = $\frac{1}{3}$ the area of its circular base times its height. We are told to use $\pi = \frac{22}{7}$. We know that the volume = $\frac{1}{3}$ the area of the base × height. Because we know the base is a circle, the area of the base is the area of a circle. The area of a circle with a radius r is πr^2. The circular base here, we are told, has a diameter of 7 ft; therefore, it has a radius of $\frac{7}{2}$ ft. The area of this circular base is approximately

$\frac{22}{7}\left(\frac{7}{2}\right)^2 = \frac{22}{7} \times \frac{7}{2} \times \frac{7}{2} = \frac{11}{7} \times \frac{7}{1} \times \frac{7}{2} = \frac{11}{1} \times \frac{1}{1} \times \frac{7}{2} = \frac{77}{2}$.

We know that the height is $2\frac{8}{11}$ ft. Let's convert that to an improper fraction. We know that 2 is $\frac{22}{11}$; therefore, $2\frac{8}{11}$ ft $= \frac{30}{11}$ ft. The volume is approximately $\frac{1}{3} \times \frac{77}{2} \times \frac{30}{11}$. A factor of 11 can be canceled from the 77 and the 11, so the volume is approximately $\frac{1}{3} \times \frac{7}{2} \times \frac{30}{1}$. Canceling a factor of 3 from 3 and 30, we have $\frac{1}{1} \times \frac{7}{2} \times \frac{10}{1} = \frac{20}{7} = 35$. The volume is approximately 35 cubic ft.

16. D

We are given the sizes of both hands of the clock, and we want to know how far the large hand covers given that the small hand travels 120°. The small hand is the hour hand. The fact that it travels 120° means that the hour hand has traveled $\frac{1}{3}$ of a revolution around the clock. One revolution to the hour hand is equal to 12 hr, therefore $\frac{1}{3}$ of a revolution to the small hand or the hour hand is equal to 4 hr. The large hand, which is the minute hand, travels one revolution each hour, therefore in 4 hr, as the small hand travels 120°, the large hand travels four revolutions. The tip of the large hand will thus travel the distance of four circumferences. We know that each circumference is equal to $2\pi r$ where r is the radius. In this case, the radius is the length of the large hand, which we are given is 21 cm. We use $\frac{22}{7}$ for π, so we know that the length of the circumference that the tip of the large hand covers is approximately $2 \times \frac{22}{7} \times 21$ cm. Seven goes into 21 three times so we get that the circumference is about $2 \times 22 \times 3$, or 132 cm. That is one circumference. We know that the tip of the large hand had to travel a distance of four circumferences because it was traveling 4 hr. With each circumference being about 132 cm, the large hand travels about 4×132 cm $= 528$ cm, which is (D).

17. A

The easiest way to do this is to convert the decimals to fractions. So $0.84 \div 0.007 = \frac{84}{100} \div \frac{7}{1000} = \frac{84}{100} \times \frac{1000}{7} = \frac{84 \times 1000}{100 \times 7}$. Dividing the numerator and the denominator by 100 and then by 7, the fraction becomes $\frac{12 \times 10}{1 \times 1} = 120$, and we're done.

18. A

The conditions of this problem can be restated as $\frac{\frac{y}{4}}{100} \times 50z = \frac{x}{3}$. Simplifying this yields the expression $\frac{y}{400} \times \frac{50z}{1} = \frac{x}{3}$, or $\frac{yz}{8} = \frac{x}{3}$. Dividing both sides by $\frac{z}{8}$ gives $y = \frac{x}{3} \times \frac{8}{z} = \frac{8x}{3z}$.

19. B

Dividing by a fraction is the same as multiplying by its inverse, so $\frac{495}{\frac{5}{9}} = 495 \times \frac{9}{5} = \frac{495}{5} \times 9 = 99 \times 9 = 891$.

20. B

One gallon is equal to 128 oz, and 1 qt is equal to 32 oz. The given question amounts to how much is $\frac{(128 + 4)\text{ oz}}{(32 + 8)\text{ oz}}$. Because the units on the bottom and the top are equal, we can cancel them out, and the problem is then merely to simplify $\frac{132}{40}$. Dividing the numerator and denominator by 4 gives us $\frac{33}{10}$.

PERIODIC TABLE OF THE ELEMENTS

1 **H** 1.0																	2 **He** 4.0
3 **Li** 6.9	4 **Be** 9.0											5 **B** 10.8	6 **C** 12.0	7 **N** 14.0	8 **O** 16.0	9 **F** 19.0	10 **Ne** 20.2
11 **Na** 23.0	12 **Mg** 24.3											13 **Al** 27.0	14 **Si** 28.1	15 **P** 31.0	16 **S** 32.1	17 **Cl** 35.5	18 **Ar** 39.9
19 **K** 39.1	20 **Ca** 40.1	21 **Sc** 45.0	22 **Ti** 47.9	23 **V** 50.9	24 **Cr** 52.0	25 **Mn** 54.9	26 **Fe** 55.8	27 **Co** 58.9	28 **Ni** 58.7	29 **Cu** 63.5	30 **Zn** 65.4	31 **Ga** 69.7	32 **Ge** 72.6	33 **As** 74.9	34 **Se** 79.0	35 **Br** 79.9	36 **Kr** 83.8
37 **Rb** 85.5	38 **Sr** 87.6	39 **Y** 88.9	40 **Zr** 91.2	41 **Nb** 92.9	42 **Mo** 95.9	43 **Tc** (98)	44 **Ru** 101.1	45 **Rh** 102.9	46 **Pd** 106.4	47 **Ag** 107.9	48 **Cd** 112.4	49 **In** 114.8	50 **Sn** 118.7	51 **Sb** 121.8	52 **Te** 127.6	53 **I** 126.9	54 **Xe** 131.3
55 **Cs** 132.9	56 **Ba** 137.3	57 **La** * 138.9	72 **Hf** 178.5	73 **Ta** 180.9	74 **W** 183.9	75 **Re** 186.2	76 **Os** 190.2	77 **Ir** 192.2	78 **Pt** 195.1	79 **Au** 197.0	80 **Hg** 200.6	81 **Tl** 204.4	82 **Pb** 207.2	83 **Bi** 209.0	84 **Po** (209)	85 **At** (210)	86 **Rn** (222)
87 **Fr** (223)	88 **Ra** 226.0	89 **Ac** † 227.0	104 **Rf** (261)	105 **Db** (262)	106 **Sg** (263)	107 **Bh** (264)	108 **Hs** (269)	109 **Mt** (268)	110 **Ds** (269)	111 **Rg** (272)	112 **Uub** (277)	113 **Uut** (284)	114 **Uug** (289)	115 **Uup** (288)	116 **Uuh** (292)	117 **Uus** (291)	118 **Uuo** (293)

*	58 **Ce** 140.1	59 **Pr** 140.9	60 **Nd** 144.2	61 **Pm** (145)	62 **Sm** 150.4	63 **Eu** 152.0	64 **Gd** 157.3	65 **Tb** 158.9	66 **Dy** 162.5	67 **Ho** 164.9	68 **Er** 167.3	69 **Tm** 168.9	70 **Yb** 173.0	71 **Lu** 175.0
†	90 **Th** 232.0	91 **Pa** (231)	92 **U** 238.0	93 **Np** (237)	94 **Pu** (244)	95 **Am** (243)	96 **Cm** (247)	97 **Bk** (247)	98 **Cf** (251)	99 **Es** (252)	100 **Fm** (257)	101 **Md** (258)	102 **No** (259)	103 **Lr** (260)

Survey of the Natural Sciences: Practice Set 2

40 questions—36 minutes

Directions: Choose the best answer for each question from the five choices provided.

1. According to the modern theory of evolution, which of the following evolved first?

   (A) Krebs cycle
   (B) Anaerobic respiration
   (C) Autotrophic nutrition
   (D) Photosynthesis
   (E) Chemosynthesis

2. Compounds from the glomerular filtrate are partially reabsorbed in the

   (A) Bowman's capsule.
   (B) glomerulus.
   (C) proximal convoluted tubule.
   (D) villi.
   (E) ureter.

3. A bacteriophage, when present within a bacterium, usually consists of

   (A) protein.
   (B) DNA.
   (C) a nucleus.
   (D) specialized cells.
   (E) other parasitic bacteria.

4. Which of the following is an INCORRECT association?

   (A) Porifera : sessile
   (B) Echinodermata : radial symmetry
   (C) Annelida : coelom
   (D) Platyhelminthes : anus
   (E) Insects : tracheal tubes

5. Intestinal nematodes evolved from a free-living to a parasitic form by the evolution of

   (A) special reproductive segments.
   (B) a symbiotic relationship with intestinal bacteria.
   (C) an external cuticle resistant to digestive enzymes.
   (D) a long digestive tube.
   (E) an intricate nervous system.

6. Which are CORRECTLY related?

   (A) White blood cell : no nucleus
   (B) Smooth-muscle cell : multinuclear
   (C) Smooth-muscle : voluntary action
   (D) Cardiac cells : protoplasmic connections
   (E) Smooth muscles : striations

GO ON TO THE NEXT PAGE

7. Motor neurons are characterized by their
   (A) dorsal root.
   (B) ventral root ganglion.
   (C) afferent activity.
   (D) ventral root.
   (E) None of the above

8. In a pond community, the greatest mass present would consist of
   (A) algae.
   (B) insects.
   (C) frogs.
   (D) fish.
   (E) fungi.

9. Phagocytosis is found in
   (A) paramecia.
   (B) erythrocytes.
   (C) hydra.
   (D) leukocytes.
   (E) flame cells.

10. Which of the following is CORRECTLY associated?
    (A) Coelenterate : mesoderm
    (B) Annelid : ventral hollow nerve cord
    (C) Mollusk : chitinous exoskeleton
    (D) Platyhelminthes : circulatory system
    (E) Chordata : dorsal hollow nerve cord

11. Venous blood, en route from the kidneys to the heart, must pass through the
    (A) iliac vein.
    (B) inferior vena cava.
    (C) liver.
    (D) hepatic vein.
    (E) pulmonary vein.

12. $ATP + 2NH_3 + CO_2 + NH_2C \rightarrow ONH_2 + ADP + P + H_2O$ will occur in the
    (A) kidney.
    (B) liver.
    (C) small intestine.
    (D) lungs.
    (E) ribosome.

13. Which of the following is (are) derived from the mesoderm?
    (A) Heart
    (B) Lung epithelium
    (C) Intestinal mucosa
    (D) Nerve
    (E) Two of the above

14. Which of the following is NOT a steroid?
    (A) Cholesterol
    (B) Vitamin D
    (C) Testosterone
    (D) Carotene
    (E) Cortisol

15. Which of the following yields 4 calories/gram upon digestion?
    (A) Glucose
    (B) Proteins
    (C) Fats
    (D) Two of the above
    (E) All of the above

16. The rate of an enzyme-catalyzed reaction can be influenced by all of the following EXCEPT
    (A) Substrate concentration
    (B) Temperature
    (C) Enzyme concentration
    (D) Rate constant
    (E) pH

GO ON TO THE NEXT PAGE

17. What is the probability of a white, long-tailed mouse from the cross of a heterozygous black, heterozygous long-tailed mouse with a homozygous recessive white, homozygous recessive short-tailed mouse?

(A) 0%
(B) 25%
(C) 50%
(D) 75%
(E) 100%

18. PGAL

(A) is considered the prime end-product of photosynthesis.
(B) can be used immediately as food.
(C) can be combined and rearranged to form glucose.
(D) can be stored as insoluble polysaccharides such as starch.
(E) All of the above

19. During what stage of meiosis does crossing over occur?

(A) Prophase I
(B) Metaphase I
(C) Anaphase I
(D) Telophase I
(E) Interkinesis

20. The blood group antigens are an example of

(A) pleiotropy.
(B) incomplete dominance.
(C) codominance.
(D) epistasis.
(E) incomplete penetrance.

21. What is the mole fraction of C_2H_5OH in an aqueous solution that is simultaneously 3.86 m C_2H_5OH and 2.14 m CH_3OH?
(Atomic weights: C = 12, H = 1, O = 16)

(A) $\frac{3.86}{61.55}$
(B) $\frac{2.14}{61.55}$
(C) $\frac{3.86}{6.00}$
(D) $\frac{2.14}{6.00}$
(E) None of the above

22. The reaction $NH_4^+ + H_2O \rightarrow NH_3 + H_3O^+$ is

(A) an electron-transfer reaction.
(B) a single replacement reaction.
(C) a double replacement reaction.
(D) a redox reaction.
(E) a proton-transfer reaction.

23. Which of the following represents the equation for positron emission by Sb?

(A) $^{120}_{51}Sb \rightarrow {}^{0}_{+1}e + {}^{120}_{51}Sn$
(B) $^{120}_{51}Sb + {}^{0}_{+1}e \rightarrow {}^{120}_{52}Te$
(C) $^{120}_{51}Sb \rightarrow {}^{0}_{+1}e + {}^{120}_{50}Sn$
(D) $^{120}_{51}Sb + {}^{0}_{+1}e \rightarrow {}^{120}_{50}Sn$
(E) None of the above

GO ON TO THE NEXT PAGE

24. An unknown nonelectrolyte dissolves in an aqueous solution to yield a solution containing 4.68 g unknown per 1,000 g H_2O. If the measured freezing point of the solution is –0.372°C, what is the molecular weight of the unknown compound in g/mol? (Freezing point depression constant for H_2O = 1.86°C)

(A) $\frac{4.68}{1{,}000}$

(B) $\frac{(4.68 \times 0.372)}{1{,}000}$

(C) $\frac{4.68}{0.2}$

(D) $\frac{(1.86 \times 0.372)}{0.2}$

(E) None of the above

25. An aqueous sulfuric acid solution is 39.2% H_2SO_4 by mass and has a specific gravity of 1.25. How many mL of this solution are required to make 100 mL of a 0.20 M sulfuric acid solution? (FW of H_2SO_4 = 98 g/mol)

(A) 1.6

(B) 3.0

(C) 4.0

(D) 5.0

(E) 6.25

26. Which of the following will be observed when a nonvolatile solute is added to a pure solvent?

I. The vapor pressure of the solvent above the resulting solution will decrease.
II. The boiling point of the resulting solution will be higher than that of the pure solvent.
III. The freezing point of the resulting solution will be lower than that of the pure solvent.
IV. The osmotic pressure will change.

(A) I only

(B) IV only

(C) I and IV only

(D) II and III only

(E) I, II, III, and IV

27. What is the mole fraction of chloride ions in a 1 *m* solution of NaCl? (Atomic weights: Na = 23, Cl = 35)

(A) $\frac{1}{3}$

(B) $\frac{1}{2}$

(C) $\frac{35}{38}$

(D) 1

(E) None of the above

28. Compute the sum of the $X_1 + X_2 + X_3 + X_4 + X_5$ in the following nuclear equation.

$${}^{26}_{X_1}\text{Mg} + {}^{X_2}_{0}\text{n} \rightarrow {}^{X_3}_{X_4}\text{He} + {}^{X_5}_{10}\text{Ne}$$

(A) 39

(B) 40

(C) 41

(D) 42

(E) 43

29. Find the K_a of HCN, given that a 0.20 M solution of HCN(*aq*) is 0.002% ionized at 25°C.

(A) 8×10^{-11}

(B) 4×10^{-8}

(C) 4×10^{-11}

(D) 8×10^{-8}

(E) 8×10^{-7}

30. A total of 100 mL of 5 M $H_2SO_4(aq)$ are diluted to 800 mL. What is the molarity of the solution after dilution?

(A) $\frac{16}{10}$ M

(B) $\frac{8}{10}$ M

(C) $\frac{10}{8}$ M

(D) $\frac{10}{12}$ M

(E) $\frac{5}{8}$ M

GO ON TO THE NEXT PAGE

31. Which of the compounds below is the strongest base?

(A) 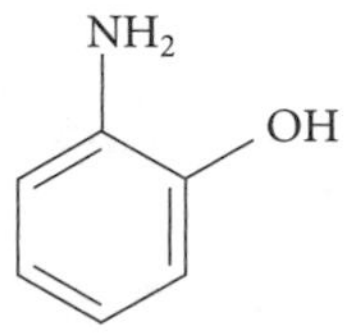

(B) 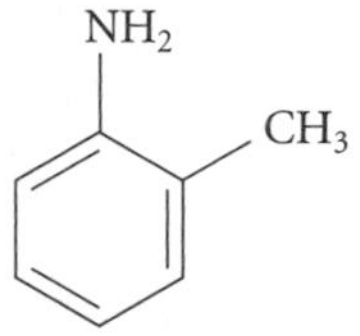

(C) 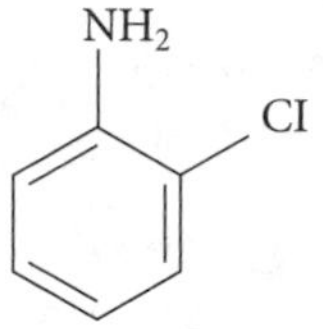

(D) 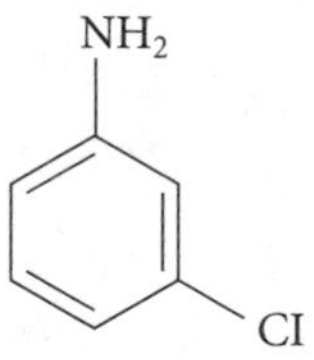

(E) 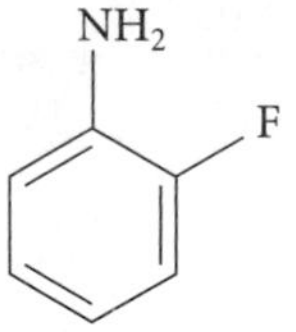

32. 3-Methyl-3-decanol can be prepared from which of the following reaction(s)?

(A) $CH_3MgBr + CH_3CH_2\overset{\overset{O}{\|}}{C}(CH_2)_6CH_3 \xrightarrow{H^{\oplus}}$

(B) $CH_3CH_2MgBr + CH_3\overset{\overset{O}{\|}}{C}(CH_2)_6CH_3 \xrightarrow{H^{\oplus}}$

(C) $CH_3(CH_2)_6MgBr + CH_3\overset{\overset{O}{\|}}{C}CH_2CH_3 \xrightarrow{H^{\oplus}}$

(D) All of the above

(E) None of the above

33. What is the product of the reaction sequence below?

$$HC{\equiv}CH \xrightarrow{NaNH_2} \xrightarrow{CH_3CH_2I} \xrightarrow{NaNH_2} \xrightarrow{CH_3CH_2CH_2I} \xrightarrow[\text{liq. } NH_3]{Na}$$

(A) 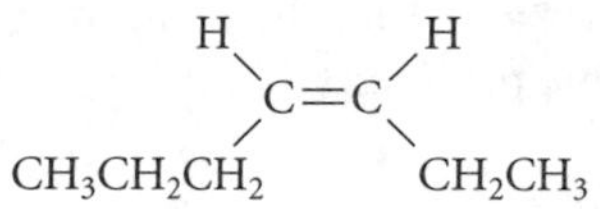

(B) 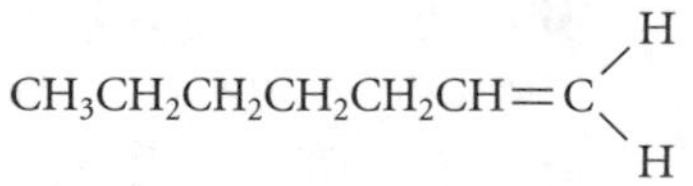

(C) $CH_3CH_2CH_2C{\equiv}CCH_2CH_3$

(D) 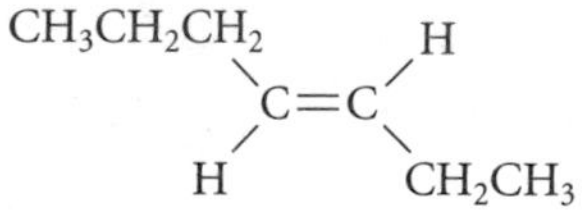

(E) $CH_3(CH_2)_5CH_3$

34. When the epoxide shown below is placed in a solution of sodium methoxide in methanol

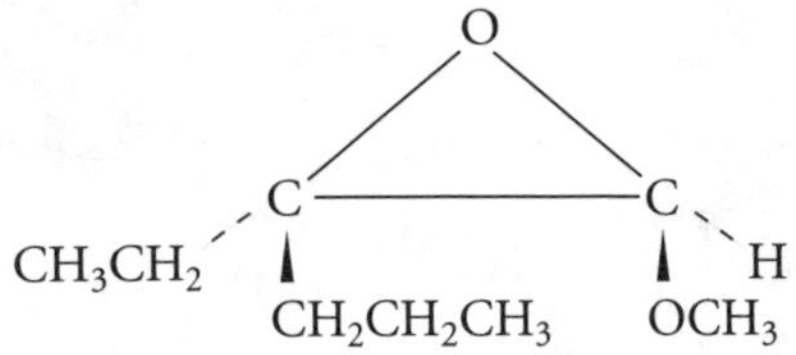

(A) no reaction ensues.
(B) the major product is a racemic mixture of peroxides.
(C) the major product formed is an acetal that contains one chiral center.
(D) the major product formed is an acetal that contains two chiral centers.
(E) the major products formed are an acetal and a peroxide, both optically inactive.

35. When the compound shown below undergoes elimination via an E1 mechanism, what would be the most stable product(s)?

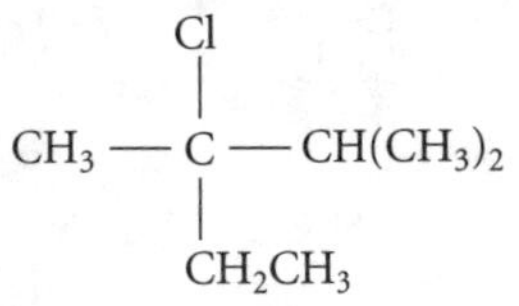

(A)

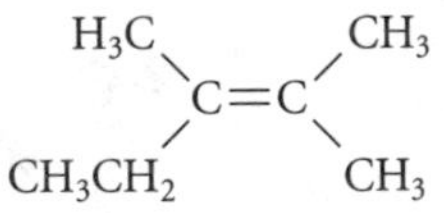

(B)

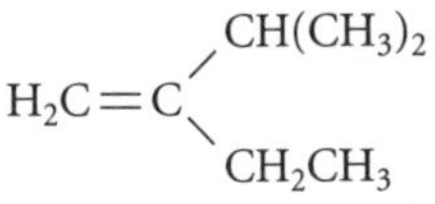

(C)

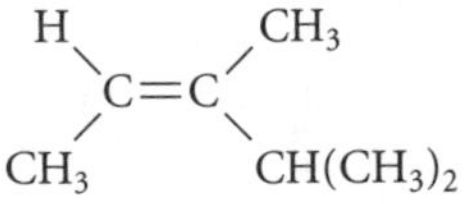

(D)

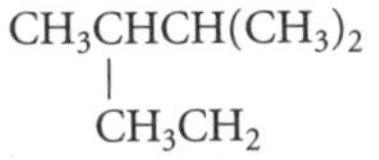

(E) All of the above

36. When the compound shown below undergoes acid-catalyzed hydration, what is the major product?

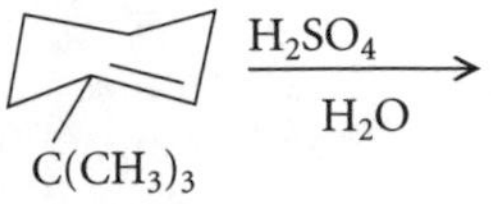

(A)

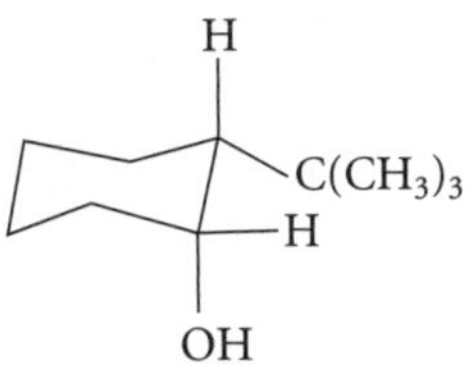

(B)

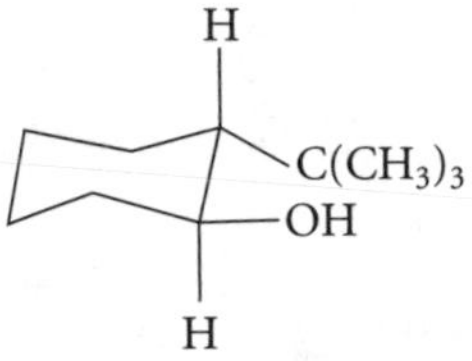

(C)

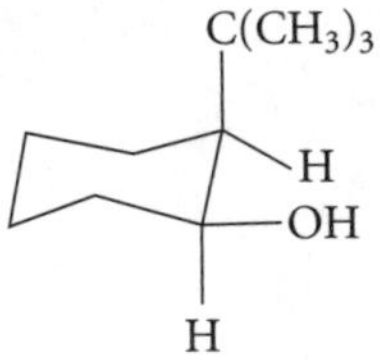

(D)

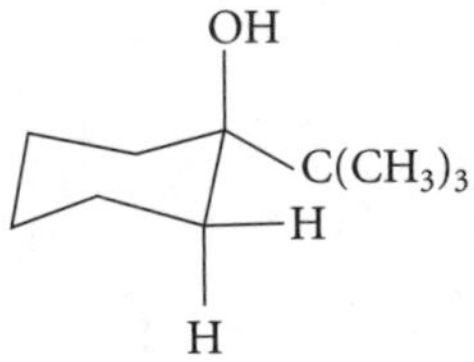

(E)

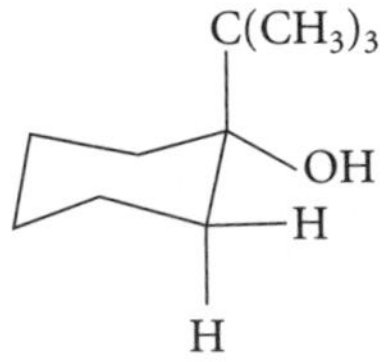

GO ON TO THE NEXT PAGE

37. Which is the anomeric carbon of glucose?

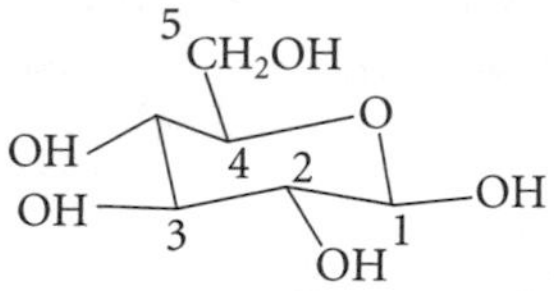

(A) 1
(B) 2
(C) 3
(D) 4
(E) 5

38. An unknown aldotetrose, when treated with $NaBH_4$, yields a single optically active compound. Which of the following structures could be the unknown aldotetrose?

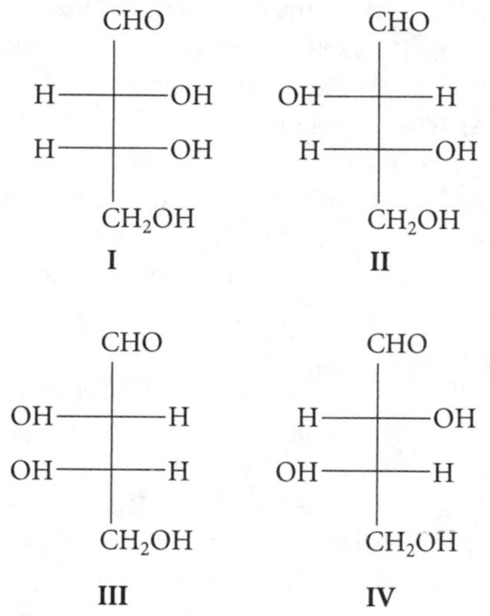

(A) I and II only
(B) I and III only
(C) II and III only
(D) II and IV only
(E) None of the above

39. Give the reagents necessary to complete the following reaction.

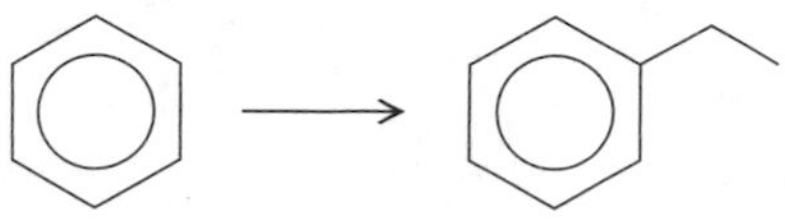

(A) CH_3CH_2Cl
(B) CH_3CH_2Cl, $AlCl_3$
(C) 1) $CH_3C(=O){-}Cl$, $AlCl_3$ 2) Zn(Hg), HCl
(D) Two of the above
(E) All of the above

40. What are the products of the following reaction?

$$CH_3{-}C(CH_3)_2{-}CH_2CH_2MgBr + H_2O \longrightarrow$$

(A) $CH_3{-}C(CH_3)_2{-}CH_2CH_2MgOH + HBr$

(B) $CH_3{-}C(CH_3)_2{-}CH_2CH_2OH + MgBrH$

(C) $CH_3{-}C(CH_3)_2{-}CH_2CH_3 + MgBrOH$

(D) (B) and (C)
(E) None of the above

IF YOU FINISH BEFORE TIME IS CALLED, YOU MAY CHECK YOUR WORK ON THIS SECTION ONLY. DO NOT TURN TO ANY OTHER SECTION IN THE TEST. **STOP**

ANSWERS AND EXPLANATIONS

1. B	11. B	21. A	31. A
2. C	12. B	22. E	32. D
3. B	13. A	23. C	33. D
4. D	14. D	24. C	34. C
5. C	15. D	25. C	35. A
6. D	16. D	26. E	36. D
7. D	17. B	27. E	37. A
8. A	18. E	28. D	38. D
9. D	19. A	29. A	39. D
10. E	20. C	30. E	40. C

1. B

According to evolutionary theory, large numbers of spontaneously formed organic molecules became simple organisms able to respire in the simplest way—anaerobically. These anaerobic heterotrophs developed first, then chemosynthetic bacteria developed. Then photosynthetic bacteria developed and released O_2 as a by-product, allowing the development of aerobic heterotrophs and the Krebs cycle.

2. C

As blood passes through the glomerulus, it is filtered by passing through the capillary walls. Only blood cells and protein remain in the blood, whereas water, salts, glucose, and amino acids are filtered into the Bowman's capsule. Resorption of amino acids, glucose, and salts occurs predominantly in the proximal convoluted tubules. The cells lining the tubules actively transport these materials out of the tubular lumen and into the peritubular capillary network. Movement of these materials produces an osmotic gradient, which drives some simultaneous passive diffusion of water out of the tubules. (D) is incorrect because villi are small projections in the walls of the small intestine that increase the surface area to facilitate absorption of nutrients. (E) is incorrect because the ureter is a duct that carries urine from the kidneys to the bladder.

3. B

A bacteriophage is a virus that infects bacteria. It is made up of either RNA or DNA and a protein coat. The protein coat injects the genetic material into a bacterium like a syringe but remains outside the cell. When the genetic material is inside the bacterium, it reproduces and forms many viral progeny. (A) is incorrect because the protein coat remains on the outside of the cell. (C) is incorrect because neither viruses nor bacteria have nuclei. (D) and (E) are incorrect because a virus is smaller than a cell and is considered noncellular. Therefore, it would be unable to consist of specialized cells or other bacteria.

4. D

Platyhelminthes are ribbonlike, bilaterally symmetrical organisms with three layers of cells including a solid mesoderm. They do not have a circulatory system, and their nervous system consists of eyes, an anterior brain ganglion, and a pair of longitudinal nerve cords. They also have a primitive excretory system containing flame cells. They do not have an anus. (A) is incorrect because Porifera are sponges that have two layers of cells, have pores, are sessile, and have a low degree of cellular specialization. (B) is incorrect because echinoderms are spiny and radially symmetrical, contain a water-vascular system, and possess the capacity for regeneration of parts. (C) is incorrect because annelids are segmented worms and possess a true body cavity, the coelom, contained in the mesoderm. Annelids have well-defined systems including nervous, circulatory, and excretory systems. (E) is incorrect because insects are arthropods and possess jointed appendages, chitinous exoskeletons, and open circulatory systems. They have three pairs of legs, spiracles, and tracheal tubes designed for breathing outside of an aquatic environment.

5. C

This development was the most important evolutionary development for internal intestinal parasites so they would not be digested by the host's acidic environment in the gut. (D) is false as they consume the already-digested food of their host so they do not need developed digestive tracts. (E) has nothing to do with parasitism, and nematodes actually have quite primitive nervous systems. (A) is incorrect because this is a characteristic of tapeworms, not roundworms. Roundworms actually reproduce by releasing eggs. (B) is incorrect because this answer has nothing to do with parasitism.

6. D

Cardiac cells have protoplasmic connections termed intercellular connections between cells. They do have some striations although they are not voluntary. (B), (C), and (E) are incorrect because smooth muscle has no striations, is mononuclear, and is involuntary. (A) is false because white blood cells have nuclei. In adult humans, red blood cells do not have nuclei to make room for more hemoglobin.

7. D

Motor neuron dendrites in the central nervous system receive signals from either sensory neurons or from other neurons in the central nervous system. Motor neuron cell bodies are found in the ventral portion of the spinal cord, their axons leave the spinal cord though the ventral root, and their axons innervate effector tissue such as skeletal muscle. (A) is incorrect because motor neurons are associated with the ventral root, not the dorsal root, and (B) is incorrect because there is no such thing as the ventral root ganglion. (C) is false because motor neurons are efferent, and (E) is incorrect because (D) is correct.

8. A

In an ecology pyramid, the primary producers (photosynthetic or chemosynthetic organisms) are always the largest population. (B) and (E) are primary consumers whereas (C) and (D) are secondary consumers.

9. D

White blood cells are part of the body's defense against pathogens and tumor surveillance. Some white blood cells, in particular macrophages and neutrophils, are able to phagocytose bacteria and cellular debris. (A) is incorrect because paramecia are members of the ciliate class of protozoa, which ingest food through an oral groove that is guided by beating cilia. The cilia direct the food into a food vacuole where it is digested, and waste is exuded through the anal pore. (B) is incorrect because red blood cells do not phagocytose; rather, their function is to carry O_2 in hemoglobin. (C) is incorrect because hydras are coelenterates that have a mouth/anus common opening. Tentacles help push food into this cavity as this organism is too large to phagocytose. (E) is incorrect because flame cells are the excretory system of flatworms. The cilia that push the waste out of the organism look like a flame.

10. E

This is the definition of chordates and helps to explain why they have such an advanced nervous system compared to other organisms. (A) is incorrect because coelenterates have a mesoglia rather than a full germ layer of mesoderm. This mesoglia is mostly gelatinous with a few scattered cells. (B) is incorrect because annelids have ventral double solid nerve cords. (C) is incorrect because mollusks are broken down into three parts: the foot, which aids in locomotion; the visceral mass; and the mantle, which typically secretes the shell. This shell is not chitinous; rather, chitinous exoskeletons are characteristic of insects. (D) is incorrect because flatworms do not have a respiratory or circulatory system, although they do have primitive excretory and reproductive systems.

11. B

Blood leaving the kidneys travels through the inferior vena cava before entering the right atrium. All of the blood from the lower half of the body is collected in the inferior vena cava. This vessel merges with the superior vena cava (that collects blood from the upper half of the body) immediately before it enters the right atrium. (A) is incorrect because the iliac veins return blood from each leg before joining and becoming the common iliac vein, which then enters the inferior vena cava. (C) and (D) are incorrect because blood enters the liver through the hepatic portal artery after absorbing monosaccharides and amino acids from the small intestine and leaves through the hepatic portal vein after filtration. (E) is incorrect because the pulmonary vein brings blood back from the lungs to the left atrium. This blood has already reached the heart via the right atrium.

12. B

The liver uses ATP to convert ammonia and CO_2 into urea so that it may be excreted in the urine. Ammonia is too toxic to be excreted in that form. (A) is incorrect because urea is excreted by the kidneys although it is formed in the liver. (C) is incorrect because food is digested in the small intestine; there is no waste accumulation as that occurs after the tissues have utilized the energy from the ingested food and produced waste by-products. (D) is incorrect because CO_2 is exhaled from the lungs without urea formation, and (E) is incorrect because ribosomes are sites of protein synthesis, not urea formation.

13. A

The ectodermal germ layers give rise to the epidermis of the skin and also the nervous system. The endodermis, or endodermal germ layer, gives rise to the lining of the digestive system, its associated glands and organs (such as the liver and pancreas), and the lungs. Most of the other organs and systems of the body are mesodermal, including the excretory system, the reproductive system, the muscular and skeletal systems, and the circulatory system. Many of the human body tissues are derived from the mesoderm. In answering questions of this type, if you review and eliminate tissues derived from the ectoderm and endoderm, you find that the remaining tissues are mesodermal. In this question, answer choices (B) and (C) are endodermal tissues. Answer choice (D), nerve, is an ectodermal derivative.

14. D

Carotene is an orange plant pigment that is the precursor of vitamin A. All of the other answer choices are steroids and belong to a class of lipid-derived molecules with a characteristic ring structure. Steroid hormones pass through the cell membrane with ease because they are lipid-soluble.

15. D

Carbohydrates, such as glucose and maltose, and proteins both yield 4 calories per gram consumed. Fats, in contrast, are very high-energy, yielding 9 calories per gram consumed.

16. D

The rate constant (k) that appears in the rate law is a temperature-dependent constant. For a given temperature, nothing will change k, so it can have no influence on an enzyme-catalyzed reaction. We can eliminate choice (A) with the understanding that if the substrate concentration increases, the reaction rate will also increase, until you hit a maximum rate (at which point the enzymes become saturated with substrate). All enzymes have an optimal temperature and pH (for most enzymes; it is body temperature and plasma pH, 37°C and 7.2 respectively) under which they operate most efficiently. If the temperature or pH is increased or decreased from the optimal point, the reaction rate will decrease, eliminating choices (B) and (E). Finally, an increase in enzyme concentration will cause an increase in reaction rate, so we are left with choice (D).

17. B

Let B = black coat color and b = white coat color and L = long tail and l = short tail. So what is the probability of a white, long-tailed mouse from the cross of BbLl x bbll?

Let's construct the Punnett square:

	Bb	bb
Ll	BbLl	bbLl
ll	Bbll	bbll

B = black
b = white
L = Long
l = short

25 percent of the offspring will be black with long tails, 25 percent of the offspring will be black with short tails, 25 percent of the offspring will be white with long tails (what we're looking for), and 25 percent of the offspring will be white with short tails.

18. E

PGAL is generally considered the prime end-product of photosynthesis, and it can be used as an immediate food nutrient; combined and rearranged to form monosaccharide sugars, such as glucose, which can be transported to other cells; or packaged for storage as insoluble polysaccharides such as starch.

19. A

During prophase I, the chromatin condenses into chromosomes, the spindle apparatus forms, and the nucleoli and nuclear membrane disappear. Homologous chromosomes come together and intertwine in a process called synapsis. Sometimes chromatids of homologous chromosomes break at corresponding points and exchange equivalent pieces of DNA; this process is called crossing over. Choice (B) is incorrect. During metaphase I, homologous pairs align at the equatorial plane, and each pair attaches to a separate spindle fiber by its kinetochore. Choice (C) is incorrect. During anaphase I, the homologous pairs separate and are pulled to opposite poles of the cell. This process is called disjunction, and it accounts for a fundamental Mendelian law. Choice (D) is incorrect. During telophase I, a nuclear membrane forms around each new nucleus. At this point, each chromosome still consists of sister chromatids joined at the centromere. The cell divides into two daughter cells, each receiving a nucleus containing the haploid number of chromosomes. Choice (E) is incorrect because interkinesis is a short rest period between the two cell divisions of meiosis during which the chromosomes partially uncoil.

20. C

The blood group antigens are an example of codominance. Codominance occurs when multiple alleles exist for a given gene and more than one is dominant. When the genotype is heterozygous for codominant alleles, the phenotype is the result of the expression of both alleles simultaneously. The classic example of codominance and multiple alleles is the inheritance of ABO blood groups in humans. Blood type is determined by three different alleles, IA, IB, and i. Only two alleles are present in any single individual, but the population contains all three alleles. IA and IB are both dominant to i. Individuals who are homozygous IA or heterozygous IAi have blood type A; individuals who are homozygous IB or heterozygous IBi have blood type B; and individuals who are homozygous ii have blood type O.

However, IA and IB are codominant; individuals who are heterozygous IAIB have a distinct blood type, AB, which combines characteristics of both the A and B blood groups. Choice (A) is incorrect because pleiotropy is the ability of a single gene to have multiple effects. Choice (B) is incorrect. Some progeny phenotypes are apparently blends of the parental phenotypes. This is known as incomplete dominance. Choice (D) is incorrect. Epistasis is a phenomenon in which one gene alters the expression of another gene that is independently inherited. Choice (E) is incorrect. Penetrance is the proportion of individuals who show the phenotype that is expected from their genotype. One example of incomplete penetrance is a type of eye tumor called retinoblastoma, which is due to a dominant allele. Not all individuals who inherit the allele develop the tumor. Furthermore, the severity of the tumor varies among those individuals who show the retinoblastoma phenotype.

21. A

Another rather involved question on concentration units, this one requires that you know how to apply the definitions of both molality and mole fraction. Once again, a glance at the answer choices indicates that full calculation is unnecessary. In fact, we can avoid most of the calculations by reasoning from the values shown in the choices. For instance, because we are asked to find the mole fraction of ethanol rather than methanol, we can eliminate (B) and (D) for using the number 2.14 rather than 3.86. Thinking about the other two numbers shown, 6.00 and 61.55, we might determine that (C) and (D) can be eliminated for ignoring the moles of water present in the aqueous solution (i.e., 6.00 is the sum of 2.14 and 3.86, the numbers of moles of the two solutes only). To decide between (A) and (E), we would have to do the math:

$$X_{ethanol} = mol_{ethanol}/mol_{total}$$

$$= mol_{ethanol}/(mol_{ethanol} + mol_{methanol} + mol_{water})$$

Because the solution is 2.14 molal in methanol and 3.86 molal in ethanol, there will be this number of moles, respectively, per kilogram of water. Assuming a solution made with exactly 1 kilogram of H_2O, or (1,000 g)/(18 g/mol) = 55.55 mol of H_2O, we can substitute into the expression above to arrive at (A):

$$X_{ethanol} = mol_{ethanol}/mol_{total}$$

$$= 3.86/(3.86 + 2.14 + 55.55) = 3.86/61.55$$

22. E

The reaction shown is an acid/base reaction in which a proton, H^+, is transferred from the NH_4^+ on the reactant side to the H_2O; as a result, H_3O^+ appears on the product side along with its newly acquired proton.

(A) and (D) can be eliminated as equivalent answer choices; besides, no electrons are transferred in the reaction so none of the oxidation numbers change.

This reaction cannot truly be thought of as a single displacement, which requires redox, nor as a double displacement, which requires that two species exchange partners. (B) and (C) are likewise incorrect.

23. C

This question on nuclear decay requires you to recognize positron emission and identify the daughter element of this decay reaction correctly. A positron is a nuclear particle with the same mass and spin as an electron but with a positive charge rather than the usual negative charge, leading to the nuclide symbol ${}^{0}_{+1}e$. To qualify as emission, the positron must arise from the decay of the parent nucleus and must, therefore, appear on the product side of the nuclear equation; (B) and (D), which actually depict positron capture rather than emission, can be eliminated for this reason. The final consideration now is to determine the identity of the daughter element; this is accomplished by summing, separately, the upper and lower numbers on the nuclide symbols. Because all the daughter elements' mass (upper) numbers are 120, this sum need not be determined. The nuclear charge (lower) numbers on the right side of (C), 1 and 50, correctly sum to the charge number on the left, 51, whereas those in (A) do not. A glance at the periodic table verifies that an atomic number of 50 does indeed correspond to the element Sn, making (C) the correct answer.

24. C

(C) is correct. This question on colligative properties utilizes the relationship between the freezing point depression and the molality of a solute in solution (i.e., $\Delta T = K_f m$). Because the freezing point depression, ΔT, is apparently 0.2 times the freezing point depression constant, K_f, the solution must be 0.2 molal. If a 0.2 molal solution is produced by dissolving 4.68 g of solute in 1 kg of solvent, it follows that 5 times as much would be required to make a 1 molal solution. Thus one mole of solute per kg of solvent is equivalent to 5 × 4.68 g of solute per kg of solvent, and the formula weight of the solute must therefore be 5 × 4.68 or, equivalently, 4.68/0.2 g/mol. As a more quantitative approach, we can set up and solve the dimensional expression:

$$\frac{4.68\ \text{g/kg}_{\text{solvent}}}{0.2\ \text{mol/kg}_{\text{solvent}}} = \frac{4.68}{0.2}\ \text{g/mol}$$

25. C

This is a question of solution stoichiometry, requiring that you convert the given mass percentage and specific gravity into molarity and then perform a dilution calculation as well. Alternatively, we could use the backsolving method on the choices offered to determine which one corresponds to the required 0.020 mol of H_2SO_4. (To make 100 mL, or 0.100 L, of 0.20 M sulfuric acid, one would need 0.020 mol of H_2SO_4.) We can proceed to find out how many mL of the more-concentrated solution will contain this number of moles of H_2SO_4. The formula weight of H_2SO_4 is given to be 98 g/mol; therefore, (0.020 × 98) g = 1.96 g of H_2SO_4 is needed. The solution contains 39.2 percent H_2SO_4 by mass. Hence, to obtain the mass of the solution containing the needed amount of H_2SO_4, we need to divide 1.96 g by this percentage: 1.96 g/0.392 = 5.0 g of solution. The specific gravity of the solution is 1.25, which means that its density is 1.25 times that of water, or 1.25 g/mL. Therefore, 5 g of the solution translates to 5.0/1.25 = 4.0 mL.

26. E

This is a question on colligative properties (i.e., physical properties of a mixture that depend on its concentration rather than on the chemical identity of the solute added). Vapor pressure depression, Statement I, is a colligative property and can be approximated by applying Raoult's law. Boiling point elevation, Statement II, and freezing point depression, Statement III, are also colligative properties, calculated via the relationship $\Delta T = Km$, where K is either the boiling point elevation constant or the freezing point depression constant as warranted, usually expressed in °C/m. Finally, osmotic pressure, Statement IV, is also a colligative property. Because all four statements correctly list colligative properties, (E) is correct.

27. E

This question on concentration units asks us to convert molality to mole fraction. Recall that molality is moles of solute per kilogram of solvent and that the mole fraction of component A in a mixture is $X_A = n_A/n_{total}$, where X_A is the mole fraction of A, n_A is the number of moles of A present in the mixture, and n_{total} is the total number of moles present.

Let us assume that the solution was produced by adding the required quantity of NaCl, 1 mol, to 1 L (= 1 kg) of water. One kilogram of water, at 18 g/mol, is about 56 mol of water. Adding in the 1 mol of Na^+ and the 1 mol of Cl^- (derived from the dissolution of 1 mol of NaCl), we have an approximate total of 58 mol present in the mixture. The mole fraction of Cl^- is thus approximately 1/58, much smaller than are any of the choices offered, making (E) the credited choice. A much less quantitative pathway to the same result would have been to realize that if there are more than 3 mol of water per mole of NaCl, then (A) is too big and that the other choices are even larger. Note that the given atomic masses of Na and Cl do not even come into play.

28. D

This question on nuclear chemistry requires you to determine the upper and lower numbers on the nuclide symbols. The sum of the nuclear charge (lower) numbers on the right side of the reaction must equal the sum of the charge numbers on the left, but each of these lower numbers corresponds to the atomic number of the associated element. Thus $X_1 = 12$ and $X_4 = 2$ can be determined directly from the periodic table. Because the mass (upper) numbers on the reactant side must sum to the same value as the mass numbers on the product side, and because a neutron has a mass number of 1 (i.e., $X_2 = 1$), we can set up an algebraic expression to solve for the desired sum:

$$26 + X_2 = X_3 + X_5$$
$$X_3 + X_5 = 27$$
$$X_1 + X_2 + X_3 + X_4 + X_5 = X_1 + X_2 + X_4 + (X_3 + X_5)$$
$$= 12 + 1 + 2 + (27) = 42$$

29. A

Calculations involving K_a, concentration, and percent ionization can be accomplished via the approximation $K_a = x^2/c_o$, where $x = [H^+]$ and $c_o = [HA]$ for dilute solutions of the weak acid HA. Because the acid is 0.002 percent (or 0.00002) ionized in a 0.20 M solution, we can find $x = [H^+]$ as:

$$x = (0.00002)(0.20) = 4 \times 10^{-6}\text{M}$$

We can safely assume that c_o – 0.002 percent $c_o = c_o =$ 0.20 M. Substituting into the K_a expression yields:

$$K_a = x^2/c_o = (4 \times 10^{-6})^2/(0.20)$$
$$= (16 \times 10^{-12})/(2 \times 10^{-1}) = 8 \times 10^{-11}.$$

30. E

This is a dilution problem for which our standard formula $V_1C_1 = V_2C_2$ can be used. Rearranging to solve for C_2 and plugging in the numbers from the stem gives $C_2 = V_1C_1/V_2 = (100\text{ mL})(5\text{ M})/(800\text{ mL}) = 5/8$ M. More intuitively, if we dilute to 8 times the volume, we will have 1/8 of the concentration.

31. A

Electron-donating substituent groups will destabilize the lone pair of electrons on nitrogen, making it more reactive (more basic). Fluorine and chlorine are both electronegative atoms that would help stabilize the electron pair, so they can be eliminated. The hydroxyl group and the methyl group are both electron donating, with the hydroxyl group much more so. The lone pair of electrons on nitrogen in compound A would therefore be most likely to grab a proton and is, hence, by definition the most basic.

32. D

Grignard reagents (magnesium alkyl bromides) are very good nucleophiles and add readily to carbonyl groups, yielding secondary (from aldehydes) or tertiary (from ketones) alcohols after treatment with aqueous acid. 3-Methyl-3-decanol must have a total chain length of 10 carbons, with a methyl attached at the third carbon (same as the OH group). In each case, the reactions depicted in choices (A), (B), and (C) will give an overall carbon chain length of 10 with a methyl group at the third position. Therefore, (D) is correct.

33. D

This answer may be inferred from the reagents used for the last step of the given synthesis, which are common reagents used to *trans*-hydrogenate the triple bond, but stopping before further reducing the alkene. The only choice with a *trans* double bond is (D). Strong bases will remove the acetylenic proton, leaving the terminal triple-bonded carbon with a lone pair of electrons, which can then act as a nucleophile. Addition to alkyl halides, with the halide acting as the leaving group, leads to chain elongation. The product of the first two steps is 1-butyne. A second round of chain elongation, with iodopropane as the substrate, leads to the formation of 3-heptyne. *Trans*-hydrogenation results in (D) rather than (A), which would be formed by *cis*-hydrogenation. (E) would be formed only if uncontrolled reduction (two molar H_2 equivalents) occurred, reducing the alkyne all the way back to the alkane.

34. C

Epoxides are inherently unstable molecules because of ring strain and are very sensitive to nucleophilic addition. The particular compound shown in the diagram can be considered a cyclic acetal because of the methoxy group attached to the carbon on the right (the acetal carbon). The methoxide ion will attack this acetal carbon, because it is both less hindered sterically and more electron-deficient (it is attached to one more electronegative oxygen atom and does not have electron-releasing alkyl groups attached). The attack by the methoxide will open up the epoxide ring. The acetal carbon will now have exchanged the oxygen of the ring for another methoxy group, thus retaining its acetal status. The left carbon in the ring will inherit the oxygen from the epoxide ring, which will then protonate to form an alcohol. Because this carbon will be bonded to four different groups, the molecule will be chiral. Thus (C), in which there is one acetal and one chiral center formed, is correct.

35. A

The first step in the elimination reaction of the compound, 3-chloro-2,3-methyl-pentane, involves the departure of the chloride ion, leaving behind the relatively stable tertiary carbocation. Subsequent extraction of a proton will occur such that the most highly substituted alkene (the most thermodynamically stable one) will be formed. In this case; the proton will be extracted from the carbon with two methyl groups attached (C2 in the straight chain), leading to the formation of a double bond between C2 and C3, corresponding to the structure shown in (A). (D), and therefore (E), are incorrect, as elimination reactions result in alkenes, not alkanes. (Even though alkanes are thermodynamically more stable than are their corresponding alkenes, the question explicitly states that the species undergoes an elimination reaction.) (B) and (C) are incorrect because they are not as stable as the alkene shown in (A), even though they are possible products of the reaction.

36. D

Acid-catalyzed hydration of an alkene follows Markovnikov's rule, because the first and rate-determining step of the reaction consists of the electrophilic addition of a proton to the double bond to form the most stable carbocation possible. In this case, the proton will attach itself to the less-substituted carbon atom, thus leaving the tertiary carbon (the one attached to the *t*-butyl group) with the positive charge and sp^2 hybridization. When the hydroxyl group adds, the most stable orientation will be with the *t*-butyl group oriented in the equatorial position, as this minimizes the steric strain, giving the axial addition of the hydroxide. Choices (A), (B), and (C) are incorrect because the hydroxide adds to the wrong carbon. (E) is incorrect because the *t*-butyl group would not occupy the axial group due to its large bulk.

37. A

This is a basic definition involving carbohydrate chemistry. The anomeric carbon is the carbon directly bonded to two oxygen atoms (i.e., the hemiacetal carbon atom). This is (A), or carbon 1. This carbon is the most reactive because it can form a double bond with the ring oxygen, forming a cationic intermediate. This intermediate is involved in the formation of glycosidic bonds.

38. D

$NaBH_4$ treatment will reduce the aldehyde group to a primary alcohol. Within the context of this problem, one should realize that the result of the reaction would be to make the two ends of each of the four molecules shown identical (a $-CH_2OH$ group on both ends). For the compound to be optically active, it must not possess a plane of symmetry. In compounds I and III, it should be obvious that after the reductive treatment, the molecule would have a plane of symmetry between the second and third carbons (i.e., the top half of the molecule would be a mirror image of the bottom half of the molecule). These are termed *meso* compounds and do not have any optical activity despite having two chiral centers. Compounds II and IV would still have two chiral centers after the indicated treatments but would not have a plane of symmetry. As such, they would retain their optical activity. The correct choice is then (D). Note, however, that an equimolar mixture of II and IV would be racemic and would not be optically active.

39. D

To attach an ethyl group to a benzene ring, two different electrophilic aromatic substitution pathways are available: Friedel-Crafts alkylation and Friedel-Crafts acylation, the latter followed by reduction. Both reactions involve the use of a Lewis acid ($AlCl_3$) to enhance the electrophilic nature of the molecule, either by extracting the halide from the alkyl or acyl halide to form a carbocation or by forming a complex with the alkyl or acyl halide in which the electron density of the carbon atom is further depleted. (B) depicts the Friedel-Crafts alkylation reaction and will lead to the product shown in the question. The first step of the reaction sequence in (C) is a Friedel-Crafts acylation and leads to the formation of acetophenone (methyl phenyl ketone). This ketone can then be reduced to yield the desired product by refluxing it with hydrochloric acid containing amalgamated zinc. This reaction is known as the Clemmensen reduction. This acylation-reduction pathway is often a much better alternative to direct alkylation, because rearrangement of the alkyl group may occur in direct alkylation, leading to undesired products.

40. C

One of the reactants shown is a Grignard reagent and as such is a strong base as well as a powerful nucleophile. It is such a strong base, in fact, that it will extract protons from hydroxyl groups and terminal alkynes, among others. In the presence of water, therefore, the only reaction that will take place is the acid-base reaction in which a proton is extracted from water to give the saturated alkane and the magnesium, bromide, and hydroxide ions. This is why in the preparation of and in reactions involving Grignard reagents, care must be taken to exclude moisture from the apparatus and anhydrous ether is used as the solvent.

Reading Comprehension: **Practice Set 2**

20 minutes—17 questions

Directions: The following practice set consists of a reading passage and questions that test your comprehension of the passage. Choose the best answer for each question from the five choices provided.

Any study of caries initiation and progression must at the very least include some discussion of enamel and dentin structure and physiology.

The entire crown surface of a tooth is covered by a variable thickness of enamel, which ranges from a maximum of 2–2.5 mm at the cusp tips to a thin veneer at the cervical margin. Enamel is the hardest tissue in the human body. In spite of this, it is relatively brittle. It has a specific gravity of 2.8 and consists primarily of inorganic material (96 percent) and a relatively small component of organic matrix and water (4 percent).

Structurally, enamel is composed of rods or prisms, rod sheaths, and interprismatic substance. The number of rods ranges from 5–12 million depending on the size of the tooth in question. The actual rod length is greater than the measurable distance from the dentinoenamel junction (DEJ) outward to the surface of the tooth due to the oblique and wavy configuration of the rods. Oriented approximately parallel to the long axis of the prism are the apatite crystals.

At the DEJ, enamel rods are perpendicular to the dentin surface. This means that in vertical areas the rods will run horizontally out to the surface of the tooth, while at the cusp tips they will run obliquely or vertically to the surface of the tooth. This change of direction is visible, in a cross-section view of the tooth, as alternating bands of dark and light strips, called Hunter-Schreger bands. The lines of Retzius, which appear in ground section of enamel as brown bands, may be likened to the concentric growth rings found in the cross section of a tree. They have been attributed to variation in basic organic structure or to periodic hypo- and hypercalcification of the rods. The importance of these lines lies in their degree of mineralization and proximity to the tooth surface.

The external surface of enamel, which is formed last, is important because it is a more highly mineralized zone of ≈ 30–40 micron thickness and is relatively caries-resistant. It has a greater hardness and different crystalline orientation than the underlying subsurface enamel.

Dentin consists of 30 percent water and organic material and 70 percent inorganic material. It is softer than enamel and more elastic. The organic matrix is composed of collagen fibers, displaying their characteristic 640 Å periodicity, interwoven in an amorphous ground substance.

Dentin crystalline orientation conforms to the pattern of the collagen fibers. While resembling those of bone and cementum, the apatite crystals of dentin bear little similarity to those of enamel. The incremental lines of Von Ebner correspond to periods of hypomineralization and hypermineralization within the dentin. Dentin mineralization usually begins in isolated areas and grows until fusion of those areas results in a uniformly calcified dentin layer. When fusion fails to occur, isolated pockets of hypomineralized dentin remain, called interglobular dentin.

GO ON TO THE NEXT PAGE

It is generally accepted that five environmental factors are of great significance in the formation of dental caries: microflora, dietary (sucrose) intake, decreased salivary flow rate and buffering capacity, fluoride, and plaque pH. As each tooth first erupts into the oral cavity, it is covered by a pellicle of precipitated salivary proteins that adhere to the tooth surface. The combination of the tooth, microbial masses, and the pellicle interposed between them creates the entity known as dental plaque, which is the basis of dental decay and periodontal disease. The composition of plaque varies with diet and with age. It is, however, about 80 percent water and 20 percent solids.

That bacteria are of importance in the evolution of caries is proven by the fact that gnotobiotic (germ-free) rats do not develop caries even when fed a cariogenic diet. The organism of primary importance in coronal plaque, and hence in the etiology of caries, is the acidogenic *Streptococcus mutans*. Somewhat less important, though numerically dominant, is *Streptococcus sanguis*.

According to the acidogenic theory, the oldest and still most widely accepted theory of caries initiation, carious lesions are produced by an acid attack on the mineralized tooth surface, followed by a second stage in which the already acid-softened protein matrix is degraded by bacterial proteolytic enzymes. The critical acid level at which this occurs is at a pH of 5.5 or below.

The two main types of caries are smooth-surface and pit and fissure caries. Smooth-surface caries penetrate through the enamel skin in a narrow front. However, after piercing this 40-micron-thick shell, the caries advance laterally roughly equally in all directions, forming a conical or hemispherical area, whose apex is oriented toward the dentino-enamel junction. Thus, selective penetration at the sites where the striae of Retzius come to the surface is possible, leaving the external enamel shell relatively intact but the subsurface enamel subject to major carious involvement.

Pit and fissure caries, while conforming to the same basic principles governing smooth-surface caries initiation, assume a different cross-sectional configuration. Enamel at the base of a fissure is very thin and is often hypocalcified or in some other way imperfect. The prisms radiate out from the base of the fissure and a carious lesion tends to assume the same triangular configuration. This time, however, the base is at the DEJ and the apex points to the deepest portion of the fissures.

Once they have reached the DEJ, both smooth-surface caries and pit and fissure caries progress identically and predictably in a rapid lateral spread, which tends to undermine the uninfected enamel above it and to infect previously healthy dentinal tubules. Simultaneously, there is a pulpward progression of the caries down the dentinal tubules resulting in death of the odontoblast and possible infection of the pulp. Once again a roughly triangular or hemispherical area is involved, with its base at the DEJ and its apex at the pulp.

Patterns of caries can be differentiated based on their speed of infiltration and infection. Acute caries, frequently found in children, is a rapidly advancing type. Chronic caries is a somewhat less rapidly advancing lesion associated mainly with older teeth.

Peak caries incidence is generally limited to individuals between the ages of 7–20 years. In fact, dental caries is the most common physical defect found in school-age children. In children suffering from Down syndrome, however, dental caries susceptibility is usually low. Forty-four percent of Down syndrome children were found to be caries-free in a study by Cunningham and Brown.

A familial pattern has been found in tooth morphology and enamel defects. Goldberg, in a study of identical twins, reported that tooth morphology, especially pit and fissure formation, apparently determined by heredity, indirectly influences the incidence of dental caries. However, parents of children with rampant or severe caries who tend to blame the condition of heredity have little scientific evidence to support their contention. The incidence of caries is more related to dietary and oral hygiene habits than to heredity. Yet evidence linking caries predisposition to genetic factors cannot be dismissed. Hunt and associates performed a series of interesting experiments in

GO ON TO THE NEXT PAGE

which they produced two distinct strains of albino rats, one caries-resistant and the other caries-susceptible. In spite of a consistent caries-producing diet, subsequent generations of caries-resistant rats remained caries-resistant.

1. Enamel consists of what percentage of inorganic material?

    (A) 30 percent
    (B) 44 percent
    (C) 70 percent
    (D) 80 percent
    (E) 96 percent

2. Dentin consists approximately of what percentage of organic material?

    (A) 30 percent
    (B) 44 percent
    (C) 70 percent
    (D) 80 percent
    (E) 96 percent

3. The rods within the subsurface enamel

    (A) run straight from the DEJ to the enamel surface.
    (B) regularly change direction as they run from the DEJ to the enamel surface.
    (C) tend to increase the likelihood of tooth fracture.
    (D) lack configuration.
    (E) are perpendicular to the apatite crystals.

4. Which of the following correctly describes some aspect of the incremental lines of Von Ebner?

    (A) They are identical in composition to the Hunter-Schreger bands.
    (B) They run parallel to the dentinal tubules.
    (C) They represent hypercalcification.
    (D) They are found just above the DEJ.
    (E) They correspond to periodic variations in dentin mineralization.

5. Which of the following correspond to the striae of Retzius found in enamel?

    (A) Hunter-Schreger bands
    (B) Lines of Von Ebner
    (C) Apatite crystals
    (D) Collagen fibers
    (E) DEJ

6. The organic matrix of dentin is composed of

    (A) apatite crystals.
    (B) collagen fibers.
    (C) cementum.
    (D) proteolytic enzymes.
    (E) calcium.

7. The external enamel surface of a tooth is

    (A) generally 50 microns thick.
    (B) harder than subsurface enamel.
    (C) especially prone to caries.
    (D) formed from collagen fibers.
    (E) similar to subsurface enamel in its crystalline orientation.

GO ON TO THE NEXT PAGE

8. The critical pH level at which enamel decalcification occurs is

   (A) 5.0.
   (B) 5.5.
   (C) 6.0.
   (D) 6.5.
   (E) 7.0.

9. The MOST important bacteria in the initiation of caries are

   (A) not identified in this article.
   (B) part of the pellicle.
   (C) *Streptococcus mutans.*
   (D) *Streptococcus sanguis.*
   (E) *Streptococcus bacteriosus.*

10. According to the article, gnotobiotic rats are

    (A) selectively bred.
    (B) caries-susceptible.
    (C) germ-free.
    (D) omnivorous.
    (E) herbivorous.

11. The passage suggests that a reduction in salivary flow will result in

    (A) decreased caries incidence.
    (B) increased caries incidence.
    (C) decreased microflora population.
    (D) increased sucrose absorption.
    (E) decreased pellicle formation.

12. Which of the following correctly describes some aspect of the enamel at the base of a fissure?

    (A) Its base reaches into the deepest portion of the fissures.
    (B) It is thicker than most surface enamel.
    (C) It is often hypocalcified.
    (D) It is often hypercalcified.
    (E) Its apex is oriented toward the DEJ.

13. Structurally speaking, subsurface enamel is

    (A) composed of equal parts organic and inorganic material.
    (B) thickest at the cervical margin.
    (C) harder than bone, but brittle.
    (D) formed entirely of rods and prisms.
    (E) harder than external enamel.

14. Goldberg's study determined that a major hereditary influence on caries formation is

    (A) the gene that causes albinism.
    (B) the gene that causes Down syndrome.
    (C) the degree of mineralization in subsurface enamel.
    (D) the percentage of interprismatic material in subsurface enamel.
    (E) the shape and structure of teeth.

15. Which of the following is/are integral to the initial formation of plaque?

    (A) Apatite crystals
    (B) The pellicle
    (C) Cementum
    (D) The striae of Retzius
    (E) Water

GO ON TO THE NEXT PAGE

16. Which of the following terms is a synonym for the type of caries characterized by swift advancement?
    (A) Pit and fissure caries
    (B) Smooth-surface caries
    (C) Peak caries
    (D) Chronic caries
    (E) Acute caries

17. According to the article, human susceptibility to caries is generally greatest
    (A) between the ages of 5 and 17.
    (B) between the ages of 7 and 20.
    (C) until the age of 21.
    (D) during periods of sucrose consumption.
    (E) during prenatal development.

IF YOU FINISH BEFORE TIME IS CALLED, YOU MAY CHECK YOUR WORK ON THIS SECTION ONLY. DO NOT TURN TO ANY OTHER SECTION IN THE TEST. STOP

ANSWERS AND EXPLANATIONS

1. E	6. B	11. B	16. E
2. A	7. B	12. C	17. B
3. B	8. B	13. C	
4. E	9. C	14. E	
5. B	10. C	15. B	

1. E

The author states on lines 10 and 11 that enamel "consists primarily of inorganic material (96 percent)." Choice (C) would have been correct had the question asked for the percentage of inorganic material found in dentin, but this answer is incorrect for enamel.

2. A

Lines 44 and 45 of the passage indicate that dentin consists of 70 percent inorganic material and 30 percent water and organic material. Choice (D) is incorrect because 96 percent is the amount of inorganic material found in enamel, not dentin.

3. B

Lines 17–20 of the passage state that the rod length is greater than the measurable distance from the outer surface of the tooth to the dentinoenamel junction due to an "oblique and wavy configuration of the rods." This statement implies that the rods regularly change direction as they run from the DEJ to the enamel surface. Therefore, rods do not run straight from the DEJ to the enamel surface as is stated in choice (A). Also, rods do have a configuration; they are described as "oblique and wavy." Therefore, choice (D) is incorrect. Choice (C) is incorrect, as paragraph 2 indicates that the rods that make up enamel engender it the "hardest tissue in the human body."

4. E

Lines 53–56 of the passage clearly state that "the incremental lines of Von Ebner correspond to the periods of hypomineralization and hypermineralization within the dentin." Choice (A) is incorrect because the Hunter-Schreger bands are made up of enamel, not dentin. The incremental lines of Von Ebner begin in isolated areas and grow until fusion, making choice (B) incorrect as well. Finally, choice (D) is incorrect because the apatite crystals, not the incremental lines of Von Ebner, are immediately adjacent to the DEJ.

5. B

According to ines 30–35 of the passage, the lines of Retzius have "been attributed to . . . periodic hypo- and hypercalcification of the rods." Because the lines of Retzius are important in mineralization, they correspond most closely to the lines of Von Ebner. The Hunter-Schreger bands correspond to enamel rods, rendering choice (A) incorrect. Apatite crystals are parallel to enamel rods, yet no mention is made of their relationship to hypo- and hypermineralization (which was not the case for the lines of Retzius and Von Ebner). Finally, collagen fibers, although oriented similarly to lines of Von Ebner, bear no similarity with regards to substance (i.e., hypo- and hypermineralization).

6. B

Line 47 of the passage clearly states that the organic matrix of dentin is "composed of collagen fibers." Therefore, apatite crystals, cementum, and proteolytic enzymes are incorrect answer choices.

7. B

Lines 41–43 of the passage indicate that the external surface of enamel "has a greater hardness and different crystalline orientation than the underlying subsurface enamel." The external surface is approximately 30–40 microns thick, making choice (A) incorrect. It is relatively caries-resistant, making choice (C) incorrect. Finally, the external surface of enamel is composed of minerals, not collagen fibers; therefore, choice (D) is incorrect. Choice (E) can be ruled out by the statement contained in the first sentence of this paragraph.

8. B

According to the acidogenic theory, carious lesions occur at a critical acid level of a "pH of 5.5 or below." Although carious lesions would occur at choice (A), or a pH of 5.0, the critical acid level is 5.5. Therefore, choices (C), (D), and (E) would also be incorrect because carious lesions would not occur at these pHs.

9. C

The author reflects that the "organism of primary importance in coronal plaque . . . is the acidogenic *Streptococcus mutans*." Although numerically dominant, the organism *Streptococcus sanguis* is less important than *Streptococcus mutans* with regards to the etiology of dental caries. Who ever heard of *Streptococcus bacteriosus*?

10. C

In lines 76 and77 of the passage, the author states that gnotobiotic rats are germ free. The passage makes no mention of the gnotobiotic rats being omnivorous—choice (D), herbivorous—choice (E), or selectively bred—choice (A). It also states that these particular rats do not develop caries, which renders choice (B) incorrect.

11. B

This can be inferred from lines 61–65, which state that a reduction in salivary flow rate will result in an increased probability of developing dental caries. The passage makes no mention of the role of saliva in decreasing the microflora population other than to say that a decrease in saliva (with a concomitant salivary pellicle formation) may predispose an individual to the development of a salivary pellicle, making choice (E) incorrect.

12. C

The passage, when describing pit and fissure caries, states that the enamel at the base of a fissure is very thin and is often hypocalcified. This answer immediately excludes choices (B) and (D). Choice (A) is incorrect because the base of the carious lesion begins at the DEJ and the apex points to the deepest portions of the fissures. Choice (E) is incorrect because the apex is oriented toward the deepest portions of the fissures, not the DEJ.

13. C

Subsurface enamel is harder than bone, but it is brittle. The beginning of the passage states that the enamel is the hardest tissue in the human body (i.e., it is harder than bone). However, in spite of this, the enamel is relatively brittle.

14. E

The passage states that Goldberg, in a study of identical twins, reported that tooth morphology, especially pit and fissure formation, apparently determined by heredity, indirectly influences the incidence of dental caries. His studies did not address the gene that causes Down syndrome, the degree of mineralization in subsurface enamel, or the percentage of interprismatic material in subsurface enamel.

15. B

The passage states that dental plaque is formed when a combination of the tooth and microbial masses are interposed by pellicles. No mention is made in the passage of the role of apatite crystals, cementum, striae of Retzius, or water in the initial formation of dental plaque.

16. E

The passage states that acute caries are rapidly advancing types of caries, whereas chronic caries are those that are less rapidly advancing and are associated with older teeth. Smooth-surface and pit and fissure caries are not associated with the rapidity with which carious lesions develop. Peak caries refers to the caries acquired by people during the age period of 7–20 years.

17. B

The passage states that the peak caries incidence is generally limited to individuals between the ages of 7 and 20 years. Therefore, although choice (C) may be true to a certain extent, it includes caries incidence between the ages of 1–6, rendering the answer an incorrect choice. The consumption of sucrose is not stated to be epidemiologically related to the peak caries incidence.

Physics: **Practice Set 2**

20 questions – 25 minutes

Directions: Choose the best answer for each question from the five choices provided.

The values for the physical constants below are to be used as needed:

Gravitational acceleration at the surface of the Earth: $g = 10\ m/s^2$

Speed of light in a vacuum: $c = 3 \times 10^8\ m/s$

Charge of an electron: $e = 2.0 \times 10^{-19}$ Coulomb

1. Two different electromagnetic waves with frequencies 3×10^{14} Hz and 2×10^{14} Hz hit a metallic surface, releasing electrons in which some electrons have twice as much kinetic energy as others. What is the minimum frequency needed to remove an electron from the metal?

(A) 1×10^{14} Hz
(B) 2×10^{14} Hz
(C) 3×10^{14} Hz
(D) 4×10^{14} Hz
(E) 5×10^{14} Hz

2. Three weights are hung from a seesaw, and a fourth of unknown mass is connected to the end of the seesaw by a pulley, as shown in the diagram below. To balance the seesaw, the mass in grams must be

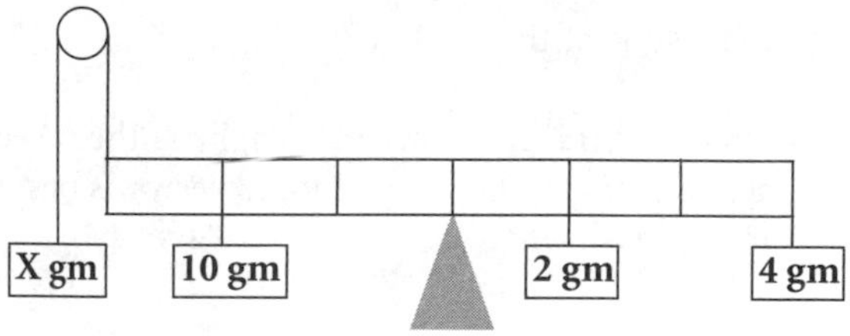

(A) $\frac{1}{3}$.
(B) $\frac{2}{3}$.
(C) 1.
(D) 2.
(E) 4.

GO ON TO THE NEXT PAGE

3. Blocks A and B are connected across a frictionless pulley by a cord of negligible weight, *W*. If block B lies on a horizontal, frictionless surface and block A hangs vertically, what can be said about the acceleration of block B?

    (A) It would accelerate at approximately 9.8 m/s^2.
    (B) It would accelerate at some constant rate other than 9.8 m/s^2.
    (C) Its rate of acceleration would increase with time.
    (D) Its acceleration would be a function of the initial velocity of block A.
    (E) It would not accelerate but rather move with constant velocity.

4. A rifle bullet is fired horizontally off the top of an ocean-based drill site. If air resistance is negligible and the vertical distance to the water below is 100 ft, what additional information is needed to determine the time required for the bullet to hit the water? (g = 32 ft/s^2)

    (A) The horizontal distance the bullet travels
    (B) The initial velocity of the bullet
    (C) The mass of the bullet
    (D) No additional information is needed.
    (E) None of the above

5. An object travels from left to right. If the object is slowing down, the applied force vector is best represented by

    (A) ←.
    (B) →.
    (C) ↑.
    (D) ↓.
    (E) a vector of magnitude zero.

6. The antinode of a standing wave is best characterized as

    (A) a point at which the displacement is zero.
    (B) a point at which the displacement takes on all values from maximum positive to maximum negative.
    (C) a point at which the displacement is always either maximum positive or maximum negative.
    (D) a point at which displacement is both maximum positive and maximum negative at the same time.
    (E) None of the above

7. Assuming that sound travels at 1,100 ft/s, the smallest resonance frequency of sound waves in a 6-inch tube closed at one end is

    (A) 275 Hz.
    (B) 550 Hz.
    (C) 1,100 Hz.
    (D) 2,200 Hz.
    (E) 4,400 Hz.

8. An object is placed near a biconcave lens as shown below. The image will form

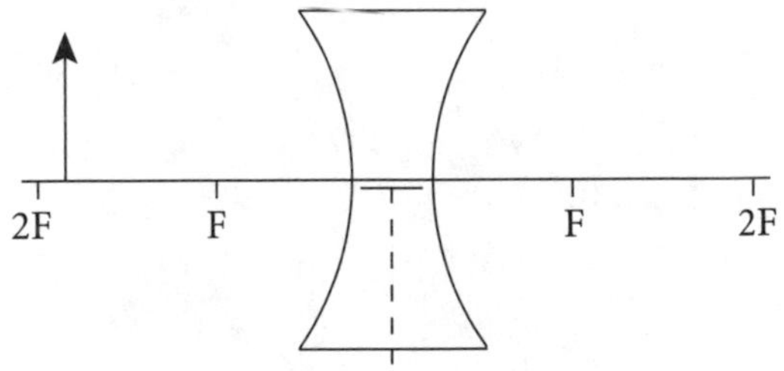

    (A) between F and 2F on the right side.
    (B) outside 2F on the right side.
    (C) between F and the lens on the left side.
    (D) between F and 2F on the left side.
    (E) outside 2F on the left side.

GO ON TO THE NEXT PAGE

9. The specific heat of a gas at constant pressure is always greater than the specific heat of a gas at constant volume because

(A) it takes more heat to expand a gas at constant pressure than at constant volume.
(B) expanding the gas at constant pressure requires heat energy.
(C) heat is conducted faster through a material under constant volume than under conditions where the material's volume is changing.
(D) the gas does work under constant volume conditions.
(E) gas molecules are attracted to each other to a greater extent under constant pressure conditions.

10. How much current passes through the 3-ohm resistor?

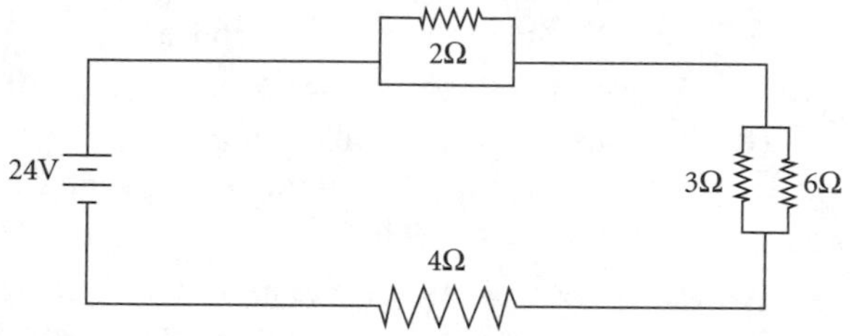

(A) 2 amps
(B) 3 amps
(C) $\frac{8}{3}$ amps
(D) 4 amps
(E) $\frac{4}{3}$ amps

11. A negatively charged particle of known magnitude q is placed in a uniform electric field of known strength E. What additional information is needed to determine the magnitude of the force on the particle?

(A) The distance from the source producing the electric field
(B) The position of the individual charges producing the electric field
(C) The magnitude of the individual charges producing the electric field
(D) The mass of the negatively charged particle.
(E) No additional information is needed.

12. An AC voltmeter reads the output of a wall socket at 110 volts AC. What is the voltage amplitude?

(A) 0 volts
(B) 80 volts
(C) 110 volts
(D) 155 volts
(E) 220 volts

13. Which of the following mirror(s) can produce a real inverted image?

(A) Convex only
(B) Concave only
(C) Plane only
(D) Convex and concave
(E) None of the above

GO ON TO THE NEXT PAGE

14. Given that the positive and negative charges shown below are of equal magnitude, where would the strength of the electric field be greatest?

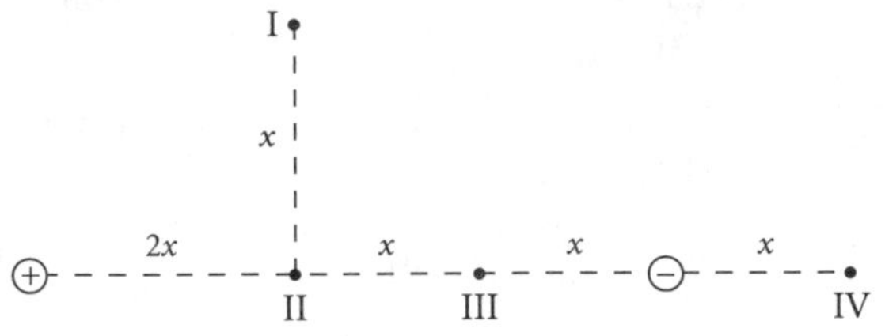

(A) I
(B) II
(C) III
(D) IV
(E) It would be the same at all four points.

15. An object is placed a distance x in front of a convex mirror of unknown focal length. What can be said about the image formed?

(A) It is real and inverted.
(B) It is real and erect.
(C) It is virtual and inverted.
(D) It is virtual and erect.
(E) It depends on the object–mirror distance x.

16. A 5-kg object is considered weightless when

(A) the object is uniformly accelerated upward at 49 m/s^2.
(B) the object is uniformly accelerated downward at 49 m/s^2.
(C) the object is uniformly accelerated upward at 9.8 m/s^2.
(D) all objects have the same weight.
(E) None of the above

17. Mass M_1 has twice the mass of M_2. M_1 and M_2 are raised from a height of 5 m to 25 m, and from 14 m to 24 m, respectively. What is the ratio of the work done on mass M_1 to that done on mass M_2?

(A) 1:4
(B) 2:1
(C) 25:12
(D) 4:1
(E) 5:1

18. Consider a marble rolling back and forth near the bottom of a curved bowl that has the shape of a hollow hemisphere. The marble exhibits simple harmonic motion as long as its maximum displacement from the center is not too great. Which of the following is true of the marble's motion?

(A) The speed of the marble is constant as it moves back and forth.
(B) The velocity of the marble is constant as it moves back and forth.
(C) The period of the marble's motion is proportional to its maximum displacement from the center of the bowl.
(D) The period of the marble's motion is independent of its maximum displacement from the center of the bowl.
(E) The direction of the normal force on the marble is constant as it rolls back and forth.

19. A person is free-falling in an elevator which itself is in free fall. At the instant that the person and elevator are falling at 2 m/s, the person lets go of a baseball that has been in her hand. After 2 s, what is the velocity of the baseball relative to the person?

(A) 0 m/s
(B) 2 m/s
(C) 9.8 m/s
(D) 19.6 m/s
(E) 21.6 m/s

GO ON TO THE NEXT PAGE

20. A car is making a trip of 40 miles. It travels half of the distance at an average speed of 20 mph. For it to have an average speed of 40 mph for the entire trip, the car would need to

(A) travel at an average speed of 40 mph for the remainder of the trip.

(B) travel at an average speed of 60 mph for the remainder of the trip.

(C) cover the remainder of the distance in no more than 15 minutes.

(D) cover the remainder of the distance in no more than 10 minutes.

(E) It is not possible for the car to have an average speed of 40 mph for the entire trip.

IF YOU FINISH BEFORE TIME IS CALLED, YOU MAY CHECK YOUR WORK ON THIS SECTION ONLY. DO NOT TURN TO ANY OTHER SECTION IN THE TEST.

STOP

ANSWERS AND EXPLANATIONS

1. A	6. B	11. E	16. E
2. D	7. B	12. D	17. D
3. B	8. C	13. B	18. D
4. D	9. A	14. C	19. A
5. A	10. C	15. D	20. E

1. A

The key equation describing the photoelectric effect is $hf = W + K$, where W is the work function (minimum energy required to liberate an electron from the surface), K is the kinetic energy of the emitted electron, f is the frequency of light, and h is Planck's constant.

Probably the best way to proceed is to consider the answer choices. (A) says the minimum frequency needed to remove an electron is 1×10^{14} Hz. The minimum frequency also means that the electrons just escape and have zero kinetic energy (i.e., $K = 0$). So we have that $W = h(1 \times 10^{14})$. When the light frequency is 2×10^{14} Hz, the electrons have kinetic energy given by $K = h(2 \times 10^{14}) - W = h(2 \times 10^{14}) - h(1 \times 10^{14})$, so $K = h(1 \times 10^{14})$. When the light frequency is 3×10^{14} Hz, the electrons have kinetic energy given by $K = h(3 \times 10^{14}) - W = h(3 \times 10^{14}) - h(1 \times 10^{14}) = 2h(1 \times 10^{14})$. So with light of frequency 3×10^{14} Hz, the electrons have twice as much energy as with light of frequency 2×10^{14} Hz. This is precisely what we're looking for. (A) is correct.

2. D

For the seesaw to balance, the net torque on it must be zero. Recall that torques can be either clockwise or counterclockwise. We'll refer to clockwise torques as positive and counterclockwise torques as negative. The clockwise torques are then due to the 2 gram, 4 gram, and x gram masses, and the only counterclockwise torque is due to the 10 gram mass. Note also that the force due to the x gram mass is simply the tension in the rope, which equals the weight of x when the system is stationary. Recalling that $t = rF\sin\theta$, we see that $\sin\theta = 1$ for all the torques considered because $\theta = 90°$. The forces are simply equal to the weights of the masses mg, so for the sum of the torques we have $2g + 12g + 3xg - 20g$, where we've used the fact that the 2 gram mass is one unit from the fulcrum, the 4 gram mass is 3 units from the fulcrum, the 10 gram mass is 2 units from the fulcrum, and the force due to x is 3 units from the fulcrum. Eliminating the common factor of g, we have $2 + 12 + 3x - 20 = 0$. Thus, $x = 2$ grams.

3. B

The safest and most direct way to solve this problem is to apply Newton's second law to each of the masses and then obtain the acceleration. The only force acting on block B is the tension in the cord, so for block B we have $T = m_B a$, where T is the tension in the cord and a is the acceleration of block B. For block A we have $m_A g - T = m_A a$, where we've chosen the downward direction as the positive direction. Notice that the acceleration of A is the same as the acceleration of B. We can substitute T from B's equation into A's equation to obtain $m_A g - m_B a = m_A a \Rightarrow a = m_A g/(m_B + m_A)$. Given that m_A and m_B are nonzero, we have that the acceleration is a constant but is different from g (i.e., different from 9.8 m/s^2). The correct answer is (B).

Let's investigate the equation for acceleration a bit more to see how it relates to another situation we know very well, namely free fall. If mass A were not attached to mass B and simply freely falling, then the acceleration would be g. Does our equation tell us this? Mass A is surely freely falling if mass B is zero (i.e., if there were no mass B). Setting $m_B = 0$, we have $a = m_A g/m_A = g$, which says mass A falls with the acceleration of gravity. What we've found above is that with a nonzero mass for B, the acceleration of A is still constant but is less than g.

4. D

A rifle bullet is a two-dimensional projectile whose initial velocity is in the horizontal direction. Recall that the motion of a projectile in the vertical direction is independent of the motion in the horizontal direction. Initial velocity only in the horizontal direction is equivalent to zero initial velocity in the vertical direction. The vertical motion of the bullet is equivalent to an object free-falling from a height of 100 ft. The equation describing its motion is then: $y = 100 - \frac{1}{2}gt^2$, where $y = 0$ is the water surface. Because we're given g in the question, we have all the information necessary to determine the time to hit the water.

5. A

An object that is slowing down experiences deceleration, which is simply acceleration in the direction opposite its motion. In this case, the acceleration will be directed toward the left. Whenever an object experiences acceleration, we know it's also being subjected to a net force. In addition, the force is in the same direction as the acceleration. Thus, the force is toward the left.

6. B

The antinode of a standing wave is a point where the displacement attains its maximum positive and negative values (i.e., a crest and a trough). The displacement at an antinode goes from maximum positive to maximum negative in half a period of the wave, then returns to maximum positive after another half period, so the displacement itself moves through all values from maximum positive to maximum negative. Although pictures of standing waves make it appear as if the crest and trough occur simultaneously, that's not the case. The crest and trough are separated by a time of a half period.

7. B

The smallest resonance frequency is also known as the fundamental frequency. To find the fundamental frequency of the tube described in the question, we'll have to remember a bit about standing waves in tubes. For a tube closed at one end and open at the other end, we'll have a node at the closed end and an antinode at the open end. Now recall that the smallest frequency also means the longest wavelength. This follows from the relation $v = f\lambda$, where λ is the wavelength, f is the frequency, and v is the wave speed, which is constant. The longest wave in a tube closed at one end and open at the other has one-quarter of a wavelength fitting inside the tube; i.e., if a quarter wavelength is inside the tube, you'll have a node at the closed end and an antinode at the open end. Thus, we have that $\lambda/4 = 6$ inches, so that $\lambda = 24$ inches $= 2$ ft. Using $v = f\lambda$ with $v = 1{,}100$ ft/s and $\lambda = 2$ ft, we have $f = 1{,}100/2 = 550$ Hz.

8. C

The system given in the problem is that of a diverging lens, and we know that diverging lenses always produce virtual images. Because virtual images are located on the same side of the lens as the object, we can immediately rule out (A) and (B), which both have the image on the other side of the lens from the object. To decide between the remaining choices, we'll need to use the equation $\frac{1}{o} + \frac{1}{i} = \frac{1}{f}$ where $f < 0$. Solving for $\frac{1}{i}$, we have $\frac{1}{i} = -\left(\frac{1}{o} + \frac{1}{|f|}\right) = -\frac{(|f| + o)}{|f|o}$. We can then invert this to give $i = \frac{-o|f|}{|f| + o} = -|f|\frac{o}{|f| + o}$. Now notice that $\frac{o}{|f| + o}$ is less than 1, which then tells us that $|i| < |f|$. In other words, we have just found that the image lies between f and the lens on the left-hand side of the lens.

9. A

Before looking at the answer choices and trying to decide which is best, let's consider the physics of the problem. First, remember that specific heat is the amount of heat required to raise the temperature of a unit mass of a substance by 1 unit of temperature, so to determine the specific heat of a gas you have to add heat. Recall that pressure is a measure of the force of the molecules on the container that holds them, which in turn depends on the speed of the molecules (faster molecules produce greater pressures). Consider a gas at constant pressure. As you add heat to a gas and require maintaining a constant pressure, you have to let the gas expand. Otherwise, the added heat will simply cause the molecules to move faster, resulting in a greater pressure. Thus, for a gas at constant pressure, some of the added heat goes into the gas doing work; and the remainder results in a temperature increase. A quick look shows that this is precisely (A).

10. C

To determine the current through the 3-ohm resistor, we'll first need to determine the current through the circuit, which in turn requires us to find the total resistance. First note that the 2-ohm resistor is in parallel with a short circuit, which means that all of the current will flow through the short circuit and none through the 2-ohm resistor. This means there's no contribution to the resistance from this part of the circuit. The effective resistance of the 3-ohm and 6-ohm combination is $\frac{1}{R} = \frac{1}{3} + \frac{1}{6} = \frac{3}{6}$, so we have

$R = 2$ ohms. Thus, the total resistance of the circuit is $2 + 4 = 6$ ohms. We then have that the total current is $I = \frac{V}{R_{tot}} = \frac{24}{6} = 4$ amps. To determine the current through the 3-ohm resistor, use the fact that the voltage drop across the 3-ohm resistor equals the voltage drop across the 6-ohm resistor. Ohm's law, $V = IR$, thus gives $3I_3 = 6I_6$, so that $I_3 = 2I_6$. From Kirchhoff's first law, $I_3 + I_6 = 4$ amps. Substituting for I_6, we have $4 = \left(\frac{3}{2}\right) I_3$, which then tells us that $I_3 = \frac{8}{3}$ amps.

11. E

The magnitude of the force on a charge q due to an electric field E is given by $F = qE$, where q and E are the magnitudes of the charge and field respectively. No other information is necessary for computing the magnitude of the electric force.

12. D

An AC voltmeter will read the root-mean-square (rms) value of the voltage, V_{rms}. Recall that $V_{rms} = \frac{V_0}{\sqrt{2}}$, so $V_o = \sqrt{2}V_{rms} = 155$ V.

13. B

To answer this question definitively, we'll use the equation $\frac{1}{o} + \frac{1}{i} = \frac{1}{f}$. For a concave (converging) mirror, $f > 0$, and for a convex (diverging) mirror, $f < 0$. First, consider a convex mirror. We then have $\frac{1}{i} = \frac{1}{f} - \frac{1}{o}$. Given that $f < 0$, we have $i < 0$. This means that all images from convex mirrors are virtual. We can then eliminate (A) and (D). Recall that plane mirrors always produce virtual images (image behind mirror), so we can eliminate (C). Now consider a concave mirror. We'll have, as before, $\frac{1}{i} = \frac{1}{f} - \frac{1}{o}$ with $f > 0$. Thus, as long as $\frac{1}{f} > \frac{1}{o}$, the image distance will be positive, which means a real image. Physically this means that the object is outside of the focal length. To determine if the image is upright or inverted, we can use the magnification $m = -\frac{i}{o}$, where $m > 0$ means upright and $m < 0$ means inverted. Given that a real image has $i > 0$ and that we always take $o > 0$, we see that $m < 0$, so the image is inverted. Thus, it's possible to produce a real and inverted image only from a concave mirror.

14. C

To answer this question, we'll need to examine the electric field at each of the given points. The electric field due to a point charge Q has strength $E = \frac{kQ}{r^2}$ at a distance of r from the charge. Recall that net electric field at a given point is the vector sum of the fields due to the individual charges. The field at II is then given by $E_{II} = \frac{kQ}{4x^2} + \frac{kQ}{4x^2} = \frac{kQ}{2x^2}$, where we've used the fact that electric fields point away from positive charges and toward negative charges and where we've chosen toward the right as positive. The electric field at III is $E_{III} = \frac{kQ}{9x^2} + \frac{kQ}{x^2} = \frac{10kQ}{9x^2}$. The electric field at IV is $E_{IV} = \frac{kQ}{25x^2} - \frac{kQ}{x^2} = -\frac{24kQ}{25x^2}$, where notice that the field due to $-Q$ is toward the left at point IV. Of the three points considered, clearly point III has the largest field strength. Now consider the field at point I. The magnitude of the field from either of the charges is $E = \frac{kQ}{5x^2}$, and the fields due to $+Q$ and $-Q$ will not be in the same direction at I. In terms of the net field at I, E_I, this implies $E_I < 2\left(\frac{kQ}{5x^2}\right)$ (i.e., the maximum resultant of $+Q$ and $-Q$ at this distance is $\frac{2kQ}{5x^2}$ and occurs when the fields are in the same direction). We then conclude that the field at point III is the strongest.

15. D

Convex mirrors are diverging mirrors. It's probably a good idea to remember that convex mirrors always produce virtual and erect images. If you don't remember that, you can always use the equation $\frac{1}{o} + \frac{1}{i} = \frac{1}{f}$ to figure it out. The image distance is found from $\frac{1}{i} = \frac{1}{f} - \frac{1}{o}$. Given that $f < 0$ for a convex mirror, we know $\frac{1}{i} < 0$, which means $i < 0$. The image is then virtual. To determine whether the image is erect or inverted, look at the sign of the magnification $m = -\frac{i}{o}$. Given that we always take $o > 0$, $i < 0$ implies $m > 0$, and $m > 0$ means an erect image. Thus, we've proven that a convex mirror always generates a virtual and erect image.

16. E

Before we look through the choices, it's probably best to review the concept of weightlessness. An object will appear weightless when it is freely falling under the influence of gravity. The idea is that if the object were placed on a scale that is also freely falling, the scale would register no weight. So we're looking for an answer that either says the object is freely falling or, equivalently, that the object is accelerating downward at the rate of 9.8 m/s^2. Looking through the answer choices, no such choice is presented. We then conclude that the correct answer is (E), none of the above.

17. D

The work done on an object in raising it is simply the change in gravitational potential energy of the object. Given that gravitational potential energy is mgh, we have that the change in potential energy is $mg\Delta h$, where Δh is the difference in initial and final heights. For mass 1, we have a change of $M_1g(20)$, and for mass 2, we have a change of $M_2g(10)$. So the ratio of the work done on mass 1 to that done on mass 2 is $\frac{M_1g(20)}{M_2g(10)} = \frac{2M_1}{M_2}$. Given that $M_1 = 2M_2$, the ratio becomes $\frac{4M_2}{M_2} = 4$.

18. D

The clue to this problem is to notice the emphasis on the concept of simple harmonic motion. Even though you're presented with a physical system that you've probably not encountered, you certainly know some general properties of systems undergoing simple harmonic motion (i.e., you've studied the motion of a simple pendulum and of a mass on a spring).

The simplest approach to this question is to read through the answer choices and try to eliminate those that are clearly incorrect. (A) states that the speed of the marble is constant as it rolls back and forth. This can't be true because the marble is instantaneously at rest when it's the farthest from the center (like the motion of a simple pendulum). (B) can then also be ruled out for the same reason. (C) and (D) deal with the relationship between the period of the marble's motion and the marble's maximum displacement from equilibrium. Recall that all systems undergoing simple harmonic motion have a period that is independent of the maximum displacement. We can then eliminate (C) and choose (D) as the correct answer.

For completeness, consider (E). The normal force is directed perpendicular to the surface of the bowl at any given point. Certainly, the direction of this force varies as the position of the marble changes because the bowl has curvature: the direction is vertical when the marble is at the center of the bowl, and it has a horizontal component at all other points

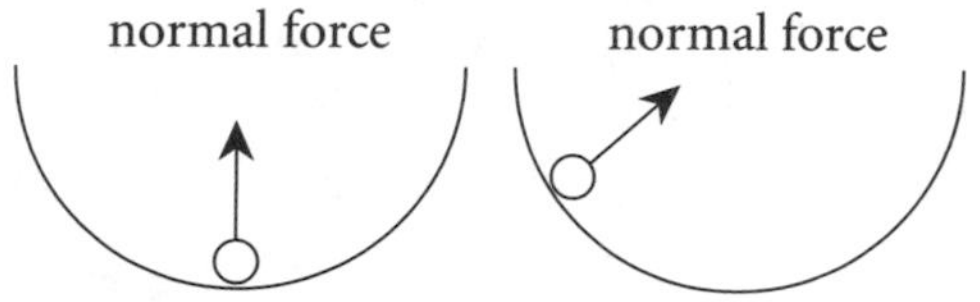

Note that the normal force is not the only force acting on the marble.

19. A

Recall that all objects in free fall have the acceleration of g (9.8 m/s^2). Because the person and the baseball are both in free fall, they both fall at the same rate. This means that the ball remains stationary with respect to the person. Thus, the velocity of the baseball relative to the person is 0 m/s.

20. E

Average speed is total distance divided by total time. Because the entire distance is 40 miles, for the speed to average out to 40 mph, the time taken, t, must satisfy:

$$40\ \frac{\text{miles}}{\text{hour}} = 40\ \frac{\text{miles}}{t}$$

$$t = 1 \text{ hour}$$

In other words, the entire trip must be covered in 1 hour.

We are told that the first half of the distance is covered at a speed of 20 mph. This distance is 20 miles (half of the total distance), and the time taken for this first half of the trip, t_1, therefore satisfies the relationship

$$20\ \frac{\text{miles}}{\text{hour}} = 20\ \frac{\text{miles}}{t_1}$$

$$t_1 = 1 \text{ hour}$$

In other words, the car has already used up all of its "allotted time" in the first half of the trip! It is not possible for the car to have an average speed of 40 mph for the entire trip.

Quantitative Reasoning: **Practice Set 2**

20 questions—18 minutes

Directions: Choose the best answer for each question from the five choices provided.

1. Which of the following is most nearly equal to $\frac{479{,}93}{0.00598}$?

   (A) 80,000
   (B) 90,000
   (C) 8,000
   (D) 9,000
   (E) 802.6

2. Find x: $\dfrac{\frac{2}{5}-1}{\frac{4}{3}-1} = \frac{5}{9}x$

   (A) $-\frac{81}{25}$
   (B) -1
   (C) $-\frac{9}{25}$
   (D) $-\frac{1}{25}$
   (E) 1

3. $\dfrac{-(2)^2 + (-2)^2 - (-2)}{\frac{1}{3}+\frac{1}{3}+\frac{1}{3}} = 6x - 6; x = ?$

   (A) $-1\frac{1}{2}$
   (B) 4
   (C) 1
   (D) $1\frac{1}{3}$
   (E) $2\frac{2}{3}$

4. It takes six workers 6 weeks to lay 1,000 feet of pipe. How long will it take eight workers to lay 400 yards of pipe?

   (A) 5.4 weeks
   (B) 3.75 weeks
   (C) 3.2 weeks
   (D) 1.8 weeks
   (E) 6.7 weeks

GO ON TO THE NEXT PAGE

5. In May of 1965, a father's age was three times the sum of the ages of his two sons. In May of 1975, the father's age was 10 years greater than the sum of his sons' ages. If the difference between the sons' ages is 4 years, how much older is the father than his older son?

(A) 23 years
(B) 13 years
(C) 33 years
(D) 27 years
(E) 40 years

6. A department store buys a case of pencils for \$25.00 and sells them at a rate of 3 for 20¢. If there are 1,000 pencils in a case, the profit is approximately what percentage of the cost?

(A) 60%
(B) 83.3%
(C) 120%
(D) 166.7%
(E) 216.2%

7. Arrange the following from least to greatest:

a) $\sqrt{\frac{1}{3}}$

b) $\frac{1}{3}$

c) $\left(\frac{1}{2}\right)\left(\frac{1}{3}\right)$

d) $\left(\frac{1}{2}+\frac{1}{3}\right)$

e) $\left(\frac{1}{3}\right)\left(\frac{1}{3}\right)$

(A) a, c, b, e, d
(B) e, c, b, a, d
(C) e, b, c, d, a
(D) e, c, a, b, d
(E) e, d, b, a, c

8. If $x = \sqrt{0.1369}$, which of the following is TRUE?

(A) $0.035 < x < 0.04$
(B) $0.11 < x < 0.12$
(C) $0.30 < x < 0.35$
(D) $0.35 < x < 0.4$
(E) $x \geq 0.40$

9. $\dfrac{106 + 26}{\frac{44}{3}} = ?$

(A) 1
(B) $1\frac{3}{4}$
(C) $6\frac{5}{11}$
(D) 9
(E) $\frac{136}{11}$

10. If 160% of $r = 2\frac{4}{5}$, $r = ?$

(A) $1\frac{2}{5}$
(B) $1\frac{3}{4}$
(C) $2\frac{1}{5}$
(D) $3\frac{1}{4}$
(E) $4\frac{12}{25}$

GO ON TO THE NEXT PAGE

11. Mr. Canine deposits $15,000 into two bank accounts. One account pays 10% interest and the other pays 5%, each compounded annually. After 1 year, he has $16,350. How much interest did the 5% account yield?

(A) $150
(B) $225
(C) $300
(D) $600
(E) $3,000

12. A model of the Earth, which has a radius of 35 inches, is to be painted. Oceans cover 75% of the total surface area and will be painted blue. If one fluid ounce of paint covers 600 square inches, how many fluid ounces of blue paint are needed? The surface area of a sphere with a radius r is given by the formula surface area = $4\pi r^2 \left(\pi = \frac{22}{7}\right)$.

(A) $2\frac{1}{5}$
(B) $19\frac{1}{4}$
(C) $25\frac{2}{3}$
(D) 77
(E) $102\frac{2}{3}$

13. Six more than $\frac{3}{5}$ of N is $\frac{2}{3}$ of the quantity 30 less than $\frac{4}{3}$ of N. What is N?

(A) $\frac{43}{13}$
(B) $\frac{1{,}170}{67}$
(C) $\frac{630}{13}$
(D) 90
(E) $\frac{1{,}170}{7}$

14. If $\frac{(100^2)(10^3)}{1{,}000^4} = (\sqrt{10})^x$, then x = ?

(A) 2
(B) 1
(C) $-\frac{5}{2}$
(D) -5
(E) -10

15. $3\frac{3}{17} \div \frac{1}{2} \bullet 2\frac{5}{6} = ?$

(A) 2
(B) $4\frac{1}{2}$
(C) 18
(D) 648
(E) $\frac{648}{289}$

16. If $\frac{22}{2x-3} - 4x = 6$, then x can be which of the following?

(A) $\frac{3}{2}$
(B) $\frac{2}{3}$
(C) $\sqrt{5}$
(D) 2
(E) $\frac{\sqrt{2}}{2}$

17. If N is any positive integer, how many consecutive integers following N are needed to ensure that at least one of the integers is divisible by another positive integer m?

(A) $m - 1$
(B) m
(C) $m + 1$
(D) $2m$
(E) m^2

GO ON TO THE NEXT PAGE

18. Stella has 3 quarters and 4 dimes. How many different amounts can she form with these 7 coins, using at least 1 coin each time?

(A) 8
(B) 19
(C) 20
(D) 21
(E) 25

19. Mrs. Parson's gross salary is $250 per week. If her employer deducts 15% from the first $10,000 earned in a year and 20% from earnings between $10,000 and $15,000 in a year, how much money does Mrs. Parson take home in 1 year (52 weeks)?

(A) $2,100
(B) $10,900
(C) $11,050
(D) $11,540
(E) $12,650

20. The prizes in a penny arcade game are worth 5¢, 50¢, and $2.00. The game costs 25¢ and pays out half that amount on the average. If one prize is awarded for each 25¢ game and there is the same number of 50¢ prizes as $2.00 prizes, how many $2.00 prizes are there in 160 drawings having the average payoff?

(A) 1
(B) 5
(C) 10
(D) 12
(E) 32

IF YOU FINISH BEFORE TIME IS CALLED, YOU MAY CHECK YOUR WORK ON THIS SECTION ONLY. DO NOT TURN TO ANY OTHER SECTION IN THE TEST. **STOP**

ANSWERS AND EXPLANATIONS

1. A	6. D	11. A	16. C
2. A	7. B	12. B	17. A
3. D	8. D	13. D	18. B
4. A	9. D	14. E	19. B
5. A	10. B	15. C	20. B

1. A

This problem requires approximation to make it manageable in the allotted time; what's more, it invites it by giving possible answers that are approximations. They are not even tightly clustered but separated out quite comfortably. At the very least, we can approximate 0.00598 as 0.006 to make our division easier. We can probably approximate 479.93 as 480 as well, but we won't, because this makes our calculation of error more complicated.

First, let's multiply top and bottom of the fraction by 1,000, making $\frac{479{,}930}{5.98}$. If we approximate 5.98 with 6.00, we are adding 0.02 to it, which is less than 1% of the original value: our degree of error stays less than 1%.

$6\overline{)479{,}930} = 79{,}988.\overline{3}$, so a 1% degree of error comes to ± 800. This means we know $79{,}188 < \frac{479{,}930}{5.98} < 80{,}788$, which is good enough to say that of the given choices, it's closest to 80,000.

It's probably overkill to calculate the quantity of error explicitly in this problem when you are under time constraints, but you should certainly try to note with every approximation you make either its percent error (in the case of multiplying) or its absolute error (in the case of adding) and make sure the spacing of the possible answers allows such approximation. If 79,900 had been one of the possible answers for this problem. we would have had to make more modest approximations.

2. A

To begin with, $\frac{2}{5} - 1 = \frac{2}{5} - \frac{5}{5} = \frac{2-5}{5} = -\frac{3}{5}$.

Second, $\frac{4}{3} - 1 = \frac{4}{3} - \frac{3}{3} + \frac{4-3}{3} = \frac{1}{3}$,

so $\dfrac{\frac{2}{5} - 1}{\frac{4}{3} - 1} = \dfrac{-\frac{3}{5}}{\frac{1}{3}} = \left(-\frac{3}{5}\right) \times \frac{3}{1} = -\frac{3 \times 3}{5 \times 1} = -\frac{9}{5}$.

According to the original equation then, $-\frac{9}{5} = \frac{5}{9} \times x$,

so multiplying both sides by $\frac{9}{5}$, we have $\frac{9}{5} \times \left(-\frac{9}{5}\right)$

$= \frac{9}{5} \times \left(\frac{5}{9} \times x\right)$.

Then $x = \frac{9}{5} \times \left(-\frac{9}{5}\right) = -\frac{9 \times 9}{5 \times 5} = -\frac{81}{25}$.

3. D

The equation is $\dfrac{-(2)^2 + (-2)^2 - (-2)}{\frac{1}{3} + \frac{1}{3} + \frac{1}{3}}$. Begin by simplifying the numerator and denominator of the fraction on the left side of the equation. First, simplify the numerator: $-(2)^2 + (-2)^2 - (-2) = -(4) + (-2)^2 + 2 = -4 + 4 + 2 = 2$. Next, simplify the denominator: $\frac{1}{3} + \frac{1}{3} + \frac{1}{3} = \frac{3}{3} = 1$. The numerator of the fraction on the left side of the equation is 2, and the denominator is 1. Our equation is $\frac{2}{1} = 6x - 6$. Now just solve this equation for x.

$$\frac{2}{1} = 6x - 6$$

$$2 = 6x - 6$$

$$8 = 6x$$

$$\frac{8}{6} = x$$

$$\frac{4}{3} = x$$

This is the same as $x = \frac{4}{3}$.

None of the answer choices is $\frac{4}{3}$. However, $\frac{4}{3} = 1\frac{1}{3}$. So $x = 1\frac{1}{3}$, and (D) is correct.

4. A

The salient idea here is that a worker-day is a *scalable unit of work*, which just means that one worker working for a certain amount of time, say a day, does the same amount of work as do two workers working half a day each or ten workers working one-tenth of a day. Multiplying the number of workers or the number of weeks by a number x, each has the same effect of increasing the amount of work done by a factor of x. So one may speak of a worker-day as a unit of work, the amount of work one worker does in 1 day, or in this case, a worker-week, the amount of work one worker does in 1 week. Thus, six workers working 6 weeks represents 36 worker-weeks, and because these workers lay 1,000 feet of pipe in that time (also a measure of work), we may make the unit conversion definition as follows:

36 worker-weeks = 1,000 feet of pipe

Taking this conversion definition, we can use it to attack the question. Because 1,000 feet of pipe equals 36 worker-weeks, 100 feet of pipe equals 3.6 worker-weeks. And because 1 yard is equal to 3 feet (a conversion factor you are expected to know for the test), 400 yards equal 1,200 feet. Thus, 1,200 feet of pipe are $12 \times 3.6 = 43.2$ worker-weeks. That is, it takes one worker 43.2 weeks to lay 400 yards of pipe, so it would take eight workers $\frac{43.2}{8} = 5.4$ weeks to lay the same amount of pipe.

5. A

Translate the information in the question into math. On May 1, 1965, the father's age was three times the sum of the ages of his two sons. Call the father's age, in years, F, and call the son's ages, in years, A and B. Then we have the equation $F = 3(A + B)$.

On May 1, 1975, the father's age was 10 years greater than the sum of his sons' ages. On May 1, 1975, the age of each of the three people was 10 years greater than it was on May 1, 1965. So on May 1, 1975, the father's age in years was $F + 10$, the age in years of one of his sons was $A + 10$, and the age in years of his other son was $B + 10$, therefore $F + 10 = (A + 10) + (B + 10) + 10$. This equation can be simplified.

$$F + 10 = (A + 10) + (B + 10) + 10$$
$$F + 10 = A + 10 + B + 10 + 10$$
$$F + 10 = A + B + 30$$
$$F = A + B + 20$$

The difference of the sons' ages is 4 years. We can let A represent the age, in years, of the older son. We then have the equation $A - B = 4$.

We want to figure out how much older the father is than his older son (i.e., we want the value of $F - A$) To find this value, we'll need the values of F and A, because there does not appear to be a quick way to obtain the value of the expression $F - A$ from the three equations. The three equations are $F = 3(A + B)$, $F = A + B + 20$, and $A - B = 4$. First, let's get rid of F by using the first two of the equations just listed and by substituting $3(A + B)$ for F into the equation $F = A + B + 20$. Then $3(A + B) = A + B + 20$. Simplify this equation.

$$3(A + B) = A + B + 20$$
$$3A + 3B = A + B + 20$$
$$2A + 2B = 20$$
$$A + B = 10$$

Now solve the equations $A + B = 10$ and $A - B = 4$ to find the values of A and B. Notice that if we add the corresponding sides of these two equations, the $+ B$ in the equation $A + B = 10$ will cancel with the $- B$ in the equation $A - B = 4$, leaving an equation with just the one unknown, A.

$$\begin{array}{rl} A + B &= 10 \\ A - B &= 4 \\ \hline 2A \quad &= 14 \end{array}$$

$$A = \frac{14}{2} = 7$$

Now we can find the value of B because $A + B = 10$, $7 + B = 10$, and $B = 10 - 7 = 3$. Now that we know that $A = 7$ and $B = 3$, the value of F can be found from the equation $F = 3(A + B)$. Thus, $F = 3(A + B) = 3(7 + 3) = 3(10) = 30$. The father's age, F, is 30, and the older son's age, A, is 7. The father is older than his older son by $F - A = 30 - 7 = 23$ years. (A) is correct.

6. D

This problem is clearly one of approximations, because the last pencil cannot be sold: after 999 are sold in groups of 3, the last one must either remain or be sold for $6\frac{2}{3}$¢! We can assume either way, but the chances are that last pencil will not be significant in the approximation. At 20¢ for 3 and 999 (or 333 sets of 3) pencils sold, the total sales are $333 \times \$0.20 = \$66.60$. The profit is therefore $\$66.60 - \$25.00 = \$41.60$. To find the percent of the cost that the profit is, divide \$41.60 by \$25.00: $\frac{\$41.60}{\$25.00} = \frac{41.60}{25} = 1.664 = 166.4\%$, which is much closer to choice (D) than to any of the others. That our answer differs simply means that the final pencil was counted in the official analysis; thus, the precise calculation is $\frac{\$41.66\overline{6}}{\$25.00} = 166.\overline{6}\% \approx 166.7\%$. Even without this further analysis, however, it's clear which answer we must choose: 166.7%.

7. B

There is a slight possibility that you remember the decimal approximation of the square root of 3, and if you do, you might be tempted to express each of the fractions as a decimal by long division. However, even if you remember this obscure bit of information, it's still probably faster to solve the problem in the following manner. The squaring function preserves the order of the positive real numbers: if a and b are positive real numbers and if $a < b$, then $a^2 < b^2$. To determine the order of the expressions, we can square each of them. First, let us find a common denominator for the rational expressions (i.e., all but the one with the square root in it). We first note that for expression (d), $\frac{1}{2} + \frac{1}{3} = \frac{3}{6} + \frac{2}{6} = \frac{5}{6}$. This being the case, we see that the least common denominator will contain the factor 3 twice and the factor 2 once, so it is $3 \times 3 \times 2 = 18$. Thus, we express (b), (c), (d), and (e) as $\frac{6}{18}, \frac{3}{18}, \frac{15}{18}$, and $\frac{2}{18}$, respectively. The squares of these are then $\frac{36}{18^2}, \frac{9}{18^2}, \frac{225}{18^2}$, and $\frac{4}{18^2}$. Furthermore, $\left(\frac{1}{\sqrt{3}}\right)^2 = \frac{1}{\sqrt{3}} \times \frac{1}{\sqrt{3}} = \frac{1}{3} = \frac{6 \times 18}{3 \times 6 \times 18} = \frac{108}{18 \times 18} = \frac{108}{18^2}$, so the squares of (a), (b), (c), (d), and (e) are $\frac{108}{18^2}, \frac{36}{18^2}, \frac{9}{18^2}, \frac{225}{18^2}$, and $\frac{4}{18^2}$. The size ordering is therefore (e), (c), (b), (a), (d).

8. D

Again, the preservation of the order of the positive real numbers under the squaring function is the key. The five conditions can then be reexpressed:

A. $(0.035)^2 < x < (0.04)^2$; that is, $0.001225 < x^2 < 0.0016$.

B. $(0.11)^2 < x^2 < (0.12)^2$; that is, $0.0121 < x^2 < 0.0144$.

C. $(0.30)^2 < x^2 < (0.35)^2$; that is, $0.09 < x^2 < 0.1225$.

D. $(0.35)^2 < x^2 < (0.4)^2$; that is, $0.1225 < x^2 < 0.16$.

E. $x^2 \geq (0.40)^2$; that is, $x^2 \geq 0.16$.

The only one of these conditions that $x^2 = (\sqrt{0.1369})^2 = 0.1369$ satisfies is D, that is, $(0.35)^2 < (\sqrt{0.1369})^2 < (0.4)^2$, so $0.35 < \sqrt{0.1369} < 0.4$.

9. D

A fraction is the same as its numerator divided by its denominator, so $\frac{106 + 26}{\frac{44}{3}} = \frac{132}{\frac{44}{3}} = 132 \div \frac{44}{3}$.

Dividing by a fraction is the same as multiplying by its inverse, so $\frac{132}{1} \div \frac{44}{3} = \frac{132}{1} \times \frac{3}{44}$. Manipulating further, $\frac{132}{1} \times \frac{3}{44} = \frac{132 \times 3}{44} = \frac{3 \times 44 \times 3}{44} = \frac{3 \times 3}{1} = \frac{9}{1} = 9$.

Therefore, the answer is 9.

10. B

Because 160% of r is the same as $1.60 \times r$, which is $1.6r$, or $\frac{8}{5}r$, the hypothesis is $\frac{8}{5}r = 2\frac{4}{5}$, which is $\frac{8}{5}r = \frac{14}{5}$. Multiplying both sides of this equation by 5 gives $8r = 14$. Dividing both sides by 2 gives $4r = 7$. Dividing both sides of this equation in turn by 4 gives $r = \frac{7}{4} = 1\frac{3}{4}$.

11. A

We have a man, Mr. Canine, who deposits $15,000 into two bank accounts. One account pays 10% interest, one account pays 5% interest, and both interest rates are compounded annually. We are given how much money he has after 1 year, and we are asked how much interest the 5% account yielded. We'll let x dollars be the amount he deposits in the account earning 10%, and we'll let y dollars be the amount he deposits in the account earning 5%. We then have the equation $x + y = 15{,}000$. Because after 1 year, he has $16,350, the amount of interest earned in that year was $16,350 – $15,000 = $1,350. The amount of interest earned in the account earning 10% is 10% of x dollars, or $0.1x$ dollars. The amount of interest earned in the account earning 5% is 5% of y dollars, or $0.05y$ dollars. This interest earned is the sum of the interests earned in the two accounts, giving the second equation $0.1x + 0.05y = 1{,}350$. Keep in mind that the question requires that we find the amount of interest earned in the account earning 5% interest, so we want the value of $0.05y$. We now have the two equations $x + y = 15{,}000$ and $0.1x + 0.05y = 1{,}350$.

Let's try to solve these two equations for the value of y, and we'll then be able to find the value of $0.05y$. Notice that the second of the equations just mentioned has $0.1x$ appearing in it. If we multiply both sides of the first equation, $x + y = 15{,}000$, by 0.1, we'll have two equations with $0.1x$ appearing in them. If we then subtract the corresponding sides of the two equations, we'll be left with one equation with just y. We can then find y and, immediately after that, $0.05y$. Multiplying both sides of the equation $x + y = 15{,}000$ by 0.1 leads to the equation $0.1(x + y) = 0.1(15{,}000)$, (i.e., $0.1x + 0.1y = 1{,}500$). Now subtract the corresponding sides of the equation $0.1x + 0.05y = 1{,}350$ from those of $0.1x + 0.1y = 1{,}500$. We then have

$$\begin{array}{r} 0.1x + 0.1y = 1{,}500 \\ -(0.1x + 0.05y = 1{,}350) \\ \hline 0.05y = 150 \end{array}$$

Notice that we don't have to calculate any further. We want the value of $0.05y$, and now we know that it equals 150. The 5% account earned $150.

Continuing the algebra, you would find that $y = \frac{150}{0.05} = \frac{15{,}000}{5} = 3{,}000$, and from the equation $x + y = 15{,}000$, it follows that $x = 12{,}000$. The sum of $12,000 and $3,000 is $15,000 and (10% of $12,000) plus (5% of $3,000) is $1,200 plus $150, or $1,350, which is the total interest earned, so our answer of $150 is indeed correct.

Notice that incorrect (E), $3,000, is the amount deposited in the 5% account, not the amount of interest earned by the 5% account. The amount of interest earned by the 5% account is 5% of $3,000, which is $150. Always read the question carefully.

12. B

This problem has to be done in several steps. The first step is to find the surface area representing the oceans. We know that the surface area of the oceans is equal to 75% of the total surface area of the Earth. We are given a formula with which to find the total surface area of a sphere. The formula is $4\pi r^2$ so therefore the surface area representing the oceans is equal to 75% of $4\pi r^2$ or $\frac{3}{4}$ of $4\pi r^2$. Thus, if r is the radius of the sphere representing the earth, the surface area representing the oceans is equal to $3\pi r^2$. We use $\frac{22}{7}$ for π, so we have $3 \times \frac{22}{7} \times r^2$. We are given that the radius is 35 inches, so r is 35. We have that the surface area representing the oceans is equal to $3 \times \frac{22}{7} \times r^2$, which is $3 \times \frac{22}{7} \times 35 \times 35$. We can now reduce this because the 7 in the denominator of $\frac{22}{7}$ goes into one of the 35s five times. The surface area representing the oceans is equal to $3 \times 22 \times 5 \times 35$, which is 11,550 square inches. Now let's find how many ounces of paint are needed to cover the 11,550 square inches. We know that one ounce of paint covers 600 square inches. Let N be the number of ounces of paint needed to cover

11,550 square inches, and then $600N = 11{,}550$.

We divide both sides by 600 and get $N = \frac{11{,}550}{600}$.

We can divide both numerator and denominator by 10 to get $N = \frac{1{,}155}{60}$. Without computing this exactly, we know that $\frac{1{,}200}{60} = 20$. Thus, $\frac{1{,}155}{60}$ must be a bit less than 20. $\frac{1{,}155}{60}$ you will find that it does in fact exactly equal $19\frac{1}{4}$.

As in some of the other problems, you can find the correct answer through estimation coupled with insightful use of your answer choices.

13. D

The problem says that if 6 more than $\frac{3}{5}$ of N is $\frac{2}{3}$ of the quantity 30 less than $\frac{4}{3}$ of N, what is N? We can write this out into an equation. Six more than $\frac{3}{5}$ of N means $\frac{3}{5}N + 6$. The quantity 30 less than $\frac{4}{3}$ of N means $\frac{4}{3}N - 30$. Therefore, $\frac{2}{3}$ of the quantity 30 less than $\frac{4}{3}$ of N means $\frac{2}{3}\left(\frac{4}{3}N - 30\right)$. Therefore, we have that $\frac{3}{5}N + 6 = \frac{2}{3}\left(\frac{4}{3}N - 30\right)$. Solve this equation for N. First, multiply out the right side using the distributive law. Then, $\frac{3}{5}N + 6 = \frac{2}{3}\left(\frac{4}{3}N\right) - \frac{2}{3}(30)$ (i.e., $\frac{3}{5}N + 6 = \frac{8}{9}N - 20$). The denominators are 5 and 9, so multiply both sides by $5 \times 9 = 45$ to get rid of the denominators, and $45\left(\frac{3}{5}N + 6\right) = 45\left(\frac{8}{9}N - 20\right)$. Multiplying out each side, $45\left(\frac{3}{5}N\right) + 45(6) = 45\left(\frac{8}{9}N\right) - 45(20)$, thus $27N + 270 = 40N - 900$. Subtracting $27N$ from both sides results in $270 = 13N - 900$. Adding 900 to each side results in $1{,}170 = 13N$. Finally, $N = \frac{1{,}170}{13} = 90$.

14. E

To simplify the expression on the right, we will express all the numbers in powers of 10. So because $100 = 10^2$,

$100^2 = (10^2)^2 = 10^{2 \times 2} = 10^4$. Likewise, $1{,}000^4 = (10^3)^4 = 10^{12}$, and so $\frac{(100^2)(10^3)}{1{,}000^4} = \frac{10^4 \times 10^3}{10^{12}} = \frac{10^{3+4}}{10^{12}} = 10^{7-12} = 10^{-5}$. Working on the other side of the equation, we note first that $\sqrt{10} = 10^{\frac{1}{2}}$, so $(\sqrt{10})^x = (10^{\frac{1}{2}})^x = 10^{\frac{1}{2}x}$. Using these equalities, we see that $10^{-5} = 10^{\frac{1}{2}x}$. Since the bases are equal, they must have equal exponents (i.e., $-5 = \frac{1}{2} \times x$, so $x = -10$).

15. C

The first order of business is to convert the compound fractions in the expression to improper fractions, which are more convenient for multiplication and division: $3\frac{3}{17} = \frac{51}{17} + \frac{3}{17} = \frac{54}{17}$ and $2\frac{5}{6} = \frac{12}{6} + \frac{5}{6} = \frac{17}{6}$. The arithmetic expression is equal to $\frac{54}{7} \div \frac{1}{2} \times \frac{17}{6}$. Remembering the order of operations, multiplication and division are done from left to right. If you were to do the order incorrectly and first multiply $\frac{1}{2}$ by $\frac{17}{6}$, and then divide $\frac{54}{7}$ by the result, you would get (E), which is incorrect.

Back to the solution. Dividing by $\frac{1}{2}$ is the same as multiplying by 2, so $\left(3\frac{3}{17} \div \frac{1}{2}\right) \times 2\frac{5}{6} = \left(\frac{54}{17} \times \frac{2}{1}\right) \times \frac{17}{6} = \frac{54 \times 2 \times 17}{17 \times 6}$. Dividing the numerator and denominator by 17 results in $\frac{54 \times 2}{6}$, and then $\frac{54 \times 2}{6} = \frac{9 \times 2}{1} = 18$.

16. C

One way to do this problem would be simply to plug in each of the five possible answers and compute. When you find one that fits, you're done. The more generally useful way is to multiply the whole expression by the denominator of the fraction, noting that this is not a valid move if $x = \frac{3}{2}$, because we don't want to multiply the whole expression by zero. The expression then becomes $-4x \times (2x - 3) = 6 \times (2x - 3)$. Simplifying this expression gives us $22 - 8x^2 + 12x = 12x - 18$. Adding 18 and

$8x^2$ to both sides and then subtracting $12x$ from both sides, we get $40 = 8x^2$. Dividing both sides by 8 gives $x^2 = 5$. Therefore, $x = \sqrt{5}$ or $x = -\sqrt{5}$. Thus, the correct answer is (C), $\sqrt{5}$.

17. A

One out of every m consecutive integers is divisible by the integer m. The wording of this question is difficult, so you might have thought the question was asking you to count N itself to get the correct answer. But it was not, so $m - 1$ consecutive integers after N plus N itself are required to ensure that one of these integers, including N, is a multiple of m.

18. B

You can simply enumerate the amounts of change you can make. We'll use two categories:

Amounts ending in zero	Amounts ending in five
10¢ (dime)	25¢ (quarter)
20¢ (2 dimes)	35¢ (quarter, dime)
30¢ (3 dimes)	45¢ (quarter, 2 dimes)
40¢ (4 dimes)	55¢ (quarter, 3 dimes)
50¢ (2 quarters)	65¢ (quarter, 4 dimes)
60¢ (2 quarters, dime)	75¢ (3 quarters)
70¢ (etc.)	85¢ (etc.)
80¢	95¢
90¢	$1.05
	$1.15

Counting all the possibilities, there are 19.
The answer is 19.

19. B

Mrs. Parson's total yearly salary before taxes is 52 × $250 = $13,000. Of the first $10,000, she takes home $10,000 – (15% × $10,000) = $10,000 – $1,500 = $8,500. Of the next $3,000, she takes home $3,000 – (20% × $3,000) = $3,000 – $600 = $2,400. Her total take is $8,500 + $2,400 = $10,900.

20. B

The average payoff of the game is 12.5¢, so on average if you play 160 times the total value of your prizes will be 160 × 12.5¢ = $20.00. On average, the number of 50¢ prizes and $2.00 prizes awarded in 160 games will be the same, so we call this number x. A prize is awarded every game, so the total number of prizes is 160. We call the number of 5¢ prizes y, and the following equation holds:

$$x + x + y = 160$$
$$y = 160 - 2x.$$

The payoff situation can be described by the following equation:

$$x \times \$2.00 + x \times 50¢ + y \times 5¢ = \$20.00$$

Manipulating this equation and substituting for y as per the equation derived above yields

$$x \times \$2.50 + (160 - 2x) \times 5¢ = \$20.00$$

Further manipulation gives us

$$x \times \$2.50 + \$8.00 - x \times 10¢ = \$20.00$$
$$x \times \$2.40 = \$12.00$$

We can now solve for x quite easily: $x = \dfrac{\$12.00}{\$2.40} = 5$. Checking back to our original assignment of variables, we see that x was the variable we used to represent the number of $2.00 prizes. (It was also the number of 50¢ prizes, but that is irrelevant now.) The answer to the question is 5.

The most reasonable incorrect answer listed is (C), 10. We could have solved this problem using one variable to represent the total number of $2.00 and 50¢ prizes and another to represent the number of 5¢ prizes. This would have simplified the prize-count equation but complicated the total-prize-money equation. Doing it this way, it would be very easy to forget that our first variable, which we would find out was equal to 10, had to be halved to get the correct answer, which is 5, and that 10 is not the answer.

| SECTION THREE |

Full-Length Practice Tests

ANSWER SHEET

MARK ONE AND ONLY ONE ANSWER TO EACH QUESTION. BE SURE TO FILL IN COMPLETELY THE SPACE FOR YOUR INTENDED ANSWER CHOICE. IF YOU ERASE, DO SO COMPLETELY. MAKE NO STRAY MARKS.

RIGHT MARK: ⬬ WRONG MARKS: ✓ ✗ ⊙

Survey of the Natural Sciences

1. A B C D E	11. A B C D E	21. A B C D E	31. A B C D E	41. A B C D E
2. A B C D E	12. A B C D E	22. A B C D E	32. A B C D E	42. A B C D E
3. A B C D E	13. A B C D E	23. A B C D E	33. A B C D E	43. A B C D E
4. A B C D E	14. A B C D E	24. A B C D E	34. A B C D E	44. A B C D E
5. A B C D E	15. A B C D E	25. A B C D E	35. A B C D E	45. A B C D E
6. A B C D E	16. A B C D E	26. A B C D E	36. A B C D E	46. A B C D E
7. A B C D E	17. A B C D E	27. A B C D E	37. A B C D E	47. A B C D E
8. A B C D E	18. A B C D E	28. A B C D E	38. A B C D E	48. A B C D E
9. A B C D E	19. A B C D E	29. A B C D E	39. A B C D E	49. A B C D E
10. A B C D E	20. A B C D E	30. A B C D E	40. A B C D E	50. A B C D E

51. A B C D E	61. A B C D E	71. A B C D E	81. A B C D E	91. A B C D E
52. A B C D E	62. A B C D E	72. A B C D E	82. A B C D E	92. A B C D E
53. A B C D E	63. A B C D E	73. A B C D E	83. A B C D E	93. A B C D E
54. A B C D E	64. A B C D E	74. A B C D E	84. A B C D E	94. A B C D E
55. A B C D E	65. A B C D E	75. A B C D E	85. A B C D E	95. A B C D E
56. A B C D E	66. A B C D E	76. A B C D E	86. A B C D E	96. A B C D E
57. A B C D E	67. A B C D E	77. A B C D E	87. A B C D E	97. A B C D E
58. A B C D E	68. A B C D E	78. A B C D E	88. A B C D E	98. A B C D E
59. A B C D E	69. A B C D E	79. A B C D E	89. A B C D E	99. A B C D E
60. A B C D E	70. A B C D E	80. A B C D E	90. A B C D E	100. A B C D E

Reading Comprehension

1. A B C D E	11. A B C D E	21. A B C D E	31. A B C D E	41. A B C D E
2. A B C D E	12. A B C D E	22. A B C D E	32. A B C D E	42. A B C D E
3. A B C D E	13. A B C D E	23. A B C D E	33. A B C D E	43. A B C D E
4. A B C D E	14. A B C D E	24. A B C D E	34. A B C D E	44. A B C D E
5. A B C D E	15. A B C D E	25. A B C D E	35. A B C D E	45. A B C D E
6. A B C D E	16. A B C D E	26. A B C D E	36. A B C D E	46. A B C D E
7. A B C D E	17. A B C D E	27. A B C D E	37. A B C D E	47. A B C D E
8. A B C D E	18. A B C D E	28. A B C D E	38. A B C D E	48. A B C D E
9. A B C D E	19. A B C D E	29. A B C D E	39. A B C D E	49. A B C D E
10. A B C D E	20. A B C D E	30. A B C D E	40. A B C D E	50. A B C D E

MARK ONE AND ONLY ONE ANSWER TO EACH QUESTION. BE SURE TO FILL IN COMPLETELY THE SPACE FOR YOUR INTENDED ANSWER CHOICE. IF YOU ERASE, DO SO COMPLETELY. MAKE NO STRAY MARKS.

RIGHT MARK: ⬬ WRONG MARKS: ⊘ ⊗ ⊙

Physics

1. Ⓐ Ⓑ Ⓒ Ⓓ Ⓔ	11. Ⓐ Ⓑ Ⓒ Ⓓ Ⓔ	21. Ⓐ Ⓑ Ⓒ Ⓓ Ⓔ	31. Ⓐ Ⓑ Ⓒ Ⓓ Ⓔ
2. Ⓐ Ⓑ Ⓒ Ⓓ Ⓔ	12. Ⓐ Ⓑ Ⓒ Ⓓ Ⓔ	22. Ⓐ Ⓑ Ⓒ Ⓓ Ⓔ	32. Ⓐ Ⓑ Ⓒ Ⓓ Ⓔ
3. Ⓐ Ⓑ Ⓒ Ⓓ Ⓔ	13. Ⓐ Ⓑ Ⓒ Ⓓ Ⓔ	23. Ⓐ Ⓑ Ⓒ Ⓓ Ⓔ	33. Ⓐ Ⓑ Ⓒ Ⓓ Ⓔ
4. Ⓐ Ⓑ Ⓒ Ⓓ Ⓔ	14. Ⓐ Ⓑ Ⓒ Ⓓ Ⓔ	24. Ⓐ Ⓑ Ⓒ Ⓓ Ⓔ	34. Ⓐ Ⓑ Ⓒ Ⓓ Ⓔ
5. Ⓐ Ⓑ Ⓒ Ⓓ Ⓔ	15. Ⓐ Ⓑ Ⓒ Ⓓ Ⓔ	25. Ⓐ Ⓑ Ⓒ Ⓓ Ⓔ	35. Ⓐ Ⓑ Ⓒ Ⓓ Ⓔ
6. Ⓐ Ⓑ Ⓒ Ⓓ Ⓔ	16. Ⓐ Ⓑ Ⓒ Ⓓ Ⓔ	26. Ⓐ Ⓑ Ⓒ Ⓓ Ⓔ	36. Ⓐ Ⓑ Ⓒ Ⓓ Ⓔ
7. Ⓐ Ⓑ Ⓒ Ⓓ Ⓔ	17. Ⓐ Ⓑ Ⓒ Ⓓ Ⓔ	27. Ⓐ Ⓑ Ⓒ Ⓓ Ⓔ	37. Ⓐ Ⓑ Ⓒ Ⓓ Ⓔ
8. Ⓐ Ⓑ Ⓒ Ⓓ Ⓔ	18. Ⓐ Ⓑ Ⓒ Ⓓ Ⓔ	28. Ⓐ Ⓑ Ⓒ Ⓓ Ⓔ	38. Ⓐ Ⓑ Ⓒ Ⓓ Ⓔ
9. Ⓐ Ⓑ Ⓒ Ⓓ Ⓔ	19. Ⓐ Ⓑ Ⓒ Ⓓ Ⓔ	29. Ⓐ Ⓑ Ⓒ Ⓓ Ⓔ	39. Ⓐ Ⓑ Ⓒ Ⓓ Ⓔ
10. Ⓐ Ⓑ Ⓒ Ⓓ Ⓔ	20. Ⓐ Ⓑ Ⓒ Ⓓ Ⓔ	30. Ⓐ Ⓑ Ⓒ Ⓓ Ⓔ	40. Ⓐ Ⓑ Ⓒ Ⓓ Ⓔ

Quantitative Reasoning

1. Ⓐ Ⓑ Ⓒ Ⓓ Ⓔ	11. Ⓐ Ⓑ Ⓒ Ⓓ Ⓔ	21. Ⓐ Ⓑ Ⓒ Ⓓ Ⓔ	31. Ⓐ Ⓑ Ⓒ Ⓓ Ⓔ	41. Ⓐ Ⓑ Ⓒ Ⓓ Ⓔ
2. Ⓐ Ⓑ Ⓒ Ⓓ Ⓔ	12. Ⓐ Ⓑ Ⓒ Ⓓ Ⓔ	22. Ⓐ Ⓑ Ⓒ Ⓓ Ⓔ	32. Ⓐ Ⓑ Ⓒ Ⓓ Ⓔ	42. Ⓐ Ⓑ Ⓒ Ⓓ Ⓔ
3. Ⓐ Ⓑ Ⓒ Ⓓ Ⓔ	13. Ⓐ Ⓑ Ⓒ Ⓓ Ⓔ	23. Ⓐ Ⓑ Ⓒ Ⓓ Ⓔ	33. Ⓐ Ⓑ Ⓒ Ⓓ Ⓔ	43. Ⓐ Ⓑ Ⓒ Ⓓ Ⓔ
4. Ⓐ Ⓑ Ⓒ Ⓓ Ⓔ	14. Ⓐ Ⓑ Ⓒ Ⓓ Ⓔ	24. Ⓐ Ⓑ Ⓒ Ⓓ Ⓔ	34. Ⓐ Ⓑ Ⓒ Ⓓ Ⓔ	44. Ⓐ Ⓑ Ⓒ Ⓓ Ⓔ
5. Ⓐ Ⓑ Ⓒ Ⓓ Ⓔ	15. Ⓐ Ⓑ Ⓒ Ⓓ Ⓔ	25. Ⓐ Ⓑ Ⓒ Ⓓ Ⓔ	35. Ⓐ Ⓑ Ⓒ Ⓓ Ⓔ	45. Ⓐ Ⓑ Ⓒ Ⓓ Ⓔ
6. Ⓐ Ⓑ Ⓒ Ⓓ Ⓔ	16. Ⓐ Ⓑ Ⓒ Ⓓ Ⓔ	26. Ⓐ Ⓑ Ⓒ Ⓓ Ⓔ	36. Ⓐ Ⓑ Ⓒ Ⓓ Ⓔ	46. Ⓐ Ⓑ Ⓒ Ⓓ Ⓔ
7. Ⓐ Ⓑ Ⓒ Ⓓ Ⓔ	17. Ⓐ Ⓑ Ⓒ Ⓓ Ⓔ	27. Ⓐ Ⓑ Ⓒ Ⓓ Ⓔ	37. Ⓐ Ⓑ Ⓒ Ⓓ Ⓔ	47. Ⓐ Ⓑ Ⓒ Ⓓ Ⓔ
8. Ⓐ Ⓑ Ⓒ Ⓓ Ⓔ	18. Ⓐ Ⓑ Ⓒ Ⓓ Ⓔ	28. Ⓐ Ⓑ Ⓒ Ⓓ Ⓔ	38. Ⓐ Ⓑ Ⓒ Ⓓ Ⓔ	48. Ⓐ Ⓑ Ⓒ Ⓓ Ⓔ
9. Ⓐ Ⓑ Ⓒ Ⓓ Ⓔ	19. Ⓐ Ⓑ Ⓒ Ⓓ Ⓔ	29. Ⓐ Ⓑ Ⓒ Ⓓ Ⓔ	39. Ⓐ Ⓑ Ⓒ Ⓓ Ⓔ	49. Ⓐ Ⓑ Ⓒ Ⓓ Ⓔ
10. Ⓐ Ⓑ Ⓒ Ⓓ Ⓔ	20. Ⓐ Ⓑ Ⓒ Ⓓ Ⓔ	30. Ⓐ Ⓑ Ⓒ Ⓓ Ⓔ	40. Ⓐ Ⓑ Ⓒ Ⓓ Ⓔ	50. Ⓐ Ⓑ Ⓒ Ⓓ Ⓔ

INSTRUCTIONS FOR TAKING THE PRACTICE TEST

Before taking the practice test, find a quiet place where you can work uninterrupted. Make sure you have a comfortable desk and several No. 2 pencils.

Use the answer grid provided to record your answers. You'll find the answer key and score conversion chart following the test.

The test consists of four sections: Survey of the Natural Sciences (90 minutes), Reading Comprehension (60 minutes), Physics (50 minutes), and Quantitative Reasoning (45 minutes). Remember, if you finish a section early, you may review any questions within that section, but you may not go back or forward a section.

Good luck.

PERIODIC TABLE OF THE ELEMENTS

1 **H** 1.0																	2 **He** 4.0
3 **Li** 6.9	4 **Be** 9.0											5 **B** 10.8	6 **C** 12.0	7 **N** 14.0	8 **O** 16.0	9 **F** 19.0	10 **Ne** 20.2
11 **Na** 23.0	12 **Mg** 24.3											13 **Al** 27.0	14 **Si** 28.1	15 **P** 31.0	16 **S** 32.1	17 **Cl** 35.5	18 **Ar** 39.9
19 **K** 39.1	20 **Ca** 40.1	21 **Sc** 45.0	22 **Ti** 47.9	23 **V** 50.9	24 **Cr** 52.0	25 **Mn** 54.9	26 **Fe** 55.8	27 **Co** 58.9	28 **Ni** 58.7	29 **Cu** 63.5	30 **Zn** 65.4	31 **Ga** 69.7	32 **Ge** 72.6	33 **As** 74.9	34 **Se** 79.0	35 **Br** 79.9	36 **Kr** 83.8
37 **Rb** 85.5	38 **Sr** 87.6	39 **Y** 88.9	40 **Zr** 91.2	41 **Nb** 92.9	42 **Mo** 95.9	43 **Tc** (98)	44 **Ru** 101.1	45 **Rh** 102.9	46 **Pd** 106.4	47 **Ag** 107.9	48 **Cd** 112.4	49 **In** 114.8	50 **Sn** 118.7	51 **Sb** 121.8	52 **Te** 127.6	53 **I** 126.9	54 **Xe** 131.3
55 **Cs** 132.9	56 **Ba** 137.3	57 **La** * 138.9	72 **Hf** 178.5	73 **Ta** 180.9	74 **W** 183.9	75 **Re** 186.2	76 **Os** 190.2	77 **Ir** 192.2	78 **Pt** 195.1	79 **Au** 197.0	80 **Hg** 200.6	81 **Tl** 204.4	82 **Pb** 207.2	83 **Bi** 209.0	84 **Po** (209)	85 **At** (210)	86 **Rn** (222)
87 **Fr** (223)	88 **Ra** 226.0	89 **Ac** † 227.0	104 **Rf** (261)	105 **Db** (262)	106 **Sg** (263)	107 **Bh** (264)	108 **Hs** (269)	109 **Mt** (268)	110 **Ds** (269)	111 **Rg** (272)	112 **Uub** (277)	113 **Uut** (284)	114 **Uuq** (289)	115 **Uup** (288)	116 **Uuh** (292)	117 **Uus** (291)	118 **Uuo** (293)

*	58 **Ce** 140.1	59 **Pr** 140.9	60 **Nd** 144.2	61 **Pm** (145)	62 **Sm** 150.4	63 **Eu** 152.0	64 **Gd** 157.3	65 **Tb** 158.9	66 **Dy** 162.5	67 **Ho** 164.9	68 **Er** 167.3	69 **Tm** 168.9	70 **Yb** 173.0	71 **Lu** 175.0
†	90 **Th** 232.0	91 **Pa** (231)	92 **U** 238.0	93 **Np** (237)	94 **Pu** (244)	95 **Am** (243)	96 **Cm** (247)	97 **Bk** (247)	98 **Cf** (251)	99 **Es** (252)	100 **Fm** (257)	101 **Md** (258)	102 **No** (259)	103 **Lr** (260)

Full-Length Practice Test I

SURVEY OF NATURAL SCIENCES

100 questions–90 minutes

Directions: This examination is composed of 100 items: Biology (1–40), General Chemistry (41–70), and Organic Chemistry (71–100). Choose the best answer for each question from the five choices provided.

1. Which of the following aspects of cellular respiration is correctly paired with the location in the cell where it occurs?

   (A) Electron transport chain–inner mitochondrial membrane
   (B) Glycolysis–inner mitochondrial membrane
   (C) Krebs cycle–cytoplasm
   (D) Fatty acid degradation–lysosomes
   (E) ATP synthesis–outer mitochondrial membrane

2. If a strand of DNA underwent four rounds of replication, what percentage of the total DNA present would be comprised of the original DNA molecule?

   (A) 0%
   (B) 3.125%
   (C) 6.25%
   (D) 12.5%
   (E) 25%

3. You discover an organism you believe to be a prokaryote. The presence of which of the following would support your hypothesis?

   (A) Photosynthetic granules
   (B) Cell wall made of peptidoglycans
   (C) mRNA
   (D) Cell wall made of cellulose
   (E) Linear DNA

4. All of the following statements about the glycolytic pathway are true EXCEPT

   (A) It occurs in the cytoplasm.
   (B) Glycolysis is anaerobic.
   (C) One molecule of glucose breaks down into one molecule of pyruvate.
   (D) One molecule of glucose results in the formation of 2 net ATP and 2 reduced molecules of NAD^+.
   (E) Glucose is partially oxidized.

GO ON TO THE NEXT PAGE

5. Which of the following is FALSE regarding DNA?
   (A) The basic unit is a nucleotide.
   (B) Adenine and guanine are pyrimidines.
   (C) The strands are antiparallel.
   (D) Guanine always binds with cytosine forming three hydrogen bonds.
   (E) The sugar molecule is deoxyribose.

6. Fats differ from carbohydrates in that
   (A) they have much more hydrogen than oxygen.
   (B) they have much more oxygen than hydrogen.
   (C) carbohydrates release more energy per gram than fats.
   (D) they are more likely to form polymers.
   (E) they contain nitrogen.

7. Which stage of embryonic development consists of a hollow ball of cells surrounding a fluid-filled center?
   (A) Zygote
   (B) Morula
   (C) Blastula
   (D) 2-layer gastrula
   (E) 3-layer gastrula

8. You isolate a membrane-bound vesicle containing hydrolytic enzymes. It is most likely a
   (A) chloroplast.
   (B) microbody.
   (C) phagosome.
   (D) vacuole.
   (E) lysosome.

9. In a population in Hardy–Weinberg equilibrium, the frequency of the dominant allele D is three times that of the recessive allele d. What is the frequency of heterozygotes in the population?
   (A) 6.25%
   (B) 25%
   (C) 37.5%
   (D) 56.25%
   (E) 75%

10. Shortly after gastrulation, a teratogen affects the development of the endoderm. You will most likely see a deformity in the
    (A) lens of the eye.
    (B) gonads.
    (C) nervous system.
    (D) bladder lining.
    (E) connective tissue.

11. Which of the following is involved in respiration and excretion and develops into the placenta in humans?
    (A) Chorion
    (B) Allantois
    (C) Amnion
    (D) Yolk sac
    (E) Fetus

12. Which component aggregates to form the initial framework of a clot?
    (A) Erythrocytes
    (B) Macrophages
    (C) T cells
    (D) B cells
    (E) Platelets

GO ON TO THE NEXT PAGE

13. Ten turns of the Calvin cycle will produce

(A) 10 CO_2.
(B) 20 PGAL.
(C) 20 RBP.
(D) 36 ATP.
(E) 5 glucose.

14. Which of the following elements is not commonly found in nucleic polymers?

(A) Sulfur
(B) Carbon
(C) Oxygen
(D) Nitrogen
(E) Phosphorus

15. The next Mars probe brings back spores from an unknown plant. You discover that the spores have 18 chromosomes. Therefore,

(A) the haploid number is 9.
(B) the diploid number is 18.
(C) the haploid number is 36.
(D) the diploid number is 36.
(E) the diploid number is 9.

16. A color-blind male X_cY is crossed with a normal female (X_fX_c), where X_f is the gene for Fragile X syndrome, and X_c is the gene for color blindness. What is the probability that a male child will be phenotypically normal?

(A) 0%
(B) 25%
(C) 50%
(D) 75%
(E) 100%

17. Which of the following is FALSE regarding the cytoskeleton?

(A) It is composed of microtubules and microfilaments.
(B) It gives the cell mechanical support.
(C) It maintains the cell's shape.
(D) It makes up the cell wall.
(E) It is functional in the cell's motility.

18. Someone turned the dial to 56°C from 37°C on the heat bath that you are using for an enzyme-catalyzed reaction you are studying. Your reaction will

(A) proceed more quickly as the increased heat increases the energy level of the system.
(B) proceed more quickly as the optimum temperature for most enzymes is 56°C.
(C) have a rapid drop in rate due to the denaturation of the proteins.
(D) have a rapid drop in rate due to too much energy in the system leading to ineffective collisions.
(E) None of the above

19. Cell division is different in plants versus animals. One difference is

(A) plant cells have centrioles.
(B) plant cells divide via a cell plate.
(C) plant cells divide with a cleavage furrow.
(D) animal cells lack centrioles.
(E) plant cell divisions have asymmetric cytokinesis.

20. One molecule of glucose is catabolized via cellular respiration. How many molecules of ATP are produced by oxidative phosphorylation?

(A) 2
(B) 4
(C) 32
(D) 36
(E) 40

GO ON TO THE NEXT PAGE

21. *Drosophila melanogaster* can have several eye colors. Red eyes are dominant over white eyes and sepia eyes. If a red-eyed fly that resulted from a mating of red-eyed and sepia-eyed parents is crossed with a sepia-eyed fly, what percentage of the offspring will have sepia eyes?

(A) 0%
(B) 25%
(C) 50%
(D) 75%
(E) 100%

22. The retina of the eye is a derivative of the

(A) endoderm.
(B) ectoderm.
(C) mesoderm.
(D) ectoderm and mesoderm.
(E) mesoderm and endoderm.

23. All of the following are characteristics of osmosis EXCEPT

(A) Passive transport
(B) Occurs with water
(C) Solvent will spontaneously move from a hypertonic environment to a hypotonic environment
(D) Solvent spontaneously moves from an area of high solvent concentration to low solvent concentration.
(E) Osmosis ≠ diffusion.

24. Natural selection that favors variants of both phenotypic extremes over the intermediate phenotypes is known as

(A) stabilizing selection.
(B) genetic drift.
(C) disruptive selection.
(D) directional selection.
(E) gene flow.

25. Which of the following is a secondary consumer?

(A) Snake that eats mice
(B) Aphid that eats wheat
(C) Fungus that grows in dead tree trunks
(D) Photosynthetic bacterium
(E) Hawk that eats the snake from (A)

26. What region of the brain controls the breathing rate?

(A) Medulla oblongata
(B) Hypothalamus
(C) Cerebrum
(D) Cerebellum
(E) Pituitary gland

27. The lysogenic life cycle of a bacteriophage

(A) replicates with the host DNA.
(B) can remain dormant indefinitely.
(C) can exist as a prophage.
(D) None of the above
(E) All of the above

28. Which of the following hormones is released from the posterior pituitary?

(A) Oxytocin
(B) FSH
(C) Glucagon
(D) Estrogen
(E) Calcitonin

29. The tick bird feeds on parasites on the skin of a rhinoceros. This is an example of which of the following relationships?

(A) Parasitism
(B) Commensalism
(C) Predation
(D) Mutualism
(E) None of the above

GO ON TO THE NEXT PAGE

30. In the Linnaean classification system, we are classified as *Homo sapiens*. The term *sapiens* refers to our

    (A) class.
    (B) family.
    (C) order.
    (D) genus.
    (E) species.

31. Which of the following is TRUE about the role of LH in the menstrual cycle?

    (A) LH inhibits the secretion of GnRH.
    (B) LH is secreted by the ovary.
    (C) LH induces the ruptured follicle to become the corpus luteum and secrete progesterone and estrogen.
    (D) LH stimulates the development and maintenance of the endometrium in preparation for implantation of the embryo.
    (E) LH stimulates milk production after birth.

32. Cardiac muscle

    (A) is innervated by the somatic motor nervous system.
    (B) is not striated.
    (C) is multinucleated.
    (D) has involuntary contraction.
    (E) does not require Ca^{2+}.

33. Which of the following is an example of a fixed action pattern?

    (A) Startle response
    (B) Removing your hand from a hot stove
    (C) Circadian rhythms
    (D) Characteristic movement of herd animals
    (E) None of the above

34. Which part of the flower produces the monoploid cells that develop into pollen grains?

    (A) Style
    (B) Petal
    (C) Sepal
    (D) Anther
    (E) Stigma

35. Which of the following is an example of a pioneer organism?

    (A) Lichens
    (B) Mosses
    (C) Ferns
    (D) Annual grasses
    (E) Birches

36. Which region of the kidney has the lowest solute concentration?

    (A) Nephron
    (B) Cortex
    (C) Medulla
    (D) Pelvis
    (E) Epithelia

37. Two species occupying similar niches will

    (A) both be driven to extinction.
    (B) be nocturnal.
    (C) evolve in a convergent direction.
    (D) compete for at least one resource.
    (E) Two species will never occupy similar niches.

38. Resting membrane potential depends on

    (A) the differential distribution of ions across the neuron's membrane.
    (B) active transport.
    (C) selective permeability.
    (D) the Na^+/K^+ pump.
    (E) All of the above.

GO ON TO THE NEXT PAGE

39. A patient is diagnosed with a tumor located in the cerebellum. You might notice which of the following symptoms?

(A) Loss of temperature regulation
(B) Change in heart rate
(C) Loss of sense of smell
(D) Loss of hunger and thirst drives
(E) Loss of hand-eye coordination

40. Which metal is complexed to chlorophyll?

(A) Zinc
(B) Copper
(C) Iron
(D) Magnesium
(E) Manganese

41. Which one of the following correctly lists elements in order of decreasing electronegativity?

(A) N, P, As, Sb, Bi
(B) Ga, Ge, As, Se, Br
(C) Hg, In, Ge, P, O
(D) Ra, Ba, Sr, Ca, Mg
(E) Rn, Xe, Kr, Ar, Ne

42. Which one of the following elements has the largest second ionization energy?

(A) Mg
(B) Ca
(C) Sr
(D) Rb
(E) Cs

43. What is the molecular geometry of PH_2Cl?

(A) Square planar
(B) Trigonal planar
(C) Tetrahedral
(D) Trigonal bipyramid
(E) Trigonal pyramid

44. A rigid container holds 3.00 moles of an ideal gas at 298K. How many moles of gas would need to be added to the container at constant temperature to increase the pressure from 1.00 atm to 1.80 atm?

(A) 73.4 moles
(B) 24.4 moles
(C) 22.4 moles
(D) 2.4 moles
(E) 0.80 mole

45. Determine the numerical value of the rate constant for the reaction $A + B \longrightarrow C$ from the experimental rate data given below.

Experiment	$[A]_0$ (M)	$[B]_0$ (M)	$rate_0$ (Ms^{-1})
1	0.181	0.148	1.87
2	0.181	0.300	1.87
3	0.543	0.148	16.83

(A) $k = \frac{1.87}{(0.181)(0.148)}$

(B) $k = \frac{1.87}{(0.181)(0.148)^2}$

(C) $k = \frac{1.87}{(0.181)^2(0.148)}$

(D) $k = \frac{(0.181)(0.148)}{1.87}$

(E) $k = \frac{1.87}{(0.181)^2}$

GO ON TO THE NEXT PAGE

46. The balanced equation below is for a nonspontaneous reaction ($\Delta H° = 131$ kJ/mol and $\Delta S° = 134$ J/mol·K). Assuming that ΔH and ΔS do not vary with temperature, at what temperature will the reaction become spontaneous?

$$C(s) + H_2O\,(l) \rightarrow CO(g) + H_2(g)$$

(A) 1,250°C
(B) 1,022°C
(C) 978°C
(D) 900°C
(E) 749°C

47. At 0°C, a mixture of neon and argon gases occupies a volume of 44.8 liters with a total pressure of 1 atm. If the mixture contains 1.5 moles of argon, how many moles of neon are present?

(A) 3.0
(B) 1.5
(C) 1.0
(D) 0.75
(E) 0.5

48. Which of the series of elements below correctly lists a halogen, an alkaline earth metal, and a transition metal, respectively?

(A) Cl, Na, Sr
(B) Br, Ca, Cr
(C) Se, Sr, Sn
(D) Rb, Ra, Rh
(E) I, Rb, Cu

49. What is the percentage of oxygen by mass in a 20 gram sample of $CuSO_4{\bullet}5H_2O$?

(A) 19.2%
(B) 30.1%
(C) 32.1%
(D) 36.1%
(E) 57.7%

50. Which of the following could be the correct electron configuration for the ground-state neutral atom of a nonmetallic element?

(A) $1s^22s^22p^63s^2$
(B) $1s^22s^22p^63s^3$
(C) $1s^22s^22p^63s^24s^2$
(D) $1s^22s^22p^63s^23p^4$
(E) $1s^22s^22p^63s^23p^7$

51. Which of the following is a stable resonance structure of N_2O_4?

(A) 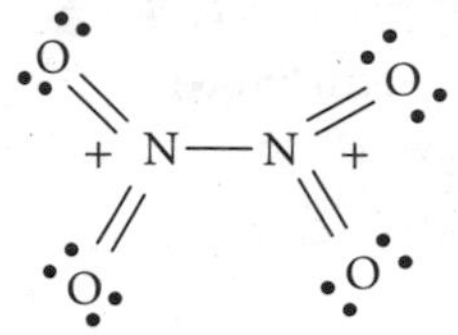

(B) 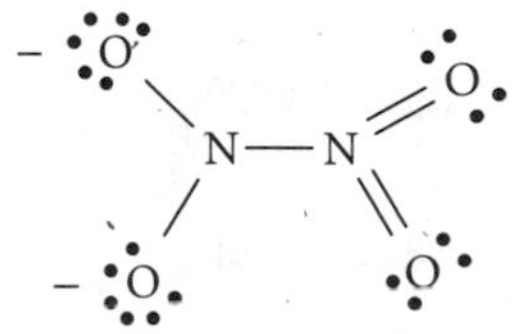

(C) 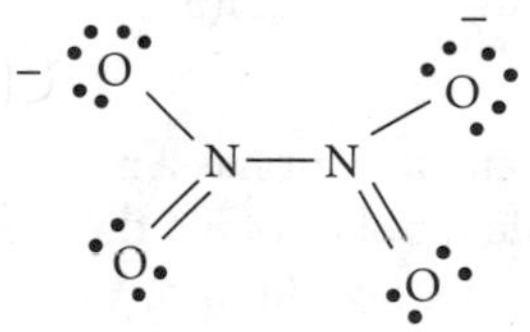

(D) 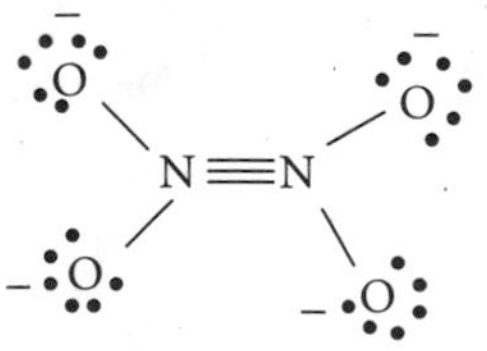

(E) 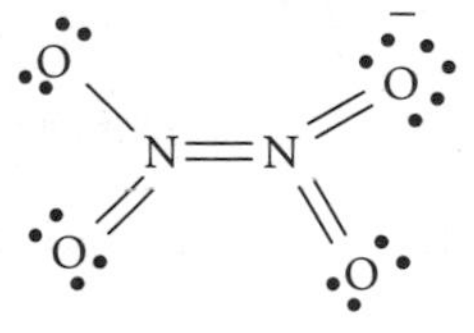

GO ON TO THE NEXT PAGE

52. Which of the following is the most polar molecular compound?

(A) BF_3
(B) CF_4
(C) CBr_4
(D) CH_2Cl_2
(E) CH_2Br_2

53. What volume of hydrogen gas, in liters, at 40°C and 763 torr can be produced by the complete reaction of 5.05 grams of zinc with excess HCl(*aq*)?

$Zn(s) + 2\ HCl(aq) \longrightarrow ZnCl_2(aq) + H_2(g)$
Note: R = 0.0821 L•atm/mol•K

(A) $\left(\frac{5.05}{65.4}\right)\left(\frac{760}{763}\right)(0.0821)(313)$

(B) $\left(\frac{5.05}{65.4}\right)\left(\frac{763}{760}\right)(0.0821)(40)$

(C) $\left(\frac{5.05}{65.4}\right)\left(\frac{760}{763}\right)(0.0821)(40)$

(D) $\left(\frac{5.05}{65.4}\right)\left(\frac{763}{760}\right)(0.0821)(313)$

(E) $(2.0)\left(\frac{5.05}{65.4}\right)\left(\frac{760}{763}\right)(0.0821)(313)$

54. If one isotope of an element has a mass number of 208 and an atomic number of 82, then another isotope of this element could have

(A) 124 neutrons.
(B) 126 neutrons.
(C) a mass number of 208.
(D) an atomic number of 80.
(E) 84 protons.

55. A sample of a pure compound is analyzed and found to contain 0.537 moles of N, 1.074 moles of H, and 0.537 moles of Cl. What is the empirical formula of this compound?

(A) NH_4Cl
(B) NH_2Cl
(C) $NHCl_2$
(D) $N_2H_2Cl_2$
(E) N_2HCl

56. Given the reactions and thermodynamic data below, calculate the ΔH°_f for C_6H_5OH in kcal/mol.

Reaction	**ΔH°(kcal)**
$C_6H_5OH + 7\ O_2 \rightarrow 6\ CO_2 + 3\ H_2O$	729.8
$C + O_2 \rightarrow CO_2$	94.4
$2\ H_2 + O_2 \rightarrow 2\ H_2O$	136.8

(A) –247.0
(B) –41.7
(C) 0.00
(D) 41.7
(E) 247.0

57. What is the percent yield if 78 g of C_6H_6 reacts and 82 g of $C_6H_5NO_2$ is formed according to the reaction below?

$C_6H_6 + HNO_3 \longrightarrow C_6H_5NO_2 + H_2O$

(A) 17%
(B) 33%
(C) 50%
(D) 67%
(E) 100%

GO ON TO THE NEXT PAGE

58. Hydrogen fluoride is a gas at room temperature, while water is a liquid. The best explanation for this observed difference in physical properties is that

(A) the difference in molecular weights indirectly accounts for the difference in boiling points because of van der Waals forces.
(B) the O–H bond dipoles of water are greater than the F–H bond dipoles of HF and account for the greater dipole–dipole interactions between water molecules.
(C) hydrogen bonding between water molecules is significantly greater than that between HF molecules.
(D) dispersion forces are significant between HF molecules but not between water molecules.
(E) water, as a universal solvent, is more likely than HF to be contaminated with impurities.

59. When 100 g of an unknown compound is dissolved in water to produce 1.00 liter of solution, the pH of the resulting solution is measured as 4.56. Which of the following statements is most likely TRUE of the unknown compound?

A. It is a strong base with a formula weight of less than 50 g/mol.
(B) It is a weak base with a pK_b of less than 5.
(C) It is a strong acid with a formula weight of less than 50 g/mol.
(D) It is a weak acid with a pK_a of more than 1.
(E) It is a weak acid with a formula weight of less than 10 g/mol.

60. If 35 mL of 0.10 M KOH is required to neutralize 50 mL of a monoprotic acid solution, the molarity of the acid solution is

(A) (35)(50)(0.10).
(B) $\left(\frac{35}{0.10}\right)(50)$.
(C) $\left(\frac{50}{35}\right)(0.10)$.
(D) $\left(\frac{35}{50}\right)(0.10)$.
(E) $\left(\frac{50}{0.10}\right)(35)$.

61. When 22.2 g of a soluble ionic compound (formula weight =111 g/mol) are added to 1.0 kg of water (K_f = 1.86°C/m), the freezing point of the resulting solution is −1.12°C. Which of the following could be the general formula of the ionic compound?

(A) MX
(B) MX_2
(C) M_2X_2
(D) MX_3
(E) M_2X_3

62. In which two compounds does sulfur have the same oxidation state?

(A) H_2S and $SOCl_2$
(B) H_2SO_4 and $SOCl_2$
(C) H_2SO_3 and $SOCl_2$
(D) H_2S and H_2SO_4
(E) H_2SO_3 and H_2SO_4

63. When carbon-14 undergoes beta decay, the daughter element is

(A) Carbon-12
(B) Carbon-13
(C) Nitrogen-14
(D) Oxygen-15
(E) Silicon-28

64. The balanced equation below is for a spontaneous oxidation-reduction reaction.

$$8\ Al(s) + 3\ NO_3^-(aq) + 5\ OH^-(aq) + 18\ H_2O\ (l) \rightarrow 8\ Al(OH)_4^-(aq) + 3\ NH_3(g)$$

Which of the following is the best oxidizing agent?

(A) $Al(s)$
(B) $NO_3^-(aq)$
(C) $NH_3(g)$
(D) $Al(OH)_4^-(aq)$
(E) $OH^-(aq)$

GO ON TO THE NEXT PAGE

65. What is the pH of a saturated aqueous solution of $Ca(OH)_2$? The K_{sp} of $Ca(OH)_2$ is 8.0×10^{-6}.

(A) 15.6
(B) 12.4
(C) 7.0
(D) 1.6
(E) 1.0

Questions 66 and 67 refer to the following diagram:

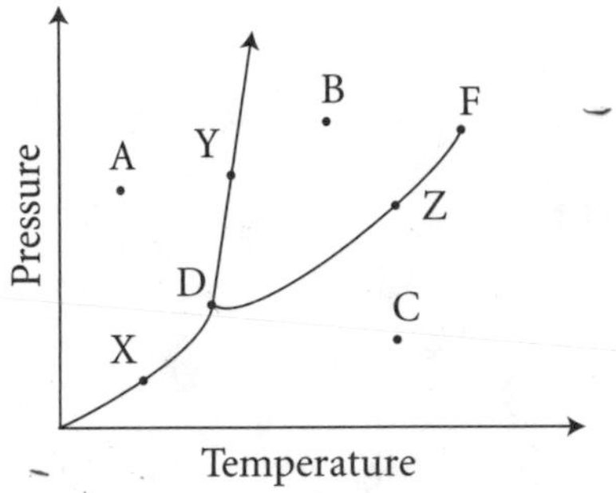

66. At which point(s) on the graph could ice, water, and water vapor exist at equilibrium together in a sealed beaker?

(A) D
(B) D and X
(C) D and Y
(D) D and Z
(E) Z

67. At which point(s) on the graph could condensation occur?

(A) D
(B) Y
(C) Z
(D) D and Y
(E) D and Z

68. Increasing the amount of liquid in a sealed container will cause the vapor pressure of the liquid to

(A) increase, regardless of the identity of the liquid.
(B) increase, if the liquid is sufficiently volatile.
(C) decrease, regardless of the identity of the liquid.
(D) remain the same, regardless of the identity of the liquid.
(E) decrease, if the liquid is sufficiently volatile.

69. Which of the following can be inferred from the heating curve shown?

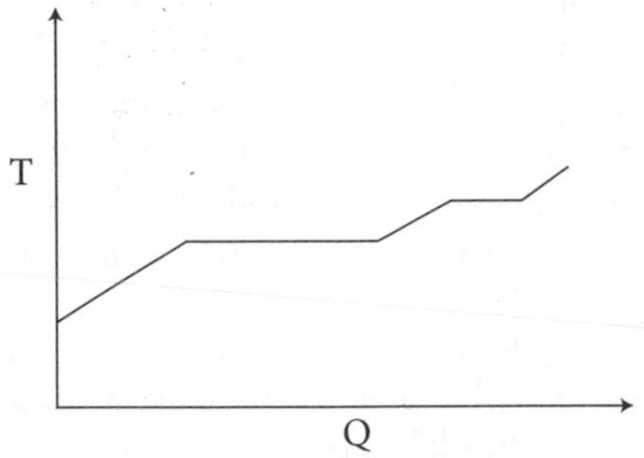

(A) The boiling point temperature is more than double the melting point temperature.
(B) The heat of vaporization is greater than the heat of fusion.
(C) The heat capacity in the gas phase is greater than that of the liquid phase.
(D) The heat capacity in the solid phase is greater than that of the liquid phase.
(E) The heat capacity in the liquid phase is greater than that of the solid phase.

70. Which of the following transformations could occur at the anode of an electrochemical cell?

(A) $Cr_2O_7^{2-} \rightarrow CrO_4^{2-}$
(B) $Cr^{2+} \rightarrow CrO_4^{2-}$
(C) $Cr_2O_7^{2-} \rightarrow Cr^{2+}$
(D) $CrO_4^{2-} \rightarrow Cr^{3+}$
(E) $Cr^{3+} \rightarrow Cr^{2+}$

GO ON TO THE NEXT PAGE

71. Which one of the following correctly matches the structure with its Fischer projection?

(A) 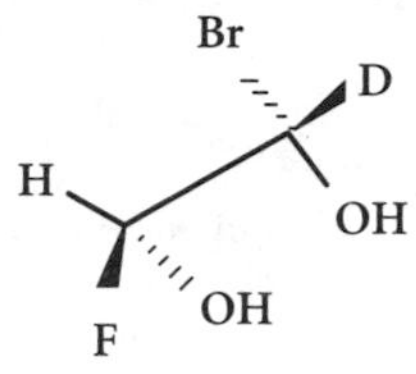 and 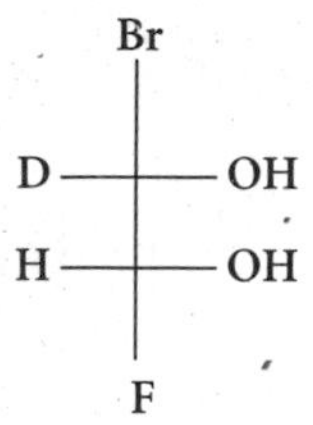

(B) 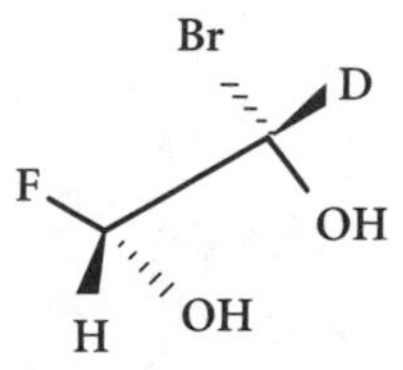 and 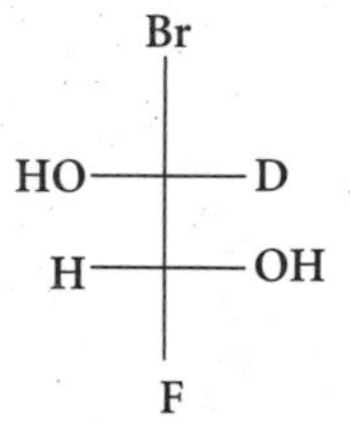

(C) 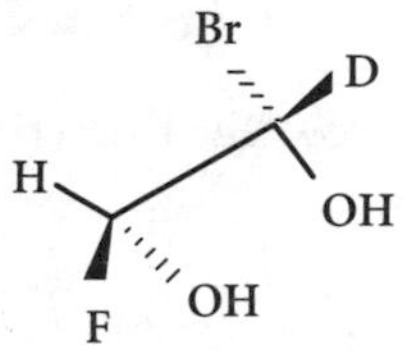 and 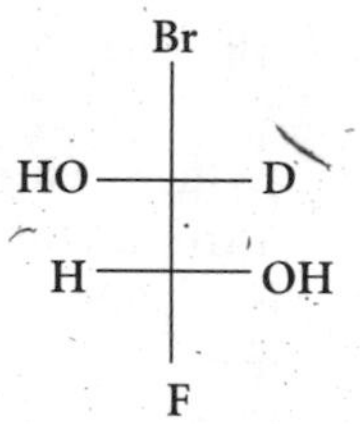

(D) 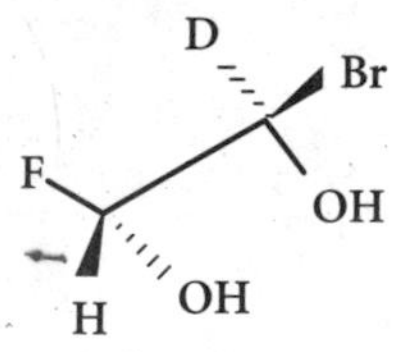 and 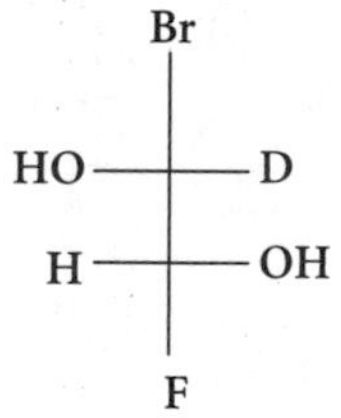

(E) 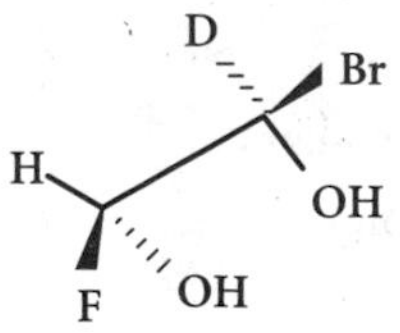 and 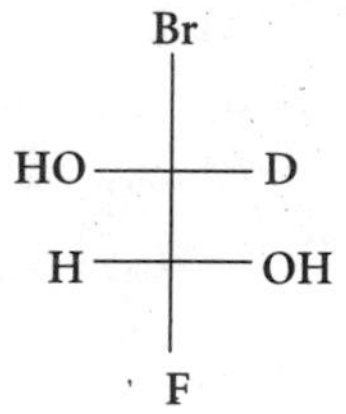

72. Which of the following alcohols is least soluble in water?

(A) 1-Propanol
(B) 2-Methyl-2-propanol
(C) 2,3-Butanediol
(D) 2-Butanol
(E) 3-Pentanol

73. What is the correct IUPAC name of the compound pictured below?

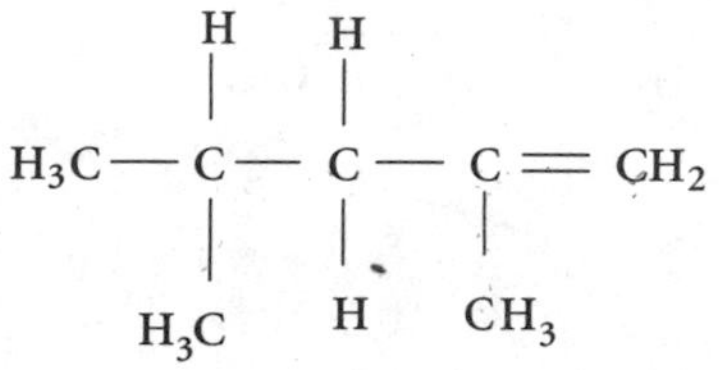

(A) 2,4-Dimethyl-1-pentene
(B) 2,4,4-Trimethyl-1-butene
(C) 1,1,3-Trimethyl-3-butene
(D) 2,4-Dimethyl-4-pentene
(E) 2-Methyl-4-methylpentane

GO ON TO THE NEXT PAGE

74. Which of the structures below has the least amount of nonbonded strain?

(A)

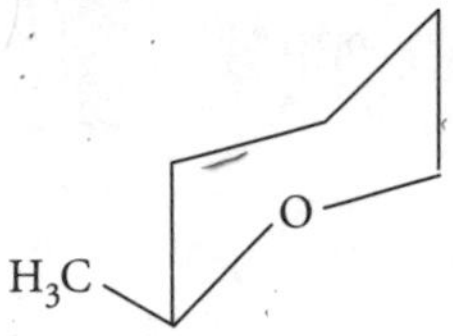

(B)

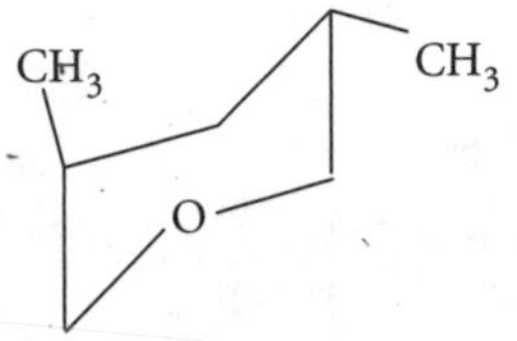

(C)

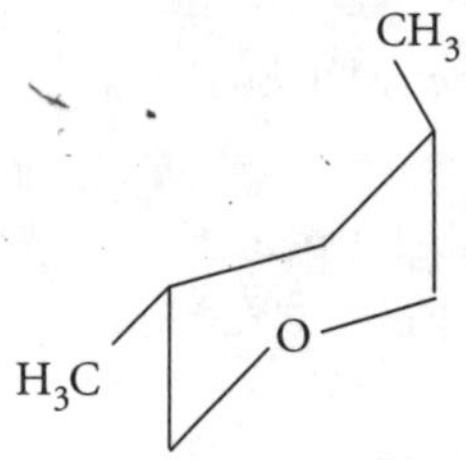

(D)

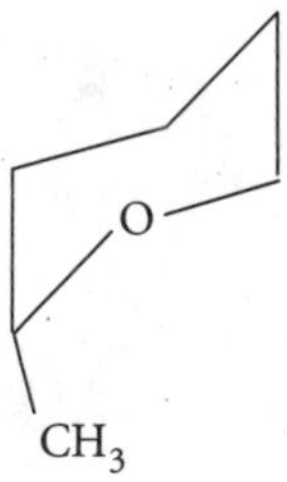

(E)

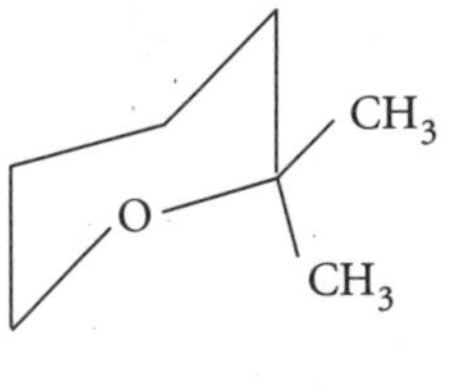

75. The Williamson ether synthesis is used to produce asymmetric ethers via an S_N2 mechanism. Which of the following pairs of compounds could be the starting materials for such a reaction?

(A) $CH_3CH_2CH_2C(=O)CH_2CH_3$ and $NaOC(=O)CH_2CH_2CH_3$

(B) $CH_3C(CH_3)(Cl)CH_2CH_2CH_3$ and $CH_3CH_2CH_2CH_2CH_2ONa$

(C) 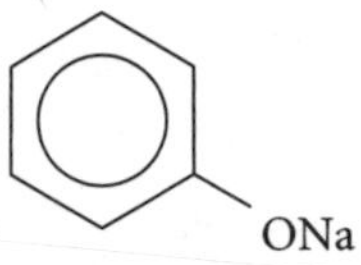 and 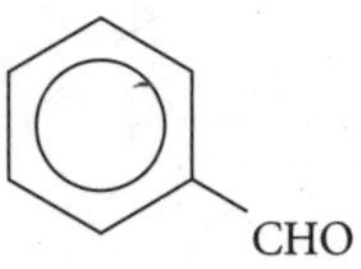

(D) CH_3CH_2ONa and $CH_3CH_2CH_2CH_2Cl$

(E) $CH_3CH_2OCH_2CH_3$ and $CH_3CH_2CH_2CH_2CH_2ONa$

76. Which of the choices below BEST describes the two structures shown?

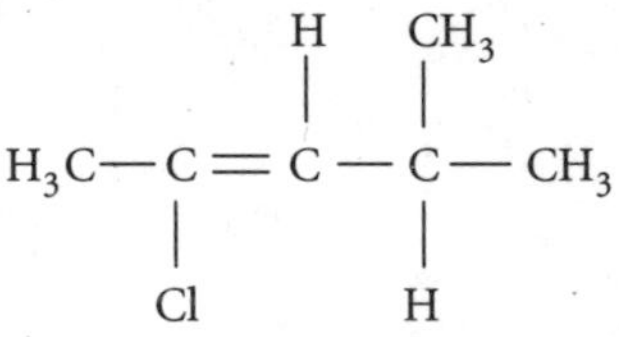

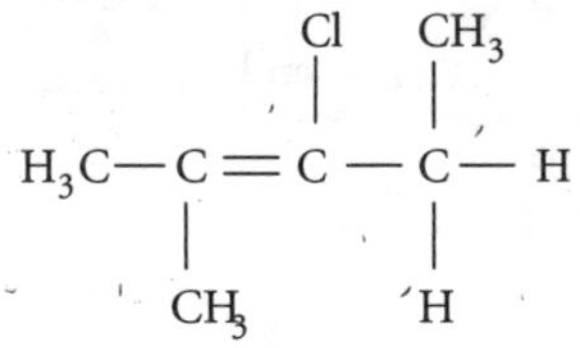

(A) Enantiomers
(B) Geometric isomers
(C) Conformational isomers
(D) Constitutional isomers
(E) Diastereomers

GO ON TO THE NEXT PAGE

77. Which of the following is a pair of structural isomers?

A. CH_3CH_2COOH and $CH_3CH_2CH_2OH$
(B) CH_3CH_2COOH and $CH_2CHCOOH$
(C) $CH_3CH_2CH_2OH$ and CH_3CH_2OH
(D) CH_3CH_2CHO and CH_3OCHCH_2
(E) $CH_3CH_2CH_2OH$ and $(CH_2CHCHO)_n$

78. Given the reaction:

$$RY + NaCN \xrightarrow{DMSO} RCN + NaY$$

Which of the following is the most likely identity of *Y*?

(A) I
(B) CH_3
(C) SH
(D) PH_2
(E) OCH_3

79. Which one of the compounds pictured below is most capable of intramolecular hydrogen bonding?

(A)
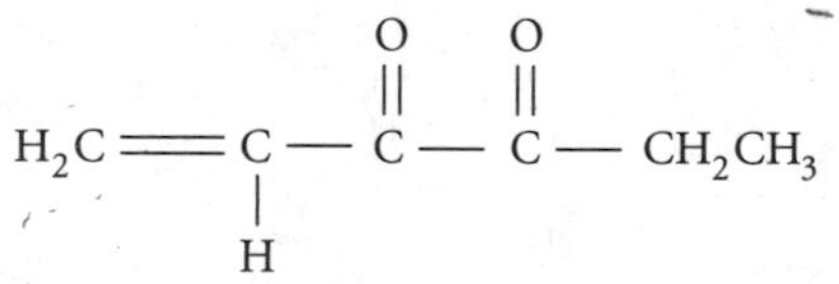

(B)
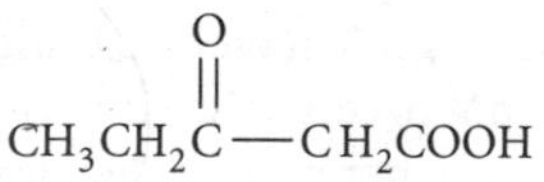

(C)
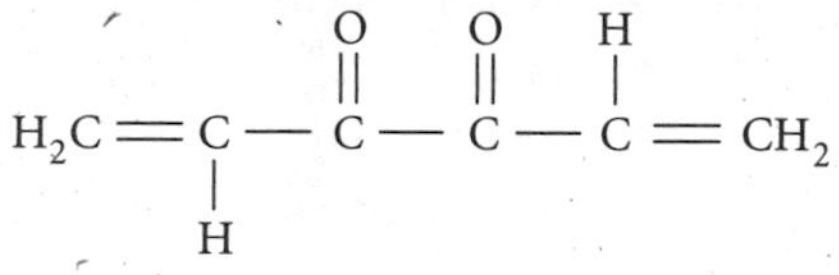

(D)
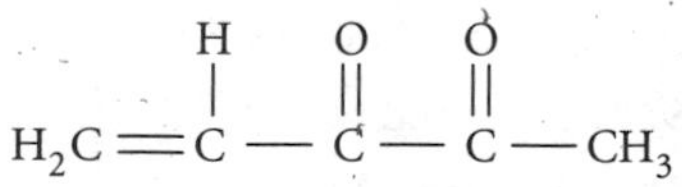

(E)
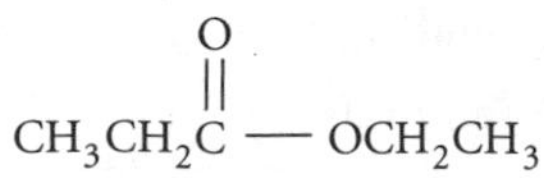

80. What is the correct IUPAC name for the compound pictured below?

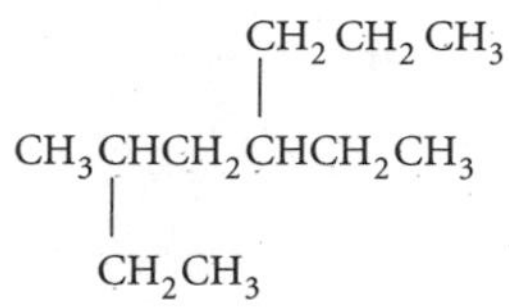

(A) 2-Ethyl-4-propylhexane
(B) 3-Propyl-5-ethylhexane
(C) 5-Ethyl-3-propylhexane
(D) 2,4-Diethylheptane
(E) 5-Ethyl-3-methyloctane

81. Which of the following is most likely to undergo an S_N1 reaction?

(A)
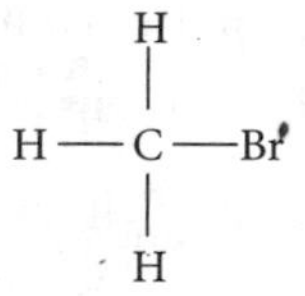

(B)
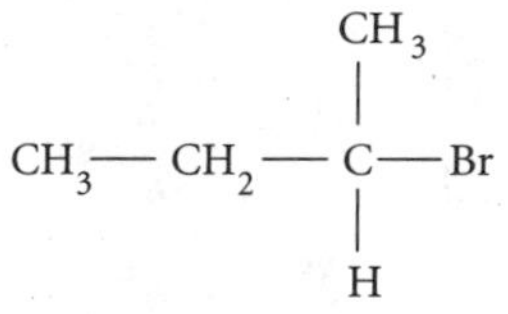

(C)
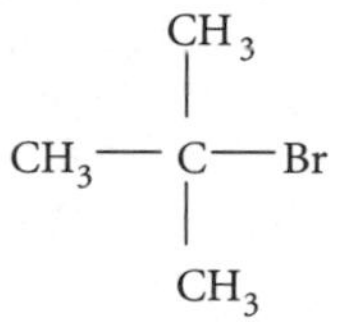

(D)
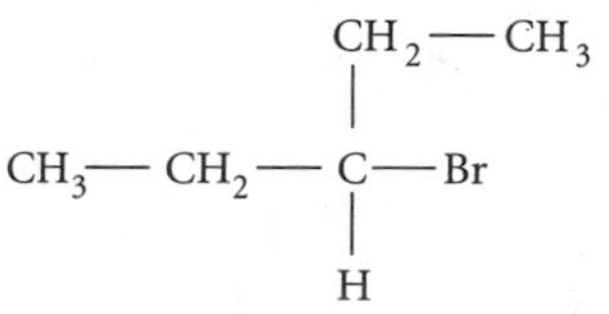

(E)
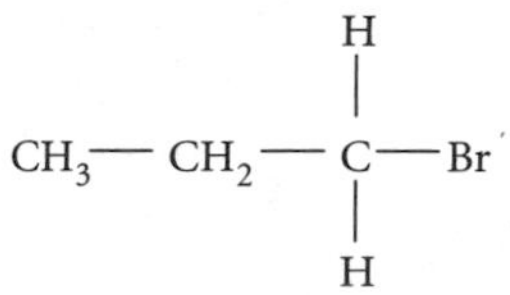

GO ON TO THE NEXT PAGE

82. The compound pictured below

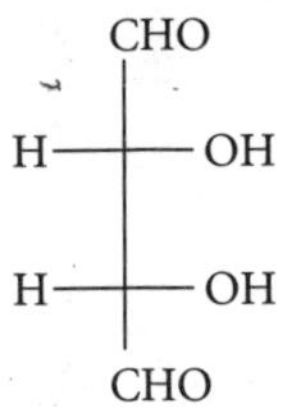

(A) has two chiral carbons and is thus optically active.
(B) is one of the four diastereomers possible for this compound.
(C) has an internal plane of symmetry and thus rotates plane polarized light.
(D) has an axis of rotational symmetry and thus rotates plane polarized light.
(E) has two chiral carbons and is optically inactive.

83. Which of the compounds pictured below is aromatic?

(A) 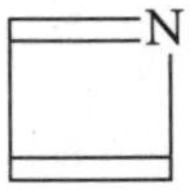

(B) 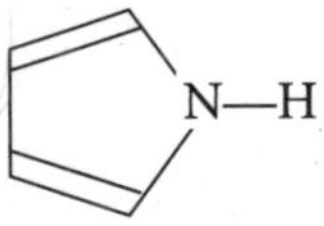

(C) 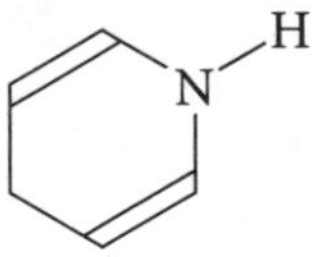

(D) 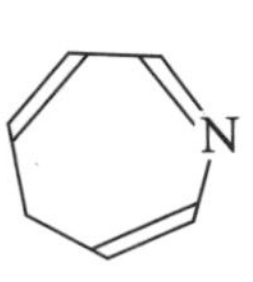

(E) 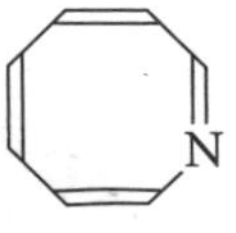

84. Which of the following structures has an E configuration?

(A) 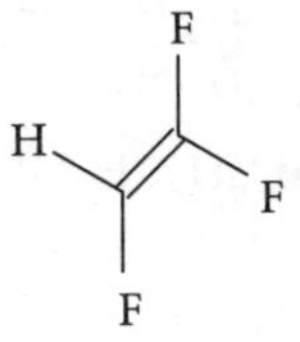

(B) 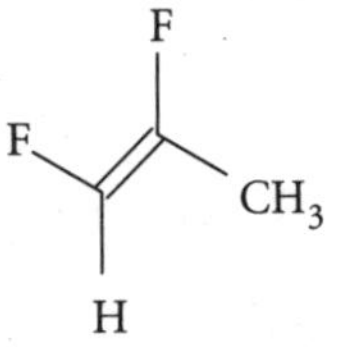

(C) 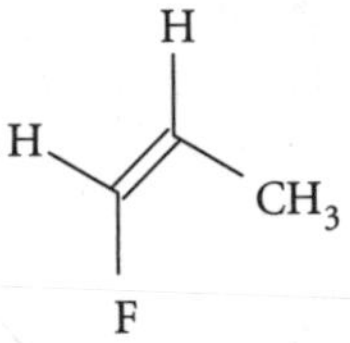

(D) 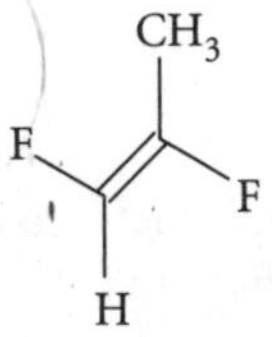

(E) 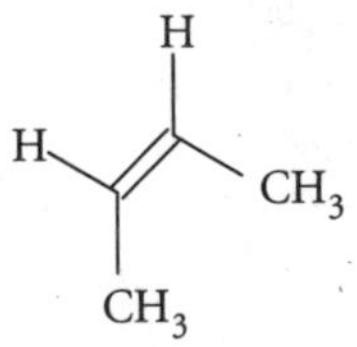

85. A portion of an organic molecule is pictured below, though not necessarily with accurate geometry. What are the approximate degree measures of angles *a*, *b*, and *c*, respectively?

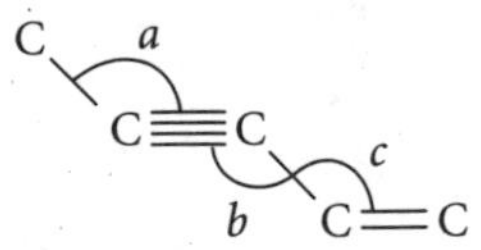

(A) 109.5°, 109.5°, and 109.5°
(B) 109.5°, 120°, and 109.5°
(C) 120°, 120°, and 120°
(D) 120°, 180°, and 120°
(E) 180°, 180°, and 120°

GO ON TO THE NEXT PAGE

86. Which of the following bromoalkanes is LEAST likely to undergo an S_N2 reaction?

(A) $CH_3CH_2CH_2CH_2Br$

(B) $CH_3CHBrCH_2CH_3$

(C)

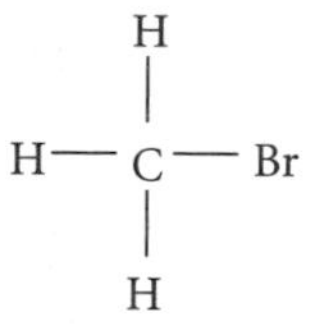

(D)

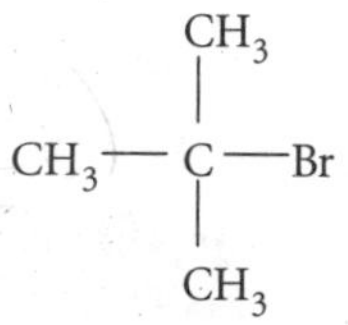

(E) CH_3CH_2Br

87. Which of the following is MOST reactive toward CH_3NH_2?

(A)

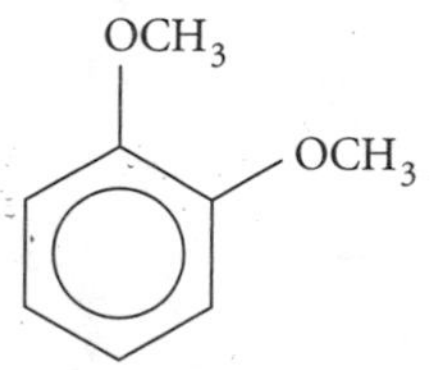

(B)

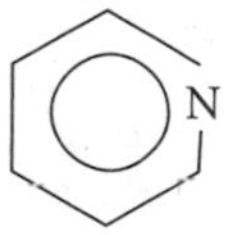

(C)

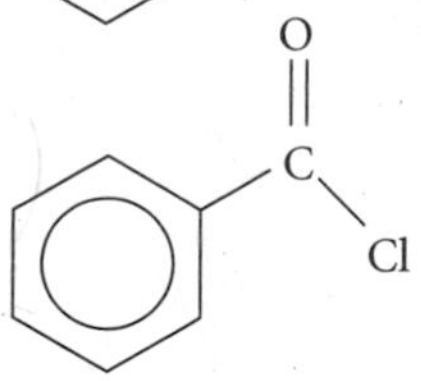

(D)

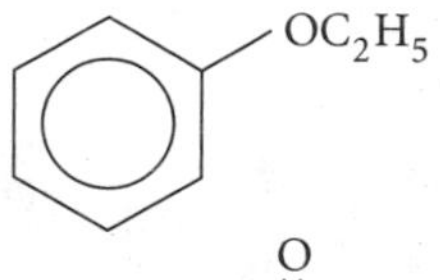

(E)

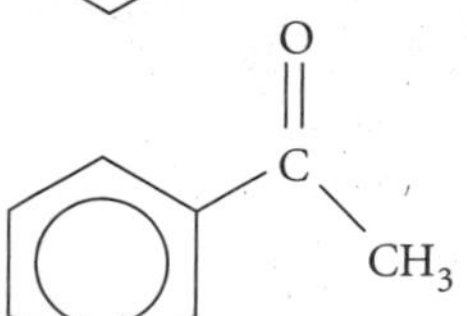

88. Which of the reagents below could be used to carry out the following conversion?

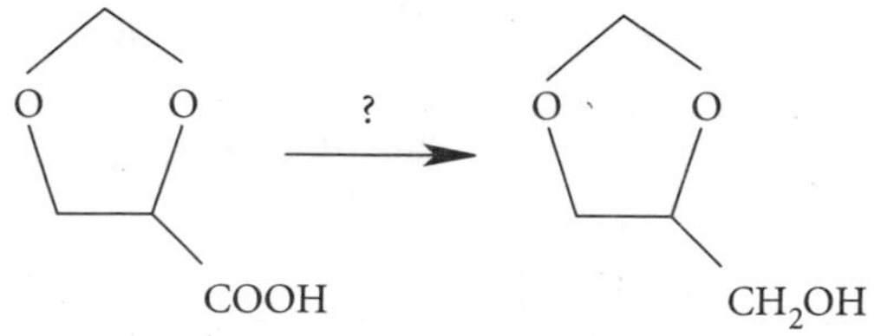

(A) $LiAlH_4$/THF, followed by H^+/H_2O

(B) aqueous $Hg(CH_3COO)_2$, followed by $NaBH_4$ and KOH

(C) KOH/C_2H_5OH

(D) BH_3/THF, followed by H_2O_2 and KOH

(E) CrO_3, H_2SO_4

89. 1,3-Cyclopentadiene reacts with sodium metal at low temperatures according to

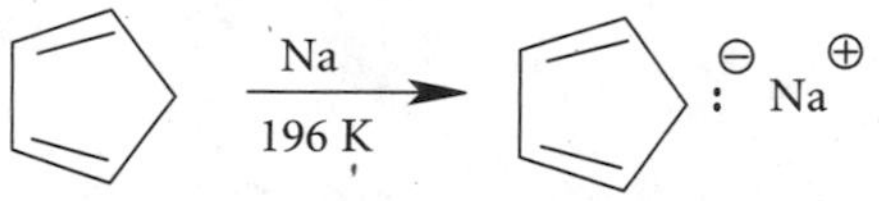

What is the BEST explanation for this observation?

(A) The reactant is more unstable at reduced temperatures.

(B) The cation formed is stabilized by aromaticity.

(C) Sodium metal is highly specific for cycloalkanes.

(D) The rehybridization of the saturated carbon atom provides additional stability to the product.

(E) The anion formed is stabilized by aromaticity.

GO ON TO THE NEXT PAGE

90. What is the final product, Z, of the synthesis below?

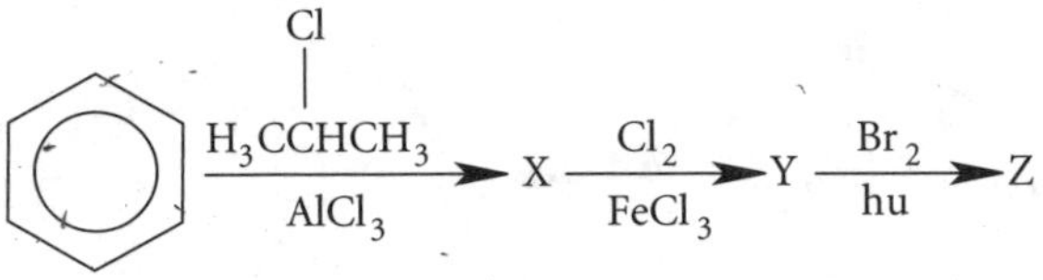

(A) 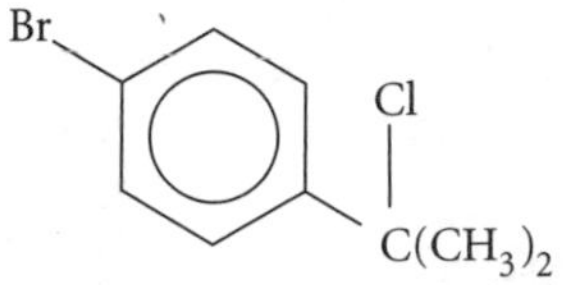

(B) 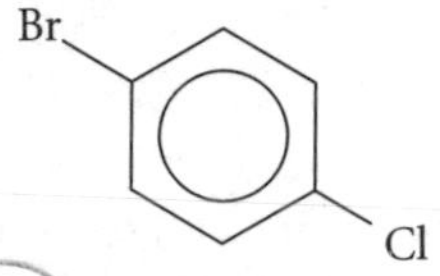

(C) 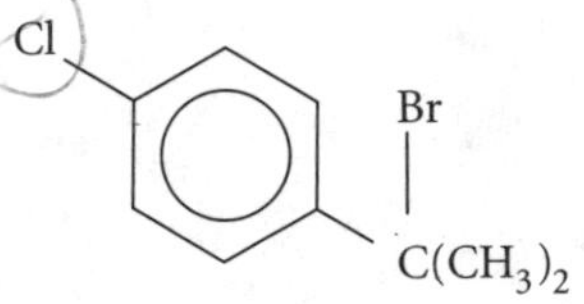

(D) 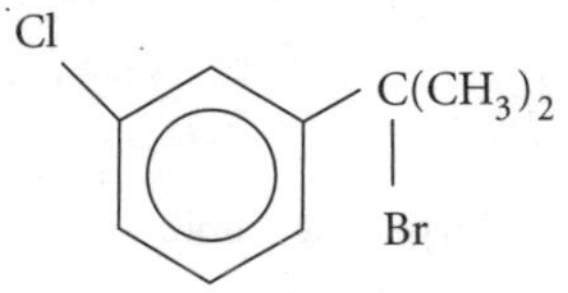

(E) 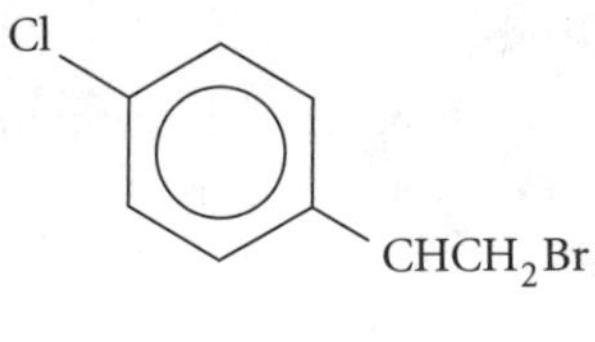

91. The compound pictured below

$$CH_3CH_2\overset{O}{\overset{\|}{C}}—OCH_2CH_3$$

(A) is optically active.
(B) can be hydrolyzed to yield acetic acid and ethanol.
(C) can be hydrolyzed to yield acetic acid and propanol.
(D) is a meso compound.
(E) can be hydrolyzed to yield propionic acid and ethanol.

92. Which of the following is an appropriate resonance form of the conjugate base of *p*-aminobenzoic acid?

(A) 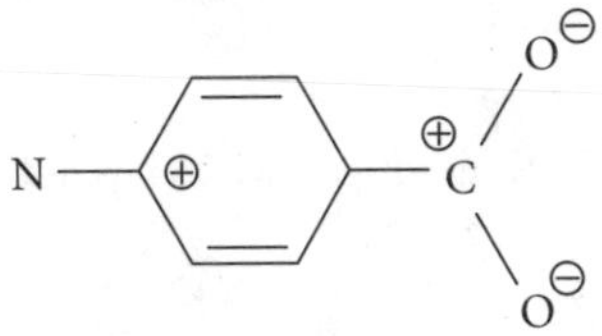

(B) 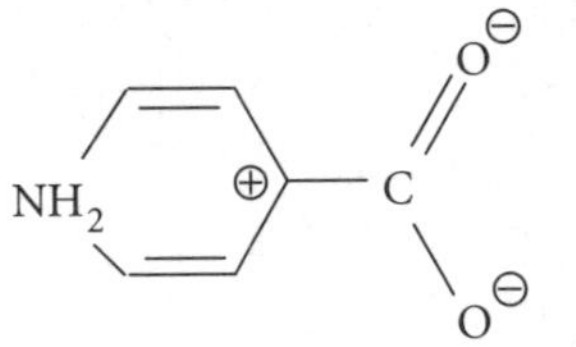

(C) 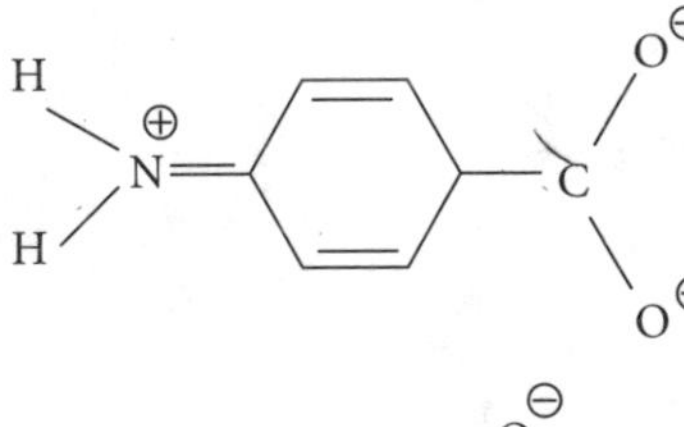

(D) 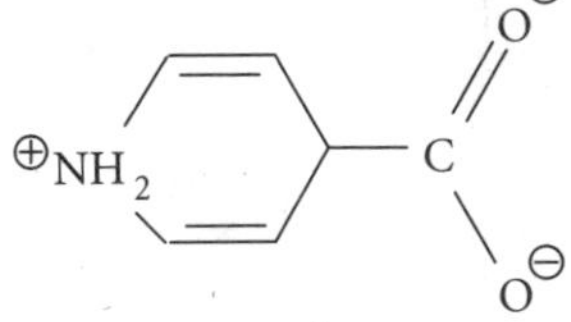

(E) 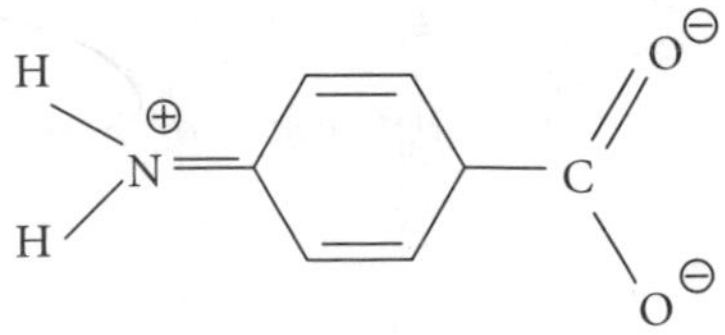

GO ON TO THE NEXT PAGE

93. What is the major organic product of the reaction below?

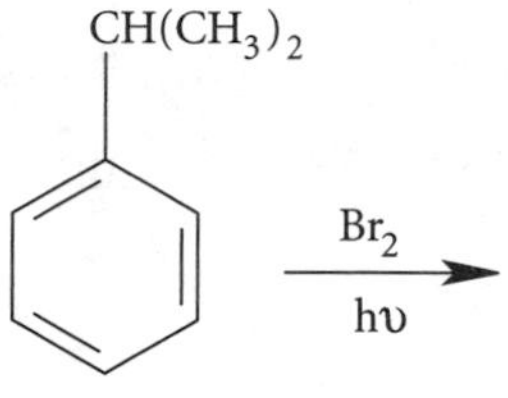

(A) 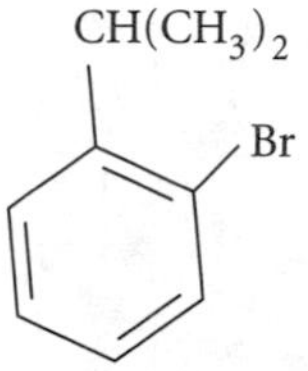

(B) 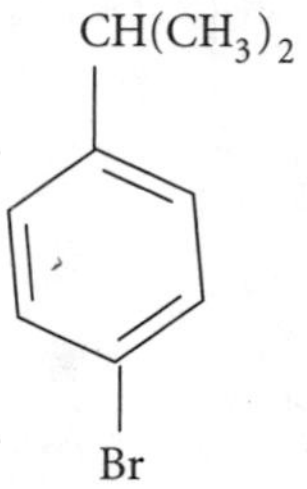

(C) 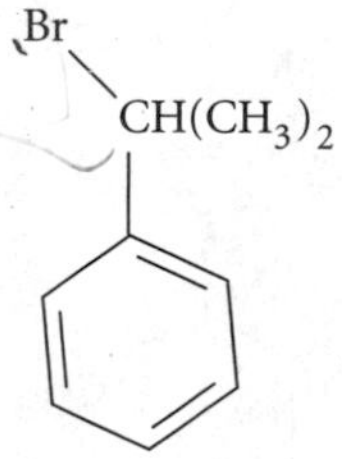

(D) 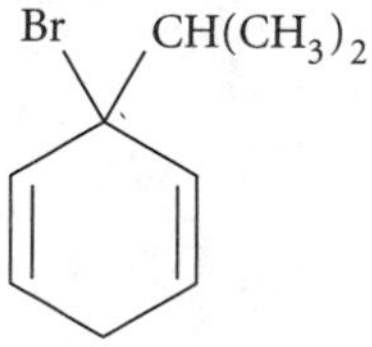

(E) 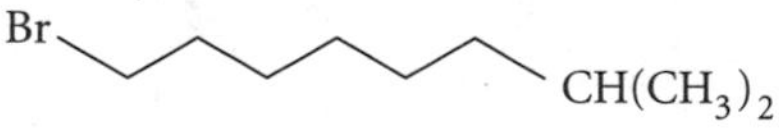

94. IR spectroscopy would be MOST useful in distinguishing between which of the following pairs of compounds?

(A) $CH_3CH_2CH_2COOH$ and $CH_3\overset{O}{\overset{\|}{C}}CH_2CH_2CH_3$

(B) $CH_3\overset{CH_3}{\overset{|}{C}}CH_2CH_2CH_3$ and $CH_3CH_2CH_2CH_2CH_2CH_3$

(C) 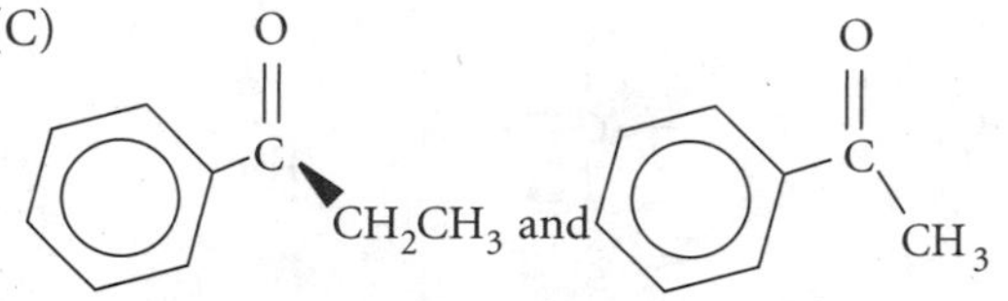

(D) $CH_3CH_2OCH_2CH_2CH_3$ and $CH_2CH_2CH_2CH_2OCH_3$

(E) $CH_3CH_2CH_2CH_2OCH_3$ and $CH_3CH_2CHOCHCH_3$

95. Which of the following is a termination step in the free radical bromination of ethane?

(A) $CH_3CH_2^{\bullet}$ + $Br^{\bullet}CH_3CH_2Br$

(B) $CH_3CH_3^{\Sigma}$ + $Br^{\Sigma}CH_3CH_2Br$ + H^{Σ}

(C) CH_3CH_3 + $Br_2CH_2BrCH_2Br$

(D) $CH_3CH_2^{\Sigma}$ + $Br^{\Sigma}CH_3CH_2Br$ + CH_3^{Σ}

(E) $CH_3CH_2^{\bullet}$ + $Br_2CH_3CH_2Br$ + $Br^{\bullet}$

96. What is the major product of the elimination reaction below?

$$CH_3 - \overset{\overset{\displaystyle H}{|}}{\underset{\underset{\displaystyle Cl}{|}}{C}} - \overset{\overset{\displaystyle H}{|}}{\underset{\underset{\displaystyle H}{|}}{C}} - \overset{\overset{\displaystyle H}{|}}{\underset{\underset{\displaystyle H}{|}}{C}} - CH_3 \quad \xrightarrow[\text{alcohol}]{\text{KOH}} \quad ?$$

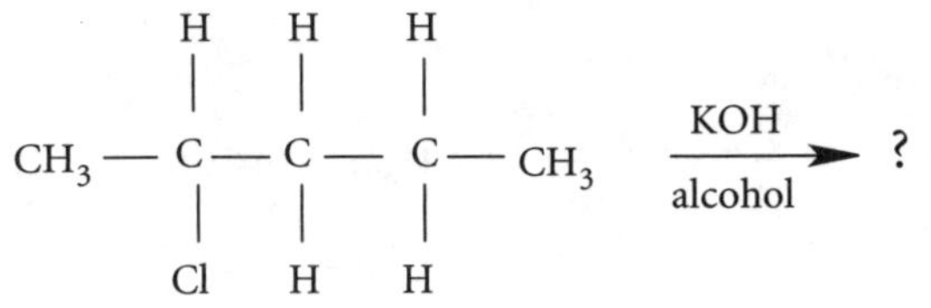

(A)

$$CH_3 - \overset{\overset{\displaystyle H}{|}}{\underset{\underset{\displaystyle Cl}{|}}{C}} = \overset{\overset{\displaystyle H}{|}}{\underset{\underset{\displaystyle H}{|}}{C}} - \overset{\overset{\displaystyle H}{|}}{\underset{\underset{\displaystyle H}{|}}{C}} - CH_3$$

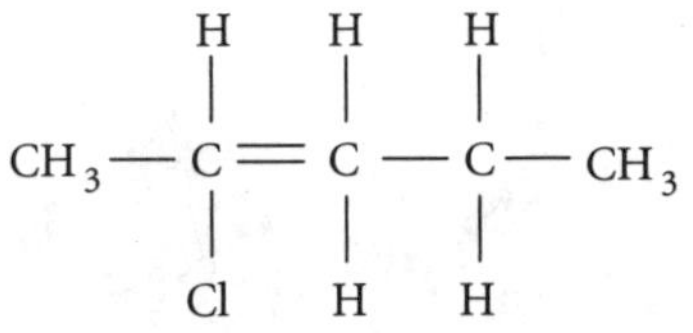

(B)

$$CH_3 - C \equiv C - \overset{\overset{\displaystyle CH_3}{|}}{\underset{\underset{\displaystyle H}{|}}{C}} - CH_3$$

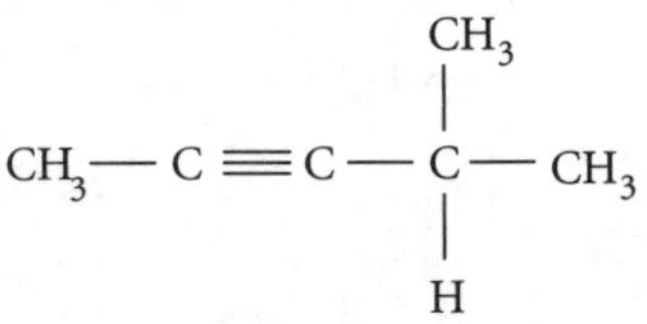

(C)

$$CH_3 - \overset{\overset{\displaystyle H}{|}}{\underset{\underset{\displaystyle Cl}{|}}{C}} = \overset{}{C} - \overset{\overset{\displaystyle CH_3}{|}}{\underset{\underset{\displaystyle H}{|}}{C}} - CH_3$$

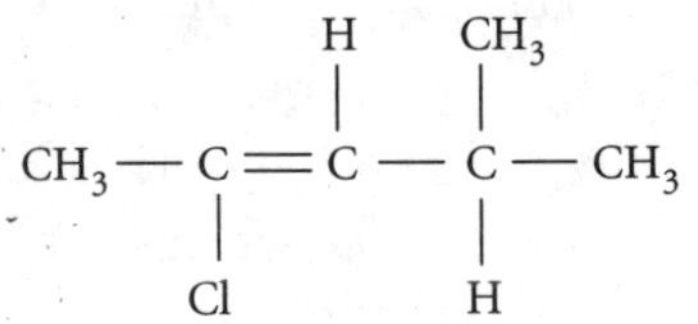

(D)

$$CH_3 - \overset{\overset{\displaystyle H}{|}}{\underset{\underset{\displaystyle Cl}{|}}{C}} - \overset{\overset{\displaystyle }{}}{\underset{\underset{\displaystyle H}{|}}{C}} = \overset{\overset{\displaystyle CH_3}{|}}{C} - CH_3$$

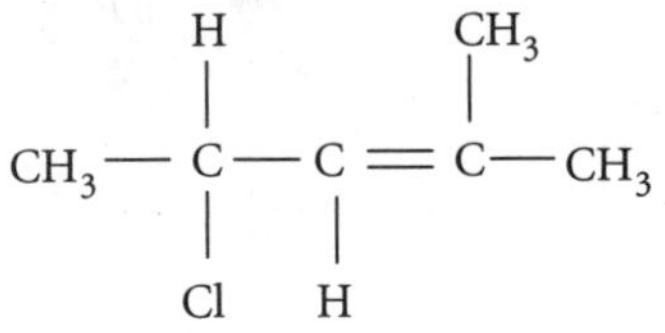

(E)

$$CH_3 - \overset{}{C} = \overset{\overset{\displaystyle H}{|}}{\underset{\underset{\displaystyle H}{|}}{C}} - \overset{\overset{\displaystyle H}{|}}{\underset{\underset{\displaystyle H}{|}}{C}} - CH_3$$

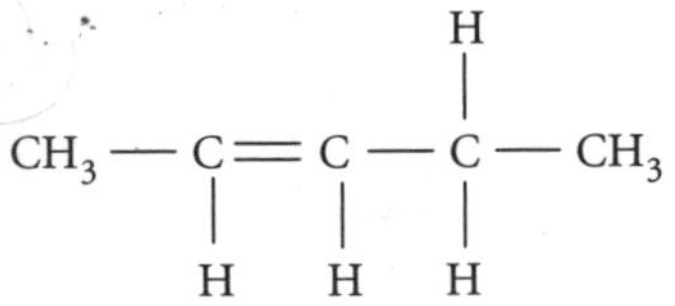

97. Which of the following is a major organic product of the reaction below?

$$\xrightarrow[\text{AlCl}_3]{\text{CH}_3\text{COCl}} \quad ?$$

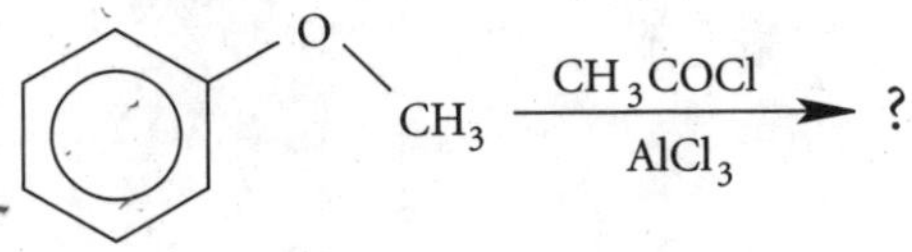

(A)

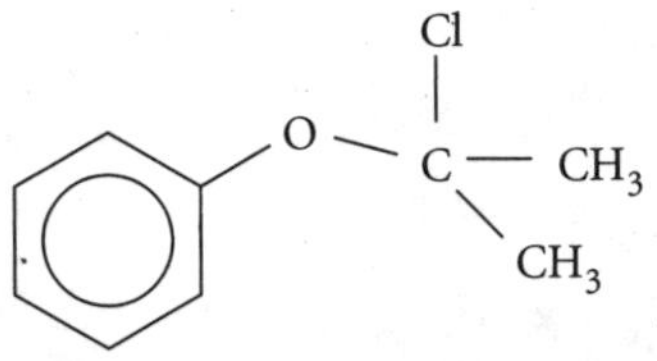

(B)

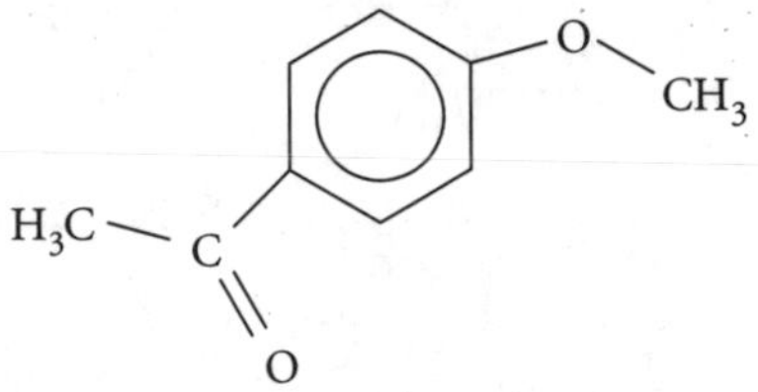

(C)

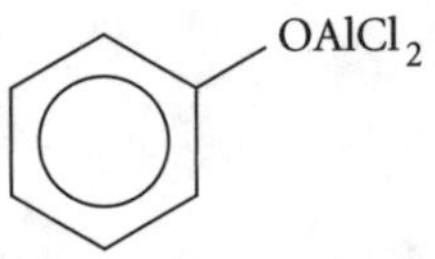

(D)

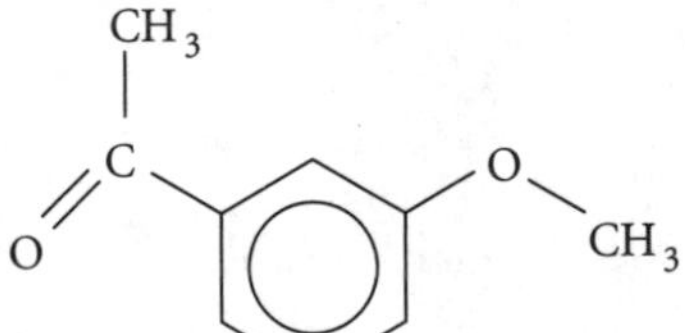

(E)

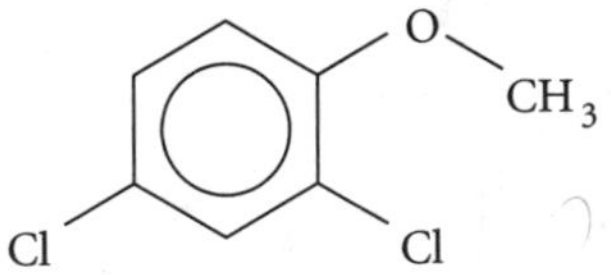

GO ON TO THE NEXT PAGE

98. Which of the following is the conjugate acid of diethylamine?

(A) $CH_3CH_2NH^-$
(B) $(CH_3CH_2)_2NH$
(C) $(CH_3CH_2)_2NH^+$
(D) $(CH_3CH_2)_2NH_2^+$
(E) $(CH_3CH_2)_2N^-$

99. What are the major products of the reaction sequence shown below?

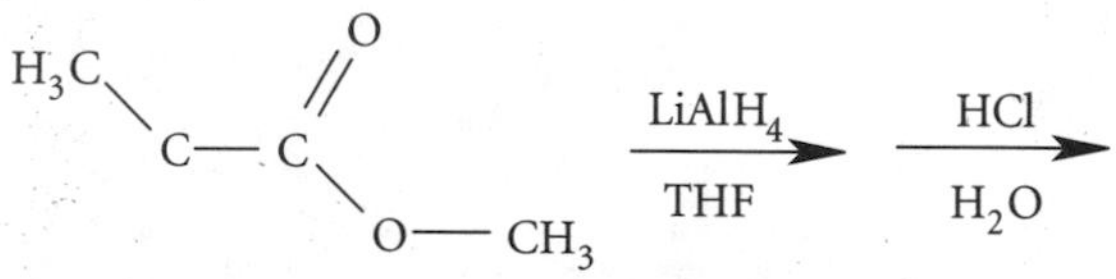

(A) CH_3CH_2COOH and CH_3OH
(B) CH_3CH_2COOH and $HCOOH$
(C) $CH_3CH_2CH_2OH$ and CH_3OH
(D) CH_3CH_2CHO and CH_3OH
(E) $CH_3CH_2CH_2OH$ and CH_2O

100. Which of the following is an organic product of the reaction sequence below?

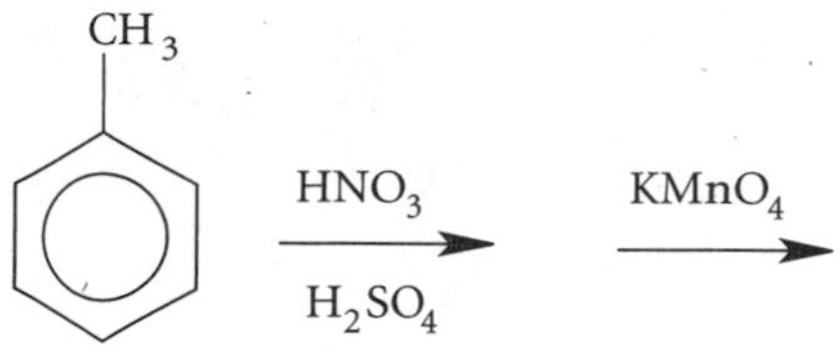

(A)

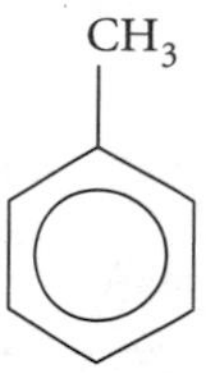

(B)

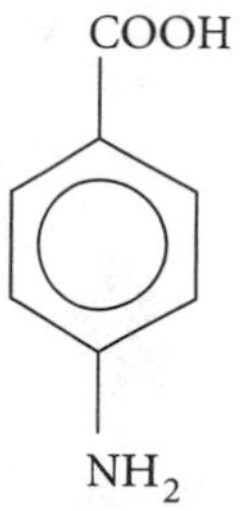

(C)

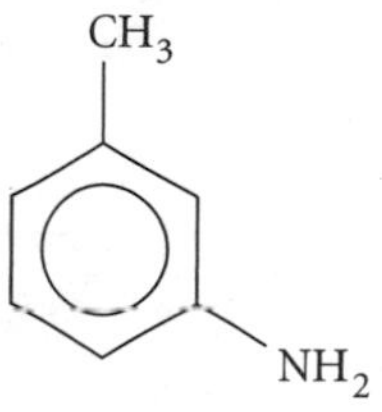

(D)

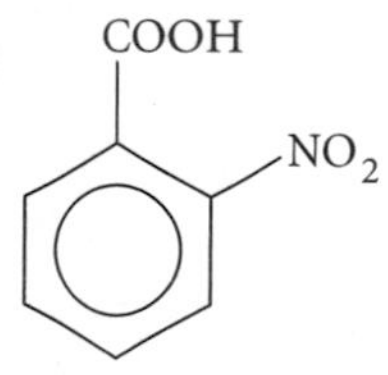

(E)

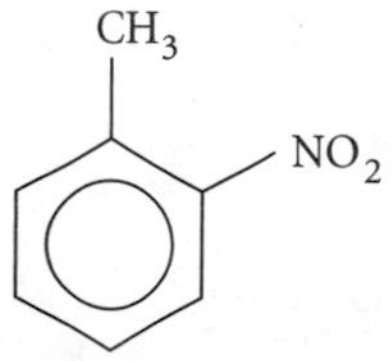

IF YOU FINISH BEFORE TIME IS CALLED, YOU MAY CHECK YOUR WORK ON THIS SECTION ONLY. DO NOT TURN TO ANY OTHER SECTION IN THE TEST.

STOP

READING COMPREHENSION

50 questions—60 minutes

Directions: The following test consists of several reading passages and questions that test your comprehension of the passages. Choose the best answer for each question from the five choices provided.

When atoms on the surface of a solid interact with molecules of a gas or liquid, they may alter the structure of the molecules ever so slightly, thereby promoting unusual chemical reactions. Indeed, by investigating the interactions between molecules and the surfaces of solids, researchers have learned to synthesize a myriad of novel substances, develop chemical processes of unprecedented efficiency, and remove pollutants from the environment. Yet the study of chemistry on solid surfaces will have the most impact . . . on the technology of catalysts—substances that increase the rates of desirable chemical reactions at the expense of others. . . .

When applying the results of surface studies to commercial catalysis, investigators face a difficult problem. The tools of surface chemistry require vacuum conditions, whereas most practical catalysis must work in a high-pressure environment. . . . Researchers need to be careful about how they apply the findings of surface chemistry to high-pressure catalytic reactions. The great disparity in pressure means a vast difference in the number of gas molecules hitting a catalyst at any one time, and therefore the kinetics of the laboratory reaction may differ from the dynamics of the high-pressure reaction. . . . [Chemists have] learned to extrapolate the behavior of high-pressure catalytic reactions from idealized surface studies.

An elegant example of how the pressure gap can be bridged is the story of a set of surface chemistry experiments aimed at improving the technology of catalytic converters for automobiles. The primary function of the converters is to remove nitric oxide (NO) and carbon monoxide (CO) from automobile exhaust. Nitric oxide reacts rapidly with air to form nitrogen-oxygen compounds (NO_x), which are harmful to the environment, notably because they contribute to acid rain. Carbon monoxide is also extremely toxic to most forms of life. . . .

A typical catalytic converter consists of particles of platinum (Pt) and rhodium (Rh) deposited on a ceramic honeycomb. The platinum and rhodium particles catalyze the reactions that remove NO_x, CO, and uncombusted hydrocarbons from car exhaust. The ceramic honeycomb and small particle size serve the dual function of maximizing the exposure of the metals to the exhaust fumes and minimizing the quantity of platinum and rhodium—two very expensive metals.

In the mid-1980s, researchers at General Motors and elsewhere set out to investigate how rhodium interacts with the nitric oxide and carbon monoxide from car exhausts. To do so, they studied reactions of NO and CO on single crystals of rhodium. Employing HREEL spectroscopy and other methods, the workers identified key steps in the breakdown of nitric oxide, and they determined how the arrangement of rhodium atoms on the surface influenced catalysis.

Yet it was not clear at first whether these results were applicable to the technology of catalytic converters: the experiments were conducted under vacuum conditions, whereas the rhodium particles used in catalytic converters are exposed to gases at high pressure. To demonstrate that practical information could be gained from the surface chemistry studies, the GM workers tested the rate of NO reduction on a rhodium surface in an environment that replicated the pressure conditions in a catalytic converter. By analyzing the action of rhodium in vacuum conditions and under high pressure, the researchers devised a mathematical model of the catalytic process. The model has allowed the results of the surface studies to be used in determining how new kinds of catalytic materials will operate under high pressures.

The GM group also found that the dissociation of NO was sensitive to the arrangement of atoms on the rhodium surface. They arrived at this conclusion by using infrared spectroscopy. This tech-

GO ON TO THE NEXT PAGE

nique is similar to HREEL spectroscopy, but it uses infrared radiation, instead of electrons, to cause molecular vibrations. Infrared spectroscopy has an advantage, however: it can be used both under vacuum conditions and at high pressures. Researchers at GM were therefore able to study, at high and low pressure, how nitric oxide interacts with irregular particles of rhodium and how it binds to a rhodium surface in which the atoms are arranged in a hexagonal pattern. Infrared spectroscopy identified differences in the vibrations of NO on the two types of surfaces, proving that surface structure influences bonding and ultimately the catalytic process. . . .

Surface chemistry has also helped researchers understand the catalytic process for removing sulfur from fossil fuels. Traces of sulfur in fossil fuels harm the environment in two ways. First, when fuel is burned in an engine, some sulfur reacts with air to form sulfur-oxygen compounds, which contribute to acid rain. Second, sulfur sticks to the platinum and rhodium in catalytic converters, thereby shutting down their activity and indirectly increasing the emission of NO and CO.

Sulfur is removed from petrochemicals at refineries as crude oil is transformed into such useful hydrocarbons as octane. Ideally, the desulfurization process should extract all the sulfur without destroying the valuable hydrocarbons. The process therefore requires a catalyst that encourages desulfurization but discourages the breakdown of pure hydrocarbons. [At the time of writing], the best catalyst for desulfurization is a mixture of molybdenum, cobalt, and sulfur itself. Because the material has a very complicated structure, chemists have had difficulty figuring out how petrochemicals interact with the catalyst. . . .

[A general model formulated by researchers at Harvard University] describes how thiols, a major class of sulfur-containing petrochemicals, interact with various molybdenum surfaces. Thiols consist of a hydrogen atom attached to a sulfur atom, which in turn is bonded to some combination of carbon and hydrogen. To study the interaction between thiols and molybdenum catalysts, they used crystals of pure molybdenum so that the atoms on the surface would form a highly ordered pattern. The regular structure limits the number of different kinds of sites available for bonding. By introducing various components to the molybdenum surface in a systematic way, the role of each component in desulfurization could be inferred.

Many years ago, chemists made an astonishing discovery about molybdenum-induced desulfurization. The performance of pure molybdenum is actually enhanced when it is contaminated with sulfur, whereas most metals lose their ability to catalyze reactions when sulfur bonds to them. To study the role of surface sulfur, researchers compared how thiols react on clean molybdenum surfaces with how they perform on molybdenum covered with an ordered array of sulfur. Thiols interact with molybdenum catalysts to produce hydrocarbons, hydrogen gas, surface carbon, and sulfur. For example, ethanethiol (CH_3CH_2SH) is broken down into sulfur and one of two hydrocarbons: ethane (CH_3CH_3) and ethene (CH_2CH_2). Ideally, the catalyst should promote only the production of hydrocarbons and the removal of sulfur; it should discourage the synthesis of surface carbon and hydrogen gas, which have little value.

The molybdenum surface coated with sulfur removes sulfur from thiols more slowly than the clean surface can, but at the same time, the sulfur on the molybdenum surface decreases the rate of reactions that lead to undesirable products, thereby increasing the yield of useful hydrocarbons. Indeed, sulfur deposited on a molybdenum surface is beneficial for the desulfurization not only of thiols but also of other petrochemicals. . . .

[The Harvard researchers] used synchrotron, infrared, and other techniques to figure out what the stages of the desulfurization are and what steps are crucial in setting the overall rate of the reaction. The first step is the cleavage of the sulfur-hydrogen bond. . . . [T]his step occurs very rapidly and is favored because both sulfur and hydrogen form strong bonds to the molybdenum surface. In subsequent steps, the carbon-sulfur bond must break, and one carbon-hydrogen bond

GO ON TO THE NEXT PAGE

is either formed or broken to yield the hydrocarbon products from the thiol. . . . [The researchers] have found evidence that for any thiol molecule, the strength of the carbon-sulfur bond determines the overall rate of the desulfurization reaction.

By using [the] general model and information about the strength of the carbon-sulfur bond, [the Harvard researchers] have been able to predict the rates of reaction and the types of products formed during the desulfurization of thiols on molybdenum surfaces. Surface-bound carbon and gaseous hydrogen—the undesirable products—are formed at a rate that depends largely on whether a carbon-hydrogen bond can be broken before the breaking of the carbon-sulfur bond. According to fundamental principles of chemistry, therefore, the fraction of thiol intermediates that lead to useful hydrocarbons is proportional to the rate of carbon-sulfur bond breaking relative to the rate of carbon-hydrogen bond breaking. Thiols with low carbon-sulfur bond strengths—that is, high rates of bond breaking—would yield a large fraction of hydrocarbons. This conclusion has been borne out by experiments.

1. It can be inferred from the passage that HREEL spectroscopy

   (A) can be used under a variety of conditions, including both high and low pressure.

   (B) uses infrared spectroscopy to cause molecular vibrations.

   (C) cannot be used at high pressures.

   (D) was developed by researchers at General Motors.

   (E) was developed by researchers at Harvard University.

2. All of the following are reasons given for why it is difficult for scientists to apply the results of surface chemistry to commercial catalysts EXCEPT

   (A) there is a large difference in the number of gas molecules colliding with the catalyst.

   (B) the rate equations for the two conditions may be vastly different.

   (C) most catalysis takes place at high pressure, whereas surface chemistry must be performed under vacuum conditions.

   (D) commercial catalysts are difficult to access and, therefore, little experimentation is performed on them.

   (E) it is necessary to extrapolate the behavior of one to the other.

3. The primary function of catalytic converters is

   (A) to prevent nitric oxide from reacting with water to generate nitrogen-oxygen compounds.

   (B) to maximize the exposure of Pt and Rh to exhaust fumes.

   (C) to regenerate Pt and Rh.

   (D) to remove nitric oxide and carbon monoxide from auto exhaust.

   (E) to clean the environment.

GO ON TO THE NEXT PAGE

4. All of the following were characteristics of the surface chemistry investigations carried out in the mid-1980s EXCEPT

   (A) HREEL spectroscopy was employed.
   (B) vacuum conditions were applied.
   (C) there was uncertainty of the applicability of the results of these investigations to catalytic converters.
   (D) the effect of the arrangement of atoms on the rhodium surface on the dissociation of NO was studied.
   (E) the rate of NO oxidation on a rhodium surface was tested at high pressure.

5. It can be inferred from the passage that the performance of a molybdenum surface is BEST assessed in terms of

   (A) the rate of reactions that produce undesirable products.
   (B) the yield of useful hydrocarbons.
   (C) the rate at which sulfur is removed from thiol.
   (D) the rate of production of surface carbon and hydrogen gas.
   (E) the rate at which sulfur is added to petrochemicals.

6. The first step in the desulfurization process is

   (A) cleavage of the carbon-sulfur bond.
   (B) formation of a carbon-hydrogen bond.
   (C) the cleavage of one carbon-hydrogen bond.
   (D) production of the hydrocarbon products from thiol.
   (E) cleavage of the sulfur-hydrogen bond.

7. The rate at which surface-bound carbon and gaseous hydrogen are produced during desulfurization is principally determined by

   (A) whether a C-H bond can be broken at all.
   (B) whether a C-H bond can be broken prior to the cleavage of the C-S bond.
   (C) the fraction of thiol intermediates present.
   (D) the properties of the molybdenum surface.
   (E) what technique is used to determine the stages of desulfurization.

8. Which of the following is a way in which traces of sulfur in fossil fuels harm the environment?

   (A) Sulfur adheres to the platinum and rhodium in catalytic converters and enhances their activity.
   (B) Sulfur produces toxic gases when released into the environment.
   (C) Sulfur reacts with air to form sulfur-oxygen compounds, which contribute to acid rain.
   (D) Sulfur in petrochemicals prevents useful hydrocarbons from being produced.
   (E) Sulfur reacts with organic compounds in the soil, reducing the pH of the soil and disrupting the organisms.

9. When thiols with high carbon-sulfur bond strengths are subjected to the desulfurization reaction, the products would include

   (A) a small fraction of useful hydrocarbons.
   (B) a large fraction of useful hydrocarbons.
   (C) a combination of hydrocarbons and carbon dioxide.
   (D) a combination of hydrocarbons and sulfur dioxide.
   (E) Cannot be determined

GO ON TO THE NEXT PAGE

10. By investigating the interactions between molecules and the surfaces of solids, researchers have made progress in all of the following areas EXCEPT

    (A) technology of catalysts.
    (B) the study of gas phase decomposition mechanisms.
    (C) the synthesis of novel substances.
    (D) the development of efficient chemical processes.
    (E) the removal of pollutants from the environment.

11. The best catalyst for desulfurization is a mixture of

    (A) iron, oxygen, and hydrogen.
    (B) carbon, nitrogen, and iron.
    (C) sulfur and cobalt only.
    (D) molybdenum, cobalt, and sulfur.
    (E) sulfur, manganese, and cobalt.

12. Pt and Rh in catalytic converters function

    (A) as coenzymes in the reactions that remove nitric acid and carbon monoxide from the car exhaust.
    (B) to coat the ceramic honeycomb in order to minimize heat loss due to friction.
    (C) to provide additional surface area for catalysis to take place.
    (D) to maximize exposure to the exhaust fumes.
    (E) to catalyze the reactions that remove nitrogen-oxygen compounds, carbon monoxide, and uncombusted hydrocarbons from car exhaust.

13. The goal of desulfurization is to

    (A) break down the hydrocarbon products, as well as remove the sulfur.
    (B) remove all the sulfur without destroying the hydrocarbons.
    (C) convert sulfur from a solid form to a gaseous form.
    (D) convert sulfur from a solid to a liquid form.
    (E) remove the hydrocarbons.

14. A thiol consists of

    (A) a hydrocarbon chain only.
    (B) two hydrogen atoms, which are bonded to alternating carbons and phosphates.
    (C) a sulfur and phosphate, which are bonded to a hydrocarbon chain.
    (D) a hydrogen atom attached to a sulfur atom, which in turn is bonded to some combination of carbon and hydrogen.
    (E) a nitrogen atom bonded to alternating sulfur and hydrogen atoms.

15. According to this passage, why is it necessary to minimize the quantity of platinum and rhodium used in a catalytic converter?

    (A) They are very expensive metals.
    (B) They are a limited resource.
    (C) They can themselves pollute the environment if used in too great a quantity.
    (D) If used in too great a quantity, they generate a large amount energy, which is difficult to dissipate.
    (E) They have a long half-life.

16. According to the passage, all of the following are harmful to the environment and/or living organisms EXCEPT

    (A) nitric oxide.
    (B) carbon monoxide.
    (C) sulfur-oxygen compounds.
    (D) nitrogen-oxygen compounds.
    (E) thiols.

GO ON TO THE NEXT PAGE

The body reacts to tissue injury through a series of remarkable vascular and cellular changes designed to isolate and destroy the cause of injury. In a relatively simple animal, such as the hydra, cells cluster around and isolate the injurious agent, which is subsequently dissolved and destroyed. Essentially the same process occurs in humans—except that it involves the vascular system and more complex reactions.

In general, inflammation can be defined as the local, protective response of living tissues to injury. Acute inflammation is usually of sudden onset and is dominated by local vascular and exudative responses. Chronic inflammation is a slow, progressive process that may be either a continuation of the acute form or a prolonged low-grade form. Acute inflammation can be a reaction to a variety of noxious stimuli, including bacteria, trauma, and chemicals. Medical observers have long recognized it as a basic pathological process. Celcus, a Roman physician in the 1st century AD, noted the four cardinal signs of inflammation as *tumor*, *calor*, *rubor*, and *dolor* (swelling, heat, redness, and pain).

The development of the microscope allowed scientists to observe the subtle vascular and cellular changes that are physiologically responsible for the outward signs of acute inflammation. In the 19th century, the German pathologist Julius Cohnheim described the changes in blood vessels during acute inflammation. Cohnheim's Russian contemporary Elie Metchnikoff added the insight that white blood cells (leukocytes) can play a key defensive role during inflammation by ingesting particulate matter, such as bacteria, in a process called phagocytosis.

Scientists now understand that inflammation develops as a series of interdependent but distinct cellular events and vascular changes, many of which affect the terminal vascular bed, a complex mesh where arterioles connect with venules via thin-wall bypass channels. The initial event, vasoconstriction, is typically a short-lived contraction of the arterioles in the immediate vicinity of the injurious agent and is rarely intense enough to result in complete ischemia (a local deficiency of blood). Vascular contraction is followed by vasodilation of the local blood vessels and a consequent increase in blood flow through the affected tissue. Blood flow initially increases through the most direct routes leading to the veins. However, as the precapillary sphincters open, increasing amounts of blood are diverted into capillary side channels, resulting in hyperemia (a local excess of blood).

In close association with increased blood flow, the permeability of the capillaries and venules increases, and plasma escapes through the widened intercellular slits of the vessels' endothelial lining. Eventually, large quantities of fluids containing fibrinogen and other proteins leak from the blood vessels into interstitial spaces. A key event in inflammation is the walling off of the affected area due to the formation of fibrinogen clots in the interspaces of the tissue.

In addition to vascular changes, an inflamed area is invaded by leukocytes and other cells. A preliminary, limited line of cellular defense involves macrophages already present in the tissue. Such cells are active in the phagocytosis of infectious or toxic agents but are relatively few in number. Macrophages, however, can play a critical role later in the inflammatory process when monocytes migrate to the injured tissue, swell, mature, and develop into macrophages capable of phagocytosis.

Some of the most important defensive cells in the acute phase of the inflammatory reaction are polymorphonuclear leukocytes (also called granulocytes), which include polymorphonuclear neutrophils, polymorphonuclear basophils, and polymorphonuclear eosinophils. Neutrophils, the most numerous of the three types, are very motile and phagocytic. They constitute slightly more than 60 percent of circulating leukocytes (an adult human normally has about 7,000 white blood cells per cubic millimeter of blood but the count can go as high as 30,000 cells/mm^3 during acute inflammation).

Within a few hours after its onset, acute inflammation is characterized by an increase in the number of

GO ON TO THE NEXT PAGE

neutrophils in the blood by as much as four-to fivefold in response to a combination of chemicals (collectively called leukocytosis-inducing factor) released from the inflamed tissue. This factor diffuses from the inflamed tissue to the blood and is carried to the bone marrow, where it mobilizes the neutrophils stored in the marrow tissue.

Enzymes, necrotic products, bacterial toxins, and chemicals released from the inflamed tissues can cause neutrophils and monocytes to move from the circulatory system to the injured tissue. These products affect the permeability of the capillaries and small venules, allowing neutrophils and monocytes to actively squeeze through the pores of the blood vessels by diapedesis. The products also can damage the capillary walls and cause large amounts of neutrophils and monocytes to adhere to the capillaries' endothelial cells, a process called margination. Margination further facilitates rapid diapedesis of the white blood cells. Neutrophils and monocytes can be drawn toward the inflamed tissues by chemotaxis.

Ranging from 10 to 12 microns in diameter, neutrophils can phagocytize particles up to 5 or 6 microns in diameter. The neutrophil projects pseudopodia around the particle, creating a chamber containing the particle. The chamber invaginates and breaks from the outer cell membrane of the neutrophil to form a free-flowing vesicle in the cytoplasm. There the particle is digested by proteolytic enzymes released from lysosomes.

Eosinophils normally make up 2 to 3 percent of all blood leukocytes. While eosinophils are phagocytic and exhibit chemotaxis, they are not nearly as efficient as neutrophils in phagocytosis. These white blood cells, however, are particularly effective in defending against relatively large quantities of histamine, bradykinin, serotonin, and a number of lysosomal enzymes. Such chemical agents can cause local vascular and tissue reactions during the allergic response.

In summary, many of the cardinal signs of inflammation first described by Celsus can be explained by the vascular and cellular events now known to occur during inflammation. *Calor* (heat) and *rubor* (redness) are due to the dilation of the blood vessels and the resulting local excess of blood. *Tumor* (swelling) is caused by the accumulation of fluid leaking from blood vessels to the damaged tissue. *Dolor* (pain) probably results from swelling that stretches tissue over inflamed areas, as well as the chemical substances released in response to injurious agents.

17. The initial vascular event in inflammation is

(A) the contraction of local vessels.
(B) vasodilation.
(C) changes in the adhesiveness of capillary walls.
(D) an increase in circulating neutrophils.
(E) ischemia.

18. Inflammation can BEST be characterized as

(A) a pathological destruction of tissue.
(B) an injury to blood vessels.
(C) the formation of cell clusters around injurious agents.
(D) a protective local response that follows tissue injury.
(E) a generalized response consisting of swelling, heat, and pain.

19. Scientists during the 19th century recognized for the first time

(A) the outward signs of inflammation.
(B) that leukocytes carry out pinocytosis.
(C) that inflammation is a pathological process.
(D) that a variety of injuries can lead to inflammation.
(E) how blood vessels change during inflammation.

GO ON TO THE NEXT PAGE

20. A local deficiency of blood in tissues is called

(A) hyperemia.
(B) acute inflammation.
(C) leukocytes.
(D) ischemia.
(E) diapedesis.

21. The opening of precapillary sphincters leads directly to

(A) an expansion of arterioles.
(B) a closing of the direct routes to the veins.
(C) increased blood in capillary side channels.
(D) edema in inflamed tissues.
(E) invasion of inflamed area by leukocytes.

22. Which of the following statements is TRUE about neutrophils?

(A) They can engulf a particle twice their own size.
(B) They are the most effective leukocytes.
(C) They are the body's first cellular line of defense against infectious agents.
(D) They use enzymes to dissolve bacteria.
(E) Eosinophils are more efficient than neutrophils in phagocytosis.

23. During phagocytosis by a neutrophil, the particle is digested in

(A) the outer wall of the cell membrane.
(B) lysosomes.
(C) the pseudopodia.
(D) local capillaries.
(E) the cellular cytoplasm.

24. After the onset of inflammation, the number of neutrophils in the blood can reach as high as

(A) 7,000 cells/mm^3.
(B) 18,000 cells/mm^3.
(C) 30,000 cells/mm^3.
(D) 75,000 cells/mm^3.
(E) 8,000 cells/mm^3.

25. The body's isolation of an inflamed area is traceable to

(A) glucose and urea diffusing out of blood vessels.
(B) crystallization around the inflamed tissues.
(C) increased leakage of proteins into interstitial spaces.
(D) clotting in local blood vessels.
(E) increased concentration of K^+ ions intracellularly.

26. Enzymes, necrotic products, bacterial toxins, and chemicals cause all of the following EXCEPT

(A) change in the permeability of the capillaries.
(B) retention of neutrophils and monocytes within the circulatory system.
(C) neutrophils and monocytes to stick to the capillaries' endothelial cells.
(D) damage to the capillary walls.
(E) margination.

27. It is now known that *tumor* is most directly caused by

(A) invasion by eosinophils.
(B) certain chemical substances.
(C) dilation of blood vessels.
(D) extensive swelling that stretches tissue over inflamed areas.
(E) the buildup of fluid leaking from blood vessels to damaged tissue.

GO ON TO THE NEXT PAGE

28. All of the following are characteristics of leukocytosis-inducing factor EXCEPT

    (A) it causes an increase in the number of neutrophils.
    (B) it is stored in the bone marrow.
    (C) it activates neutrophils stored in marrow tissue.
    (D) it is ultimately transported to the bone marrow.
    (E) it is released initially from inflamed tissue.

29. Which of the following was not considered one of the cardinal signs of inflammation according to Celcus?

    (A) *Tumor*
    (B) *Calor*
    (C) Cancer
    (D) *Rubor*
    (E) *Dolor*

30. One of the primary functions of eosinophils is

    (A) to carry out chemotaxis on other foreign cells.
    (B) to mark cells that contain foreign antigens so neutrophils can carry out phagocytosis on these cells at a later point.
    (C) to lyse cells containing foreign antigens on their surface.
    (D) to carry out phagocytosis on any foreign bacteria.
    (E) to defend against chemical agents that cause vascular and tissue reactions during an allergic response.

31. The author of this passage would MOST likely agree with which of the following statements?

    (A) The mechanism by which humans respond to tissue injury is unique to them.
    (B) Little progress has been made in elucidating the mechanisms underlying the symptoms associated with inflammation.
    (C) Most of the cardinal signs of inflammation as first described by Celcus are now better understood, since they can be explained by underlying vascular and cellular events.
    (D) To completely understand the vascular and cellular events associated with inflammation, a large amount of further research is needed.
    (E) Inflammation is maladaptive response that is widespread in the animal kingdom.

32. It can be inferred from the passage that macrophages

    (A) develop from monocytes.
    (B) are generated only when tissue is inflamed.
    (C) include neutrophils, basophils, and eosinophils.
    (D) are responsible for the process of margination.
    (E) constitute about 30 percent of circulating leukocytes.

33. Which of the following is NOT a step in the process of phagocytosis by neutrophils?

    (A) Release of proteolytic enzymes
    (B) Projection of pseudopodia
    (C) Formation of vesicle in cytoplasm
    (D) Movement toward inflamed tissue via chemotaxis
    (E) Invagination of particle-containing chamber

GO ON TO THE NEXT PAGE

Lesch-Nyhan syndrome (LNS) was first described 32 years ago by Lesch and Nyhan. Lesch-Nyhan syndrome appears to be distributed evenly among different geographic locations and occurs in approximately 1 in every 380,000 births. The disease is characterized by hypoxanthine-guanine phosphoribosyltransferase (HPRT) deficiency. The syndrome is a neurologic disorder characterized by cerebral palsy manifested in the form of bilateral involuntary movements preceded by generalized hypotonia and delayed motor development, spasticity, and compulsive self-mutilation, mainly in the form of biting away lips and the ends of fingers. There has been some debate over whether these children are mentally retarded. Nyhan originally wrote that "a severe degree of mental retardation is one of the cardinal features of the disease." However, he and others since 1977 have observed that many patients with LNS appear more intelligent than test scores indicate. The severe disabilities combined with self-abusive tendencies and the need for physical restraints complicate the testing process. In a survey study done with 42 patients, Anderson et al. concluded that "most individuals with Lesch-Nyhan syndrome are not mentally retarded." In 1995, Matthews et al. performed the first systematic study to assess the cognitive functioning of Lesch-Nyhan patients. On the Stanford Binet Intelligence Scale, scores in each of the four domains assessed by this battery, as well as the general composite score, ranged from moderately mentally retarded to low average intelligence. Areas of weakness included attention, the manipulation of complex visual images, the understanding of complex or lengthy speech, mathematical ability, and multistep reasoning.

At birth, children with LNS appear normal. The first indication that something is wrong may be the passage of brown-red/orange color sand in the diaper and extreme irritability of the infant. Until six to eight months of age, gross motor milestones may be reached appropriately. Between eight and 24 months of age, however, choreoathetosis develops and a loss of early milestones is seen. At first the infants are hypotonic, but later they develop hypertonia and hyperreflexia. Pyramidal symptoms consisting of increased deep tendon reflexes, a sustained ankle clonus, scissoring of the lower extremities, and extensor plantar responses are usually present by one year of age. By four years of age, many of the children are beginning to exhibit the classic manifestation of LNS: self-mutilation. By eight to ten years of age, almost all children exhibit self-injurious behavior and demonstrate the neurologic manifestations of the disorder, including spasticity, choreoathetosis, opisthotonos, and facial dystonia. The development of communication is hindered by poor articulation due to pseudobulbar palsy and obstructed airflow. However, most affected children appear to comprehend quite well. The motor and physical development of affected children is grossly impaired with subnormal height and weight. Severely affected children are never able to walk. The life span of patients is usually less than 20 years. Patients usually die by the third decade from infection or renal failure secondary to crystal nephropathy due to decrease in lymphocyte and IgG levels.

A compulsive aggressiveness and self-mutilation, usually beginning by three years of age, are the most variable features of Lesch-Nyhan disease. These children are capable of feeling pain and would in most cases prefer to be restrained so they are unable to hurt themselves. Behavioral abnormalities can be highly variable.

In 1994, a study was performed on 40 male patients with Lesch-Nyhan, ranging in age from 2 to 32 years. Twenty-six different types of self-injury were reported by the parents. Biting some part of the body was the most common type of self-injury, followed by throwing an arm, leg, or head out as they were wheeled through a doorway. In addition, aggression against others, both physical and verbal, was as common as self-injury. There was considerable intra-individual fluctuation in the severity of the self-injurious behavior. All patients had episodes ranging from a few days to a few weeks when the self-injury was much worse than at other times. These periods of high self-injury were related to stressful physical and

GO ON TO THE NEXT PAGE

emotional events. When the patients were calm, enjoying themselves, and free from illness or pain, the tendency to self-injure was low. In addition, it was found that in general, the patient had control over self-injury and when/how restraints should be used. Most patients wanted to be restrained most of the time and were happiest when restrained in a way that made self-injury impossible. However, during certain activities or during low-stress periods, they requested that the restraints be removed. There was a correlation between the severity of self-injury and the age when a physical problem was first noticed by the parents. The earlier the physical problem, the worse the self-injury eventually became.

Aggressive behavior against others is also included in the behavior of these children. This can be in the form of hitting, spitting, or kicking. Verbal aggression is also present in some cases occurs. Although such behavior may be expected to alienate others, these children are actually very charming and responsive, being fully aware and sensitive to their environment. They have a good sense of humor and smile and laugh easily. In some cases, their personality attributes make them seem more intelligent than actually indicated by intelligence tests.

The disease is interesting in that an exact metabolic error leads to a complex set of clinical manifestations, and in addition, despite all the behavioral and neurologic abnormalities, autopsies on these patients have shown no anatomical abnormalities in the brain. However, a defect of neurotransmitter function has been found with a decrease of all functional aspects of dopamine-neuron terminals when compared to control values in the striatum. There is also a dopamine deficit in the mouse model.

Prior to 1996, the strongest support for a dopaminergic dysfunction was from the postmortem findings of a deficit in dopamine, homovanillic acid, and dopa decarboxylase in the basal ganglia of three patients with Lesch-Nyhan disease. However, in a later study by Ernst et al., the brain was able to be visualized, and dopa decarboxylase activity was able to be measured, using the tracer 6-fluorodopa F 18, the precursor of dopamine, in conjunction with positron-emission tomography to measure presynaptic accumulation of fluorodopa F 18 tracer in the dopaminergic regions of the brain. The study population consisted of 15 healthy subjects and 12 male patients with Lesch-Nyhan disease. The fluorodopa F 18 ratio was significantly lower in the putamen (31 percent of control), caudate nucleus (39 percent), frontal cortex (44 percent), and ventral tegmental complex (substancia nigra and ventral tegmentum, 57 percent) in the patients with Lesch-Nyhan disease than in the controls. Uptake of the tracer was abnormally low even in the youngest patients tested, with Lesch-Nyhan subjects having values 31 to 57 percent of those in normal subjects; and there was no overlap between the two groups. The conclusion was made that patients with Lesch-Nyhan disease have abnormally few dopaminergic nerve terminals and cell bodies. The abnormality involves all dopaminergic pathways and is not restricted to the basal ganglia. These dopaminergic deficits are pervasive and appear to be developmental in origin, which suggests that they may contribute to the characteristic neuropsychiatric manifestations of the disease.

Lesch-Nyhan is a rare X-linked recessive disorder of purine synthesis. The primary abnormality is found in a structural gene on the X chromosome coding for the synthesis of the enzyme hypoxanthine-guanine phosphoribosyltransferase (HPRT), which is virtually absent in this disorder. Patients show a striking degree of phenotypic and genotypic variation, with a prevalence of single DNA base substitutions.

The enzyme is composed of four identical subunits, each containing 217 amino acids, not counting the N-terminal methionine with a molecular mass of 24.47 kDa. The enzyme has several substrates: magnesium phosphoribosylpyrophosphate (PRPP), hypoxanthine, and guanine. HPRT is encoded by a single copy of an X-linked gene composed of nine exons spanning about 44 kb of DNA

GO ON TO THE NEXT PAGE

in position Xq26-27. Several mutations have been identified in the gene in patients with Lesch-Nyhan disease. These mutations result in virtually a complete loss of function of the enzyme HPRT, which normally catalyzes the conversion of hypoxanthine and guanine to their respective nucleotides, inosinic acid and guanylic acid. These purine nucleotides are the building blocks of DNA and RNA and are thus essential for the normal activity of the cell.

The enzyme HPRT is normally expressed in all cells of the body, with the highest activity found in cells of the basal ganglia and testes. If the basal ganglia is damaged, problems with movement can occur, and failure of sexual maturation and atrophic testes can result from problems in the testes. In some patients, HPRT activity is absent in all cells, and in others, the HPRT activity in dialyzed erythrocyte lysates may range from less than 0.01 to 10 percent or 20 percent of the normal. In addition to the decrease in activity of HPRT in patients with a severe deficiency, there is also an increase in the activity of adenine phosphoribosyltransferase in erythrocytes but not fibroblasts, which convert adenine to its nucleotide. HPRT activity in fibroblasts of affected children is higher than is found in their erythrocytes with values of around 1 to 3 percent of the activity found in normal fibroblasts. The amount of residual activity in fibroblasts correlates inversely with the severity of clinical symptoms.

HPRT and its companion, adenine phosphoribosyltransferase, reuse preformed purine bases that result from cell turnover and metabolism through a salvage pathway. If HPRT and this salvage pathway are missing, PRPP synthetase activity increases, and PRPP accumulates within the cell, giving rise to accelerated purine production de novo, which results in overproduction of uric acid, which leads to increased blood concentrations of uric acid (hyperuricemia), increased amounts of uric acid in the urine (3–4 times that of normal individuals), tophaceous gouty arthritis, urinary tract calculi, and urate nephropathy (disease of the kidney).

34. Carrying out intelligence testing in individuals with Lesch-Nyhan syndrome is difficult because

(A) these individuals frequently refuse to cooperate.
(B) these individuals can act very charming and be very responsive to both others and their environment.
(C) of their inability to speak.
(D) of their tendency to self-injure themselves and because of their disabilities.
(E) of their tendency to be aggressive toward others.

35. In the 1994 study of patients with Lesch-Nyhan syndrome, it was found that

(A) there was little variation in the type of self-mutilation behavior done by these individuals.
(B) self-mutilation behavior fluctuated in severity over time.
(C) environmental events had little influence on the severity of self-abusive behavior.
(D) most patients resisted when restraints were applied.
(E) these patients have an increased pain threshold.

36. All of the following were found to be areas of weakness in individuals with Lesch-Nyhan syndrome according to the Stanford Binet Intelligence Scale EXCEPT

(A) ability to comprehend difficult language.
(B) mathematical skills.
(C) perceptual ability involving basic visual images.
(D) attention span.
(E) multistep reasoning.

GO ON TO THE NEXT PAGE

37. Individuals with Lesch-Nyhan syndrome are often perceived as being more intelligent than they really are. According to the passage, what is the BEST explanation for this?

(A) Individuals with Lesch-Nyhan syndrome are very creative.
(B) Individuals with Lesch-Nyhan syndrome have the ability to devise intricate plans to self-mutilate themselves.
(C) Individuals with Lesch-Nyhan syndrome can carry out planned acts of aggression toward others.
(D) Individuals with Lesch-Nyhan syndrome have a relatively large vocabulary.
(E) Individuals with Lesch-Nyhan syndrome have very likable personality traits.

38. In the Ernst et al. study, dopa decarboxylase activity was studied by

(A) examining basal ganglia of deceased Lesch-Nyhan patients.
(B) measuring the level of dopa decarboxylase in the synapses in the dopaminergic regions of the brain.
(C) measuring the activity of 6-fluorodopa F 15 in dopaminergic regions of the brain.
(D) measuring the presynaptic accumulation of fluorodopa F 18 tracer in dopaminergic regions of the brain.
(E) measuring the postsynaptic buildup of fluorodopa F 18 in dopaminergic regions of the brain.

39. At birth, infants with Lesch-Nyhan syndrome typically display

(A) hypertonia.
(B) hyperreflexia.
(C) hypotonia.
(D) clinodactyly.
(E) hyperactivity.

40. Which of the following are examples of purine nucleotides?

I. hypoxanthine
II. guanine
III. inosinic acid
IV. guanylic acid

(A) I and II only
(B) III and IV only
(C) All of the above
(D) I and III only
(E) II and IV only

41. In severely affected patients with Lesch-Nyhan syndrome, which of the following is TRUE?

(A) They have a decrease in activity of adenine phosphoribosyltransferase.
(B) They have an increase in activity of HPRT.
(C) They have an increase in activity of adenine phosphoribosyltransferase only in erythrocytes.
(D) They have an increase in activity of adenine phosphoribosyltransferase only in fibroblasts.
(E) Activity of HPRT is decreased uniformly in all cells.

42. Children with Lesch-Nyhan syndrome typically begin to engage in self-mutilating behavior

(A) before the age of 2.
(B) around the ages of 3 and 4.
(C) around the ages of 4 and 5.
(D) around the ages of 6 and 7.
(E) between the ages of 8 and10.

43. What type of inheritance pattern is found in Lesch-Nyhan syndrome?

(A) Mitochondrial inheritance
(B) Autosomal recessive
(C) Autosomal dominant
(D) X-linked dominant
(E) X-linked recessive

GO ON TO THE NEXT PAGE

44. All of the following were conclusions reached as a result of the Ernst et al. study EXCEPT

(A) dopaminergic deficits may contribute to the neuropsychiatric characteristics of Lesch-Nyhan disease.

(B) dopaminergic deficits appear to be developmental in origin.

(C) regions affected in this disorder include only the putamen and caudate nucleus.

(D) individuals with Lesch-Nyhan syndrome have only a small number of dopaminergic nerve terminals and cell bodies.

(E) all dopaminergic pathways are involved in Lesch-Nyhan syndrome.

45. Children affected with Lesch-Nyhan syndrome typically display all of the following symptoms EXCEPT

(A) poor communication skills.

(B) poor ability to comprehend speech.

(C) below average height and weight.

(D) difficulty with walking.

(E) shortened life span.

46. What is the most common type of mutation found in individuals with Lesch-Nyhan syndrome?

(A) A single base substitution

(B) A deletion

(C) An insertion

(D) A frameshift mutation

(E) An inversion

47. Overproduction of uric acid in patients with Lesch-Nyhan syndrome results from

(A) decreased de novo production of inosinic acid and guanylic acid.

(B) the conversion of hypoxanthine and guanine into inosinic acid by HPRT.

(C) accumulation of HPRT in the cells.

(D) decreased activity of PRPP.

(E) increased activity of magnesium phosphoribosylpyrophosphate synthetase.

48. Pyramidal symptoms include all of the following EXCEPT

(A) scissoring of lower extremities.

(B) extensor plantar responses.

(C) increased deep tendon reflexes.

(D) dysmorphic facial features.

(E) sustained ankle clonus.

49. Which of the following is NOT mentioned as an example of aggressive behavior of children with LNS?

(A) Projectile vomiting

(B) Hitting

(C) Verbal abuse

(D) Lip biting

(E) Kicking

50. The salvage pathway mentioned in the passage

(A) increases PRPP synthetase activity.

(B) allows preformed purine bases to be reused.

(C) accelerates de novo purine production.

(D) increases blood concentration of uric acid.

(E) All of the above

IF YOU FINISH BEFORE TIME IS CALLED, YOU MAY CHECK YOUR WORK ON THIS SECTION ONLY. DO NOT TURN TO ANY OTHER SECTION IN THE TEST. **STOP**

PHYSICS

40 questions – 50 minutes

Directions: Choose the best answer for each question from the five choices provided.

The values for the physical constants below are to be used as needed:

Gravitational acceleration at the surface of the Earth: $g = 10\ m/s^2$

Speed of light in a vacuum: $c = 3 \times 10^8\ m/s$

Charge of an electron: $e = 2.0 \times 10^{-19}$ Coulomb

1. Blocks A and B below are of equal mass and are released from rest down the frictionless inclines shown. What is the ratio of the velocity of block A to the velocity of block B at the bottom of the incline?

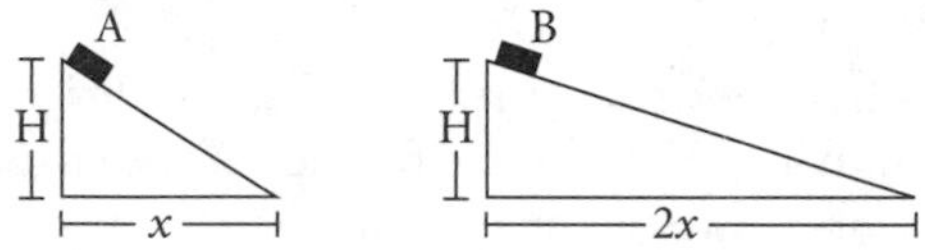

(A) 1:1
(B) $\sqrt{2}$:1
(C) $\sqrt{3}$:1
(D) 2:1
(E) 4:1

2. An air bubble in a liquid is rising to the surface with a constant velocity. If a net downward force is placed on the air bubble, after reaching a stop it will

(A) travel downward with increasing velocity.
(B) travel downward with constant velocity.
(C) rise to the surface with increasing velocity.
(D) remain stationary in the liquid.
(E) None of the above

3. A bullet is fired into the air with initial velocity V_0. Given V_0 and the gravitational acceleration g, what additional information is needed to determine the horizontal distance covered by the bullet at the instant it reaches its maximum height?

(A) Mass
(B) Time to reach the maximum height
(C) Maximum height
(D) Momentum
(E) No additional information is needed.

4. Three blocks are connected with springs of equal spring constant on a frictionless surface. A force of 8 lb pushes on block A, and a force of 3 lb pulls on block C. If the masses of blocks A, B, and C are m_A, m_B, and m_C, respectively, what is the acceleration of block B?

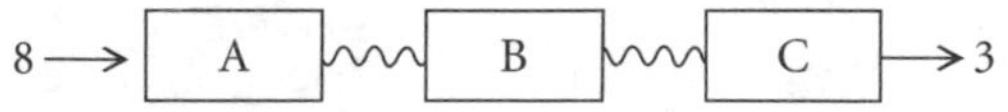

(A) $0\ ft/s^2$
(B) $\frac{11}{(m_A + m_B + m_C)}\ ft/s^2$
(C) $\frac{5}{(m_A + m_B + m_C)}\ ft/s^2$
(D) $\frac{5}{m_B}\ ft/s^2$
(E) $\frac{11}{m_B}\ ft/s^2$

GO ON TO THE NEXT PAGE

5. If the displacement from the center of oscillation of a vibrating spring is plotted against time, what sort of graph is obtained?

(A) Hyperbolic
(B) Parabolic
(C) Linear
(D) Exponential
(E) Sinusoidal

6. Two objects, A and B, are traveling with equal kinetic energies. If the velocity of A is tripled, the ratio of the kinetic energy of A to that of B will be

(A) 1:3
(B) 3:1
(C) 1:9
(D) 9:1
(E) Cannot be determined from the information given.

7. The mechanical energy of a body is defined as

(A) the mechanical force acting on the body for a given distance.
(B) the difference between the kinetic and potential energies of the body.
(C) the sum of the kinetic and potential energies of the body.
(D) the product of the mass and the velocity of the object.
(E) the product of the coefficient of friction and the weight of the body.

8. A go-cart is placed on top of a frictionless circular track and starts down from rest. When the velocity of the cart is 8 ft/s, what is the vertical distance of the cart from the point at which it started its descent? ($g = 32$ ft/s^2 in British units)

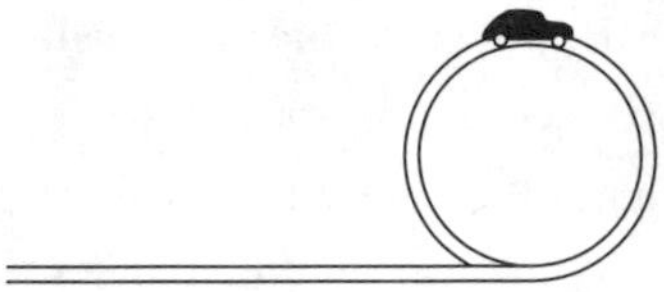

(A) 0.25 ft
(B) 1 ft
(C) 2 ft
(D) 4 ft
(E) Cannot be determined from the information given.

9. A 4-horsepower engine lifts 200 lb to a height of 11 ft in 4 s. What is the efficiency of the engine? (A horsepower is equal to 500 ft·lb/s.)

(A) 12.5%
(B) 25%
(C) 50%
(D) 75%
(E) 100%

10. The pendulum has its greatest velocity at point

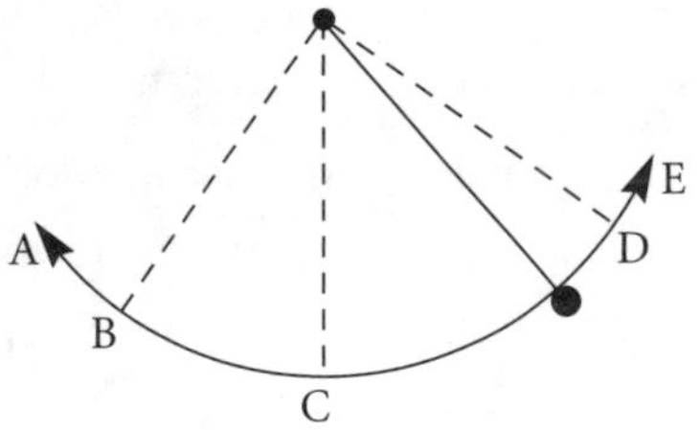

(A) A
(B) B
(C) C
(D) D
(E) E

GO ON TO THE NEXT PAGE

Questions 11–13 refer to the following scenario:

A car is traveling at 50 mph on a level road when the driver steps on the brake and holds it down so that the brake exerts a constant force.

11. The kinetic energy of the car

    (A) decreases linearly with time.
    (B) decreases nonlinearly with time.
    (C) remains the same with time.
    (D) increases linearly with time.
    (E) increases nonlinearly with time.

12. The momentum of the car

    (A) decreases linearly with time.
    (B) decreases nonlinearly with time.
    (C) remains the same with time.
    (D) increases linearly with time.
    (E) increases nonlinearly with time.

13. The temperature of the brake shoes

    (A) decreases linearly with time.
    (B) decreases nonlinearly with time.
    (C) remains the same with time.
    (D) increases linearly with time.
    (E) increases nonlinearly with time.

14. Two objects have the same mass and velocity. For which of the following do they also have the same value?

    (A) Gravitational potential
    (B) Momentum
    (C) Density
    (D) Acceleration
    (E) Radius

15. A rocket descends from an altitude 32,000 miles above the Earth's surface to an altitude of 5,000 miles. Assuming that the Earth has a radius of 4,000 miles and a mass of 6×10^{24} kg, the percent increase in the weight of a man in the rocket is

    (A) 100%.
    (B) 200%.
    (C) 400%.
    (D) 1,500%.
    (E) 1,600%.

16. Two objects with equal mass are released from the same height. One of the objects falls freely whereas the other slides down an inclined plane. Neglecting the effects of air resistance and friction, the sliding body will

    (A) reach the ground sooner.
    (B) reach the ground at the same time as the other object.
    (C) strike the ground with a lower speed.
    (D) have a lower kinetic energy at the bottom.
    (E) have the same speed as the free-falling body at any given height.

17. When $^{238}_{92}U$ radioactively decays to $^{234}_{92}U$, it undergoes three distinct decays with the intermediates $^{234}_{91}Pa$ and $^{234}_{90}Th$, but not necessarily in that order. In what sequence do these decays occur?

    (A) β, α, β
    (B) β, β, α
    (C) α, β, β
    (D) α, α, β
    (E) Any of the above

GO ON TO THE NEXT PAGE

18. Light is an electromagnetic wave, while sound is a mechanical wave. This difference is quite apparent in which of the following pairs of characteristics of these waves?

    (A) Sound waves contain energy, while light waves do not.
    (B) The speed of sound equals the wavelength times the frequency, while the speed of light is a constant at 3×10^{10} m/sec.
    (C) Sound requires medium through which to travel, while light can travel in a pure vacuum.
    (D) Light travels in packets of energy, while sound travels by the transfer of energy between molecules.
    (E) Two of the above

19. A bubble of air is released from an air tank that rests at the bottom of a lake 30 meters deep. The bubble is observed to increase in volume from 0.25 L to 1.0 L upon reaching the surface. If the temperature at the surface and bottom are equal, what is the average density of the lake water?

    (1 atm = 1.01×10^5 Pa)

    (A) 0.1 g/cm^3
    (B) 1,000 kg/m^3
    (C) 1,000 kg/L
    (D) 10 g/mL

20. When an electron falls from n = 3 to n = 2 in a hydrogen atom, what is the value of the energy released, given that A is the energy needed to remove an electron from the ground state of a hydrogen atom to an infinite distance from the atom?

    (A) 0.14A
    (B) 0.17A
    (C) 1.00A
    (D) 5.00A
    (E) 7.00A

21. A Boeing 737 aircraft has a mass of 150,000 kg and a cruising velocity of 720 km/hr. Its engines can create a total thrust of 200,000 N. If air resistance, change in altitude, and fuel consumption can be ignored, how long does it take for the plane to reach its cruising velocity starting from rest?

    (A) 100 s
    (B) 150 s
    (C) 540 s
    (D) 1,944 s
    (E) 3,000 s

22. If the pK_a of a weak acid is 5, the pH will be 6

    (A) when the concentration of dissociated acid is one-tenth the concentration of undissociated acid.
    (B) when half the acid is dissociated.
    (C) when the concentration of dissociated acid is ten times the concentration of undissociated acid.
    (D) only after a base has been added.
    (E) None of the above

23. A certain metal plate is completely illuminated by a monochromatic light source. Which of the following would increase the number of electrons ejected from the surface of the metal?

    I. Increasing the intensity of the light source
    II. Increasing the frequency of the light source
    III. Increasing the surface area of the metal plate

    (A) I only
    (B) I and II only
    (C) I and III only
    (D) II and III only
    (E) I, II, and III

GO ON TO THE NEXT PAGE

24. A ball is dropped from a height h meters above the surface of a planet and takes 10 s to fall to the planet's surface. If the planet's mass were doubled while its radius remained unchanged, how long would it now take the ball to fall to the surface from the same height?

 (A) $10\sqrt{2}$ seconds
 (B) 20 seconds
 (C) 5 seconds
 (D) $5\sqrt{2}$ seconds
 (E) 10 seconds

25. Two children of equal weight W are sitting on opposite ends of a seesaw at equal distances D from the fulcrum. The torques they exert about the fulcrum are

 (A) equal in magnitude and acting in the same direction.
 (B) equal in magnitude and acting in opposite directions.
 (C) of uncertain relative magnitude and acting in the same direction.
 (D) of uncertain relative magnitude and acting in opposite directions.
 (E) Cannot be determined from the information given.

26. A very energetic monkey with a mass of 45 kg is climbing up a massless rope that is capable of holding a maximum weight of 530 Newtons. Can the monkey climb with an acceleration of 2.5 m/s^2 without the rope snapping?

 ($g = 9.8\ m/s^2$)

 (A) Yes.
 (B) No.
 (C) It will snap but only when the monkey reaches a velocity of 2.5 m/s.
 (D) It will snap but only when the monkey reaches a velocity of 9.8 m/s.
 (E) Cannot be determined from the information given.

27. The ability of rockets to accelerate in the approximate vacuum of interstellar space is a demonstration of

 (A) conservation of energy.
 (B) conservation of momentum.
 (C) conservation of angular momentum.
 (D) Newton's first law.
 (E) None of the above

28. The acceleration of a certain 10-kg object is given by the equation $a = (0.34B)t^{-1/2} + A$, where A and B are positive constants. How does the acceleration vary with time?

 (A) It increases linearly.
 (B) It increases nonlinearly.
 (C) It decreases linearly.
 (D) It decreases nonlinearly.
 (E) It is constant with time.

Questions 29 and 30 refer to the following scenario:

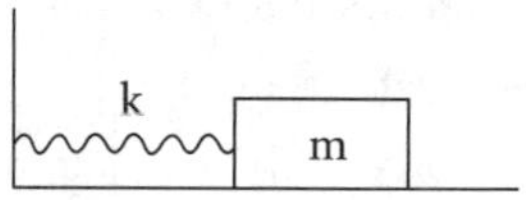

An oscillating spring-mass system is shown above. The mass glides along a horizontal frictionless surface. The spring reaches a maximum length of 4 m. When completely relaxed, the spring is 2 m long. The mass of the block is 10 kg, and the spring constant k is 5 N/m.

29. When the spring is stretched to a length of 3 m

 (A) the system's potential energy is greater than its kinetic energy.
 (B) the system's kinetic energy is greater than its potential energy.
 (C) the system's kinetic energy and potential energy are both equal to zero.
 (D) the system's kinetic energy and potential energy are both negative.
 (E) the relationship between the system's potential energy and its kinetic energy cannot be determined.

GO ON TO THE NEXT PAGE

30. The maximum velocity reached by the block in the course of its oscillations is

(A) $\frac{1}{2}$ m/s.

(B) $\frac{\sqrt{2}}{2}$ m/s.

(C) 1 m/s.

(D) $\sqrt{2}$ m/s.

(E) 2 m/s.

31. Objects A and B are on a horizontal surface. Object A exerts a force on object B, and, in accordance with the laws of motion, generates a reaction force. Motion occurs despite the fact that these two forces are equal in magnitude and opposite in direction

(A) because of the friction between the two objects.

(B) because of the friction between object A and the surface.

(C) if the mass of A is greater than the mass of B.

(D) if the mass of B is greater than the mass of A.

(E) because the action force and the reaction force act on different objects.

32. In the equation $V = \frac{Fd}{\eta x}$, η is the viscosity, F is the force, V is the velocity, and d is the distance. What must x be to make the equation correct? (Unit of viscosity = $N{\cdot}s/m^2$)

(A) Area

(B) Acceleration

(C) Pressure

(D) Mass

(E) None of the above

33. A train starts from rest and, accelerating uniformly, travels a distance D in a time T. How long, in terms of T, does the train take to travel the first half of this distance?

(A) $T - \frac{T}{\sqrt{2}}$

(B) $\frac{T}{\sqrt{2}}$

(C) $\frac{T}{2}$

(D) $\frac{T}{\sqrt{2}} - \frac{T}{2}$

(E) $\frac{T}{3}$

34. An automobile is moving at speed v along a straight and horizontal road. The driver applies the brakes, causing a constant deceleration until the car comes to rest over a distance d, called the stopping distance. If the initial speed is doubled while the deceleration remains the same, what would be the new stopping distance?

(A) $\frac{d}{4}$

(B) $\frac{d}{2}$

(C) d

(D) 2d

(E) 4d

35. A person weighs 800 N when standing on the surface of the Earth. What is the magnitude of the force exerted by this person on the Earth?

(A) 0 N

(B) Nonzero but essentially negligible

(C) 800 g/N

(D) 800 N

(E) –800 N

GO ON TO THE NEXT PAGE

36. An elevator has a downward acceleration of 1 m/s^2. A person, having a weight of 800 N as measured by a scale at rest on the ground, steps on a scale in the elevator. What does the scale read?

    (A) 0 N
    (B) Approximately 80 N
    (C) Between 80 N and 800 N
    (D) 800 N
    (E) Greater than 800 N

37. An object of mass m experiences a gravitational force of 100 N at the surface of the Earth. What is the gravitational force on this same object if the object is at a distance of one Earth radius above the surface?

    (A) 25 N
    (B) 50 N
    (C) 100 N
    (D) 200 N
    (E) 400 N

38. Which of the following quantities can be expressed dimensionally as $M{\cdot}L^2/T^2$, where M is mass, L is length, and T is time?

    I. Torque
    II. Work
    III. Energy

    (A) I only
    (B) I and II only
    (C) II and III only
    (D) III only
    (E) I, II, and III

Questions 39 and 40 refer to the following:

A 10-kg mass on a horizontal tabletop is being swung circularly in a counterclockwise direction (see diagram) and is being slowed down by the frictional force. The coefficient of friction is 0.2.

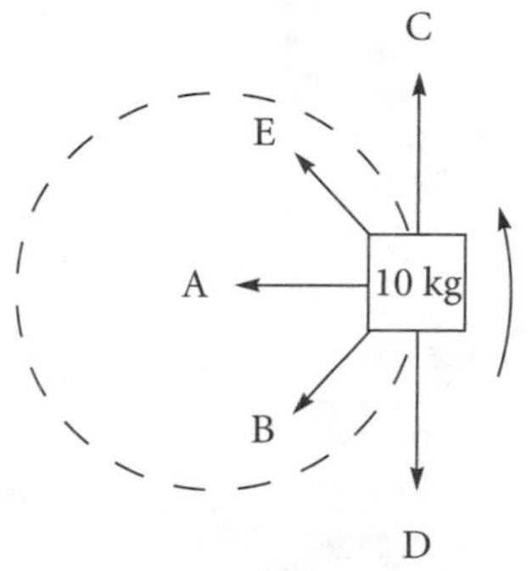

39. The net force on the mass, when it lies in the position shown, points toward

    (A) A.
    (B) B.
    (C) C.
    (D) D.
    (E) E.

40. To keep the mass from slowing down, energy must be added to the system. How great a power input would be required to maintain a speed of 2 m/s?

    (A) 4 W
    (B) 200 W
    (C) 200 J
    (D) 40 W
    (E) 40 J

IF YOU FINISH BEFORE TIME IS CALLED, YOU MAY CHECK YOUR WORK ON THIS SECTION ONLY. DO NOT TURN TO ANY OTHER SECTION IN THE TEST. STOP

QUANTITATIVE REASONING

50 questions—45 minutes

Directions: Choose the best answer to each question from the five choices provided.

1. The ratio of boys to girls in a class is 5:3. If there are 120 students, how many girls are there?

   (A) 75
   (B) 72
   (C) 45
   (D) 48
   (E) 200

2. What percent of $\sqrt{0.005}$ is $\sqrt{2}$?

   (A) 0.05%
   (B) 5%
   (C) 20%
   (D) 200%
   (E) 2,000%

3. An architect draws a blueprint so that $3\frac{1}{8}$ inches represent 125 feet. How many square inches are used to represent the area of a room 20 feet by 20 feet?

   (A) $\frac{1}{4}$
   (B) $\frac{5}{64}$
   (C) $\frac{1}{2}$
   (D) $\frac{2}{5}$
   (E) $\frac{625}{64}$

4. The Joneses' living room floor measures 10 ft. × 15 ft. If one carpeting firm charges $0.80 per square foot and another $7.50 per square yard, how much will the Joneses save by hiring the cheaper firm to do the job?

   (A) $5
   (B) $10
   (C) $12
   (D) $120
   (E) $125

5. A car travels at the rate of 60 miles per hour. Find the car's rate in feet per second. (5,280 feet = 1 mile)

   (A) 8
   (B) 10
   (C) 30
   (D) 60
   (E) 88

6. Given the information shown, find angle *PQT*.

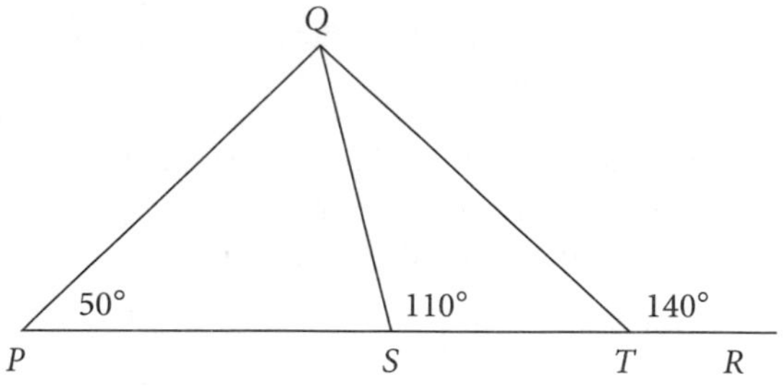

   (A) 50°
   (B) 80°
   (C) 90°
   (D) 110°
   (E) 140°

GO ON TO THE NEXT PAGE

7. What is the length, in feet, of a ladder that is 45 feet from the foot of a building and reaches up 24 feet along the wall of the building?

(A) 24
(B) 38
(C) 45
(D) 51
(E) 69

8. Given three externally tangent circles as shown, if the diameters of the circles are d, d_1, and d_2, respectively, what is the perimeter of the triangle formed by joining their centers?

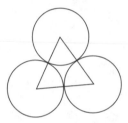

(A) $\frac{1}{2}(d + d_1 + d_2)$
(B) $\frac{1}{3}(d + d_1 + d_2)$
(C) $2(d + d_1 + d_2)$
(D) $d + d_1 + d_2$
(E) $3d$

9. Six people went shopping. Five spent $16 each, and the sixth spent $5 more than the average of all six. How much did the last person spend?

(A) $20
(B) $21
(C) $22
(D) $23
(E) $24

10. An express train leaves a station 3 hours after a freight train. The express train travels at 60 miles per hour and after 2 hours finds that it is still 20 miles behind the freight train. At what rate is the freight train traveling?

(A) 20 mph
(B) 24 mph
(C) 28 mph
(D) 30 mph
(E) 32 mph

11. A motorist travels 50 miles at 20 mph. He returns the same distance at 50 mph. What is his average rate for the entire trip?

(A) $24\frac{2}{7}$
(B) $28\frac{4}{7}$
(C) $29\frac{6}{7}$
(D) 30
(E) $32\frac{2}{7}$

12. Billy walks to school in 3 minutes. The school is 3 blocks from his house, and each block is 528 feet. What is Billy's average speed, in miles per hour? (5,280 feet = 1 mile)

(A) 0.3
(B) 0.6
(C) 3
(D) 5
(E) 6

GO ON TO THE NEXT PAGE

13. A test consists of 60 problems to be done in 1 hour. A student does 30 problems in 20 minutes. How much time can she use for each of the remaining problems?
    (A) $\frac{1}{2}$ min
    (B) $\frac{3}{4}$ min
    (C) $1\frac{1}{4}$ min
    (D) $1\frac{1}{3}$ min
    (E) $1\frac{1}{2}$ min

14. A man bought 8 books at an average price of \$6.00 and 10 books at an average price of \$2.40. Find the average cost of the books.
    (A) \$3.60
    (B) \$4.00
    (C) \$4.20
    (D) \$6.00
    (E) \$7.20

15. Fifteen movie theaters average 600 customers per day. If six are shut down, but the same number of people still attend the movies, what is the new average attendance for the movies that remain open?
    (A) 66
    (B) 100
    (C) 500
    (D) 1,000
    (E) 1,500

16. Solve for x in the equation $\frac{32 - 10\sqrt{5x}}{3} = 4$.
    (A) $\frac{2\sqrt{5}}{5}$
    (B) $\frac{1}{5}$
    (C) $\frac{2}{5}$
    (D) $\frac{\sqrt{2}}{5}$
    (E) $\frac{4}{5}$

17. When the expression $\sqrt{1 + \frac{9}{16}}$ is simplified, which

    of the following is obtained?
    (A) $\frac{5}{8}$
    (B) $\frac{\sqrt{17}}{4}$
    (C) $1\frac{3}{4}$
    (D) $1\frac{1}{4}$
    (E) $\frac{\sqrt{17}}{16}$

18. Put the following in increasing order:
    I. $\frac{\sqrt{2}}{3}$
    II. $\frac{\sqrt{3}}{4}$
    III. $\frac{\sqrt{5}}{5}$

    (A) I, II, III
    (B) I, III, II
    (C) II, I, III
    (D) II, III, I
    (E) III, I, II

19. 15 is 6% of what number?
    (A) 250
    (B) $\frac{9}{10}$
    (C) 25
    (D) 90
    (E) 900

GO ON TO THE NEXT PAGE

20. From the charts below, what percent of the world's coal is produced in Ohio?

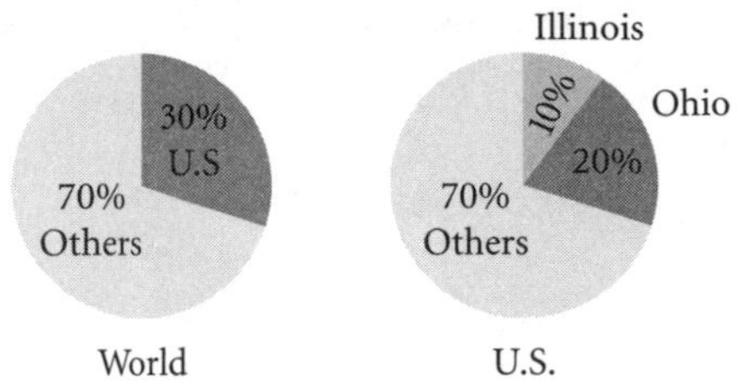

(A) 0.3%
(B) 1.2%
(C) 3.6%
(D) 4%
(E) 36%

21. The circumference of a circle is increased by 20%. Find the percent of increase in the area.

(A) 40%
(B) 44%
(C) 10%
(D) 22%
(E) 400%

22. If the diameter of a cylinder is increased by 20% and the height is decreased by $16\frac{2}{3}\%$, by what percent is the volume changed?

(A) −10%
(B) +10%
(C) +20%
(D) +24%
(E) $+83\frac{1}{3}\%$

23. The numerator of a fraction is doubled, and the denominator is halved. The value of the fraction is

(A) divided by 2.
(B) divided by 4.
(C) multiplied by 2.
(D) multiplied by 4.
(E) unchanged.

24. The length of a rectangle is twice the width. If the perimeter of a square equals the perimeter of the rectangle, what is the ratio of the area of the rectangle to the area of the square?

(A) 1:1
(B) 1:4
(C) 4:1
(D) 2:3
(E) 8:9

25. A railroad must pay a tax of 6% on all revenue exceeding $50,000. How much tax must be paid on $150,000 of revenue?

(A) $6,000
(B) $9,000
(C) $10,000
(D) $12,000
(E) $12,500

26. A picket fence is 60 feet long. Its pickets are $1\frac{1}{2}$ feet apart. If the fence is extended to 80 feet, without adding any pickets, what is the new distance, in feet, between pickets?

(A) $1\frac{1}{8}$
(B) 2
(C) $\frac{8}{9}$
(D) $2\frac{1}{8}$
(E) 3

27. A rectangular swimming pool 24 feet × 16 feet is filled to a height of 1 foot. How high would the same amount of water reach in a pool 20 feet × 8 feet?

(A) $\frac{5}{12}$ ft
(B) $\frac{3}{5}$ ft
(C) $\frac{5}{6}$ ft
(D) $2\frac{2}{5}$ ft
(E) $2\frac{3}{5}$ ft

GO ON TO THE NEXT PAGE

28. $x + y + 3z = 7$; $3x + 6y + 6z = 8$. What is the numerical value of $(y - z)$?

(A) $-\frac{13}{3}$

(B) -6

(C) 13

(D) $\frac{29}{3}$

(E) $-\frac{22}{3}$

29. *A*, *B*, and *C* have 24 marbles between them. *A* has more marbles than *B* and *B* has more marbles than *C*. What is the largest number of marbles that *B* can have?

(A) 8
(B) 9
(C) 10
(D) 11
(E) 12

30. Line ℓ is perpendicular to the line with the equation $y = -\frac{1}{5}x$, and the point $(3, -10)$ is on line ℓ. Which of the following is an equation of line ℓ ?

(A) $y = -\frac{1}{5}x - \frac{47}{5}$

(B) $y = 5x - 25$

(C) $y = 5x$

(D) $y = 5x - 5$

(E) $y = \frac{1}{5}x - \frac{53}{5}$

31. Which of the following is equal to cos 59°?

(A) sin 31°
(B) cos 31°
(C) sin 59°
(D) $\cos\left(\frac{1}{59}\right)^\circ$
(E) $\sin\left(\frac{1}{59}\right)^\circ$

32. Which of the following is true for all values of x such that $0 < x < \frac{\pi}{2}$?

(A) $\sin x = \cos^2 x + 1$

(B) $\tan x = (\sin x)(\cos x)$

(C) $\tan x = \frac{\cos x}{\sin x}$

(D) $\sin^2 x = 1 - \cos^2 x$

(E) $\sin x = \frac{1}{\cos x}$

33. Suppose that $-4 \le x \le 2$ and $3 \le y \le 5$. Which value for x and which value for y in their respective ranges will make $(x^2 - 6)(y + 7)$ its largest possible value?

(A) $x = 2$ and $y = 5$
(B) $x = 2$ and $y = 3$
(C) $x = 1$ and $y = 4$
(D) $x = -4$ and $y = 3$
(E) $x = -4$ and $y = 5$

34. What is the length of side *AB* in equilateral triangle *ABC* if the length of altitude *AD* is 12?

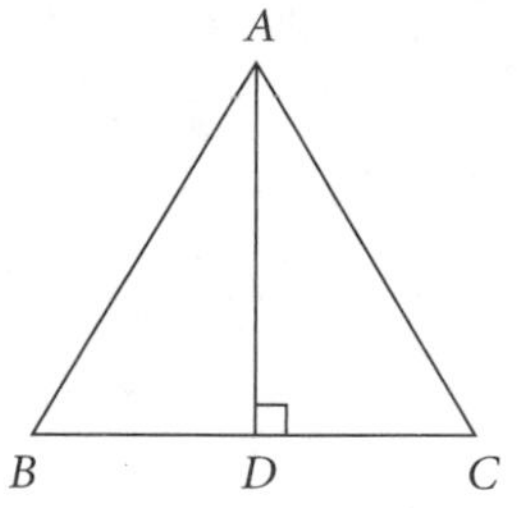

(A) $8\sqrt{3}$
(B) $10\sqrt{2}$
(C) 18
(D) $12\sqrt{3}$
(E) 24

GO ON TO THE NEXT PAGE

35. Evaluate the expression $\frac{6 \times 10^{-4}}{30 \times 10^{5}}$.

(A) 2×10^{-1}
(B) 5×10^{-10}
(C) 2×10^{-10}
(D) 5×10^{-9}
(E) 2×10^{-9}

36. Five students taking an exam have to sit one behind the other. How many different ways can they arrange themselves?

(A) 5
(B) 20
(C) 50
(D) 60
(E) 120

37. There are 5 purple marbles and 6 yellow marbles in a bag. If two balls are drawn at random (one after the other without replacement), what is the probability of selecting two purple marbles?

(A) $\frac{20}{121}$
(B) $\frac{25}{121}$
(C) $\frac{2}{11}$
(D) $\frac{5}{11}$
(E) $\frac{25}{36}$

38. Anne has a total of $34 in nickels, dimes, and quarters. If she has 3 times as many dimes as quarters and 2 times as many nickels as dimes, how many dimes does she have?

(A) 12
(B) 40
(C) 51
(D) 60
(E) 120

39. What is the distance between (–6, –9) and (3, 3)?

(A) $3\sqrt{5}$
(B) 15
(C) 3
(D) $\sqrt{21}$
(E) 21

40. What is the average of 3, 5, 5, 11, and 13?

(A) $7\frac{2}{5}$
(B) 8
(C) $6\frac{2}{5}$
(D) $9\frac{1}{4}$
(E) 5

41. If x, y, and z are all positive and $(0.04)x = 5y = 2z$, then which of the following is TRUE?

(A) $x < y < z$
(B) $x < z < y$
(C) $y < x < z$
(D) $y < z < x$
(E) $z < y < x$

42. The cos 45° is equivalent to

(A) sin 90°.
(B) sin 45°.
(C) tan 90°.
(D) cos 90°.
(E) tan 45°.

43. For how many positive integers x is $\left(\frac{130}{x}\right)$ an integer?

(A) 8
(B) 7
(C) 6
(D) 5
(E) 3

GO ON TO THE NEXT PAGE

44. A wire is cut into three equal parts. The resulting segments are then cut into 4, 6, and 8 parts, respectively. If each of the resulting segments has an integral length, what is the minimum length of the wire?

(A) 24
(B) 36
(C) 48
(D) 54
(E) 72

45. What is the average (arithmetic mean) of n, $n + 1$, $n + 2$, and $n + 3$?

(A) n
(B) $n + 1$
(C) $n + 1.5$
(D) $n + 2$
(E) $n + 6$

46. An alloy of tin and copper has 6 pounds of copper for every 2 pounds of tin. If 200 pounds of the one alloy are made, how many pounds of tin are required?

(A) 25
(B) 50
(C) 100
(D) 125
(E) 150

47. A 25-ounce solution is 20% alcohol. If 50 ounces of water are added to it, what percent of the new solution is alcohol?

(A) 5%
(B) 6.67%
(C) 8.5%
(D) 10%
(E) 20%

48. $(\sqrt{5} - \sqrt{4})(\sqrt{5} + \sqrt{4}) =$

(A) 1
(B) 3
(C) 9
(D) $9 - 4\sqrt{5}$
(E) $9 + 4\sqrt{5}$

49. Which of the following is NOT equal to 0.0675?

(A) 67.5×10^{-3}
(B) 6.75×10^{-2}
(C) 0.675×10^{-1}
(D) 0.00675×10^{2}
(E) 0.0000675×10^{3}

50. If $\frac{2}{(3b)} = 12c$, what is the value of b in terms of c?

(A) $\frac{1}{(36c)}$
(B) $\frac{1}{(18c)}$
(C) $8c$
(D) $18c$
(E) $36c$

IF YOU FINISH BEFORE TIME IS CALLED, YOU MAY CHECK YOUR WORK ON THIS SECTION ONLY. DO NOT TURN TO ANY OTHER SECTION IN THE TEST. STOP

Full-Length Practice Test I: **Answer Key**

Survey of the Natural Sciences

1. A
2. C
3. B
4. C
5. B
6. A
7. C
8. E
9. C
10. D
11. B
12. E
13. B
14. A
15. D
16. A
17. D
18. C
19. B
20. C
21. C
22. B
23. C
24. C
25. A
26. A
27. E
28. A
29. D
30. E
31. C
32. D
33. D
34. D
35. A
36. B
37. D
38. E
39. E
40. D
41. A
42. D
43. E
44. D
45. E
46. E
47. E
48. B
49. E
50. D
51. C
52. D
53. A
54. A
55. B
56. D
57. D
58. C
59. D
60. D
61. B
62. C
63. C
64. B
65. B
66. A
67. E
68. D
69. B
70. B
71. D
72. E
73. A
74. A
75. D
76. D
77. D
78. A
79. B
80. E
81. C
82. E
83. B
84. D
85. E
86. D
87. C
88. A
89. E
90. C
91. E
92. E
93. C
94. A
95. A
96. E
97. B
98. D
99. C
100. D

Reading Comprehension

1. C
2. D
3. D
4. E
5. B
6. E
7. B
8. C
9. A
10. B
11. D
12. E
13. B
14. B
15. A
16. E
17. A
18. D
19. E
20. D
21. C
22. D
23. E
24. B
25. C
26. B
27. E
28. B
29. C
30. E
31. C
32. A
33. D
34. D
35. B
36. D
37. E
38. D
39. C
40. B
41. C
42. B
43. E
44. C
45. B
46. A
47. E
48. D
49. D
50. B

Physics

1. A
2. A
3. E
4. B
5. E
6. D
7. C
8. B
9. B
10. C
11. B
12. A
13. E
14. B
15. D
16. E
17. C
18. E
19. B
20. A
21. B
22. C
23. C
24. D
25. B
26. B
27. B
28. D
29. B
30. D
31. E
32. A
33. B
34. E
35. D
36. C
37. A
38. E
39. B
40. D

Quantitative Reasoning

1. C
2. E
3. A
4. A
5. E
6. C
7. D
8. D
9. C
10. C
11. B
12. E
13. D
14. B
15. D
16. E
17. D
18. D
19. A
20. C
21. B
22. C
23. D
24. E
25. A
26. B
27. D
28. A
29. D
30. B
31. A
32. D
33. E
34. A
35. C
36. E
37. C
38. E
39. B
40. A
41. D
42. B
43. A
44. E
45. C
46. B
47. B
48. A
49. D
50. B

Answers and Explanations

1. A	21. C	41. A	61. B	81. C
2. C	22. B	42. D	62. C	82. E
3. B	23. C	43. E	63. C	83. B
4. C	24. C	44. D	64. B	84. D
5. B	25. A	45. E	65. B	85. E
6. A	26. A	46. E	66. A	86. D
7. C	27. E	47. E	67. E	87. C
8. E	28. A	48. B	68. D	88. A
9. C	29. D	49. E	69. B	89. E
10. D	30. E	50. D	70. B	90. C
11. B	31. C	51. C	71. D	91. E
12. E	32. D	52. D	72. E	92. E
13. B	33. D	53. A	73. A	93. C
14. A	34. D	54. A	74. A	94. A
15. D	35. A	55. B	75. D	95. A
16. A	36. B	56. D	76. D	96. E
17. D	37. D	57. D	77. D	97. B
18. C	38. E	58. C	78. A	98. D
19. B	39. E	59. D	79. B	99. C
20. C	40. D	60. D	80. E	100. D

1. A

The electron transport chain (ETC) is a series of integral proteins that generates ATP via oxidative phosphorylation and occurs in the inner mitochondrial membrane. Choice (B) is incorrect because glycolysis is the oxidative breakdown of glucose into two molecules of pyruvate and it occurs in the cytoplasm. Choice (C) is incorrect because the Krebs cycle occurs in the mitochondrial matrix. The Krebs cycle begins when acetyl-CoA combines with OAA to form citrate. Then a complicated series of reactions follows that results in the release of 2 CO_2 and the regeneration of OAA. Choice (D) is incorrect because fatty acid degradation occurs in microbodies called peroxisomes, which break down fat into smaller molecules to use as fuel. Choice (E) is incorrect because ATP synthesis occurs in the matrix (Krebs cycle), inner mitochondrial membrane (ETC), and in cytoplasm (glycolysis).

2. C

With each round of replication, the original DNA material gets halved. After four rounds of replication, the amount of original DNA will $= \left(\frac{1}{2}\right)^4 = \frac{1}{16} = 6.25\%$.

The original strand of DNA is comprised of two sister strands. After four rounds of replication, you would have 16 strands of DNA comprised of 32 sister strands. The two original sister strands are 6.25% of the 32 sister strands that you have at the end of the replication.

3. B

The prokaryotic cell wall is composed of peptidoglycans, which are polysaccharides cross-linked by short peptide (protein) chains. The cell walls in plants, which are eukaryotes, are not composed of peptidoglycans. Choice (A) is incorrect because photosynthetic granules (grana) are components of the eukaryotic chloroplast. The granules are stacks of thylakoid membranes within the chloroplast. Choice (C) is incorrect because mRNA is not unique to prokaryotes. mRNA (messenger RNA) is found in both prokaryotes and eukaryotes and transports genetic information from the DNA to the ribosome. Choice (D) is incorrect because cell walls made of cellulose are found in plants, which are eukaryotes. Choice (E) is incorrect because linear DNA, bundled on histones and packaged as chromosomes, is only found in eukaryotes. Prokaryotes have circular DNA.

4. C

The statement in choice (C) is false. One molecule of glucose (6-carbon sugar) breaks down into two molecules of pyruvate (pyruvate is a 3-carbon molecule). Hence, this is the choice we are looking for. Choice (A) is a true statement and therefore NOT the correct response: glycolysis occurs in the cytoplasm. Choice (B) is also true. Glycolysis is anaerobic and occurs in both eukaryotes and prokaryotes. In anaerobic conditions or in anaerobic bacteria, it is the first step in fermentation. In eukaryotes, pyruvate is reduced to lactic acid, and in prokaryotes, it is reduced to ethanol. Choice (D) is an accurate statement. In glycolysis, one molecule of glucose is broken down, and 4 ATP are formed. However, due to the initial investment of 2 ATP, the net production of ATP is 2. Also, two molecules of

NAD^+ are reduced to NADH. These molecules will later enter the electron transport chain to produce ATP.

5. B

Adenine and guanine are purines, while cytosine, uracil, and thymine are pyrimidines. Choice (A) is an accurate statement. The basic unit of DNA is a nucleotide that is made up of a phosphate group, a deoxyribose sugar, and a nucleic acid. Choice (C) is also a true statement: DNA strands are antiparallel; that is, one strand has a $5' \rightarrow 3'$ polarity, and its complementary strand has a $3' \rightarrow 5'$ polarity. Choice (D) is correct. Guanine always bonds with cytosine via three hydrogen bonds. Adenine will bond with either thymine or uracil with two hydrogen bonds. Choice (E) is correct. The sugar molecule in DNA is deoxyribose while in RNA it is ribose.

6. A

Carbohydrates have a H:O ratio of 2:1 while fats have a H:O ratio much greater than 2:1, meaning that they have much more hydrogen than oxygen. Choice (B) is incorrect because as implied above, the opposite is true. Choice (C) is incorrect: carbohydrates release 4 kcal/g while fats release 9 kcal/g. Choice (D) is incorrect because lipids do not form polymers. Carbohydrates form polymers known as polysaccharides that are chains of repeating monosaccharide subunits. Choice (E) is incorrect because neither carbohydrates nor lipids contain nitrogen. Proteins and amino acids contain nitrogen.

7. C

Blastulation begins when the morula develops a fluid-filled cavity called the blastocoel, which, by the fourth day of human development, will become a hollow sphere of cells called the blastula. Choice (A) is incorrect because the zygote is the diploid (2N) cell that results from the fusion of two haploid (N) gametes. Choice (B) is incorrect: the morula is the solid ball of cells that results from the early stages of cleavage in an embryo. Choices (D) and (E) are incorrect. The gastrula is the embryonic stage characterized by the presence of epiblast, hypoblast, the blastocoel, and the archenteron. The early gastrula is two-layered; later a third layer, the mesoderm, develops.

8. E

The lysosome is like the stomach of the cell and is characterized as a membrane-bound organelle that stores hydrolytic enzymes. Choice (A) is incorrect because chloroplasts are found only in algae and plant cells. They contain chlorophyll and are the site of photosynthesis. Chloroplasts contain their own DNA, and ribosomes and may have evolved by symbiosis. Choice (B) is incorrect because microbodies are synthetic and catabolic membrane-bound organelles specialized as containers for metabolic reactions. Choice (C) is incorrect because phagosomes are vesicles that are involved in the transport and storage of materials that are ingested by the cell through phagocytosis. Choice (D) is incorrect. Vacuoles are membrane-bound sacs involved in the transport and storage of materials that are ingested, secreted, processed, or digested by the cells. Vacuoles are larger than vesicles and are more likely to be found in plant cells.

9. C

If the frequency of the dominant allele is three times that of the recessive allele, then $p = 3q$. According to Hardy–Weinberg equilibrium, $p + q = 1$ so $3q + q = 1$. Solving for q, we get $4q = 1$; $q = 0.25$ and $p = 0.75$. Again according to Hardy–Weinberg, the frequency of the heterozygotes is equal to $2pq$. Substituting in our values for p and q we have the equation $2(0.75)(0.25)$ which equals 0.375 or 37.5%.

10. D

The endoderm develops into the endothelial linings of the digestive and respiratory tracts; parts of the liver, pancreas, thyroid; and the bladder lining. Choice (A) is incorrect because the lens of the eyes develops from the ectoderm. Choice (B) is incorrect because the gonads are developed from the mesoderm. Choice (C) is incorrect because the nervous system develops from the ectoderm. Choice (E) is incorrect because the connective tissue develops from the mesoderm.

11. B

The allantois is a saclike structure involved in respiration and excretion. It contains numerous blood vessels to transport O_2, CO_2, water, salt, and nitrogenous wastes. Later during development, the vessels enlarge and become the umbilical vessels, which will connect the fetus to the placenta. Choice (A) is incorrect because the chorion lines the inside of the embryo and is a moist membrane that permits gas exchange. Choice (C) is incorrect because the amnion is the membrane that encloses the amniotic fluid. Amniotic fluid provides an aqueous environment that protects the developing embryo from shock. Choice (D) is incorrect because the yolk sac encloses the yolk. Blood vessels in the yolk sac transfer food to the developing embryo. Choice (E) is incorrect because the placenta and the umbilical cord are outgrowths of the four previous membranes. This system allows the fetus to receive oxygen and nutrients while removing carbon dioxide and metabolic wastes.

12. E

Platelets are anucleate cell fragments involved in clot formation. Choice (A), erythrocytes, are the oxygen-carrying components of the blood. Choice (B), macrophages, carry out phagocytosis of foreign particles and bacteria, digest them, and present the processed fragments on their cell surface. Choices (C) and (D) are both components of the immune system involved in cell-mediated and humoral (antibody-mediated) immunity, respectively.

13. B

In ten turns of the Calvin cycle, 20 PGAL are formed from 6 carbon dioxide and 6 RBP molecules.

14. A

Sulfur is sometimes found in proteins but never in nucleic acids. The famous Hershey-Chase experiment took advantage of this fact to determine whether proteins or nucleic acids carried the genetic information of the cell. The other choices are incorrect: Nucleic acids contain the elements C, H, O, N, and P. They are polymers of subunits called nucleotides, and they code all the information needed by an organism to produce proteins and replicate.

15. D

In plants, spores are haploid and generate into the haploid gametophyte generation. Therefore, since they have 18 chromosomes, that would be the haploid number. The diploid number would be 36.

16. A

Any male born will receive an X chromosome from his mother and a Y from his father. The X he receives will carry either fragile X syndrome or color blindness, so he has a 50% chance of having fragile X syndrome and a 50% chance of being color blind, neither of which are phenotypically normal.

17. D

The cell wall of bacteria is made of peptidoglycans, whereas the cell wall of plants and fungi is made up of cellulose. All the other choices are true of the cytoskeleton: the cytoskeleton is composed of microtubules and microfilaments and gives the cell mechanical support, maintains its shape, and functions in cell motility.

18. C

Choice (A) is incorrect. Up to approximately 40°C, the rate of enzyme action increases; after that, the protein will denature. Choice (B) is incorrect because the optimum temperature for most enzymes is 37°C, physiological temperature. Some enzymes can work at higher temperature, but those will be in specialized organisms, such as the bacteria that thrive in hot springs. Choice (D) is incorrect because an increase in energy in the system will increase effective collisions until the temperature becomes so high as to denature the enzyme.

19. B

Plant cells are rigid and cannot form a cleavage furrow. They divide by the formation of a cell plate, an expanding partition that grows outward from the interior of the cell until it reaches the cell membrane. Choice (A) is incorrect because plant cells lack centrioles. The spindle apparatus is synthesized by microtubules organizing centers, which are not visible. Choice (C) is incorrect: cytokinesis in animal cells proceeds through formation of a cleavage furrow. Choice (D) is incorrect because animal cells have centrioles from which the spindle apparatus arises. Choice (E) is incorrect because most cell divisions have equal cytokinesis except for cells such as yeast that bud.

20. C

32 ATP are produced by the electron transport chain and oxidative phosphorylation. Ultimately, 1 molecule of glucose will be catalyzed to produce 36 ATP (32 from oxidative phosphorylation, 2 from the citric acid cycle, and 2 from glycolysis).

21. C

Before considering the Punnett square for the offspring, we will determine the phenotype of the parents. A red-eyed fly with red-eyed and sepia-eyed parents must be heterozygous, because its sepia-eyed parent can only contribute the recessive sepia allele. If this heterozygous fly is crossed with a homozygous recessive (sepia) eyed fly, half the offspring will be red-eyed because they will receive the red, dominant allele from the heterozygous fly. The Punnett square will look like this:

red-eyed parent	R	r
sepia-eyed parent r	Rr (red)	rr (sepia)
r	Rr (red)	rr (sepia)

22. B

The retina develops from the ectoderm. The ectoderm develops into the nervous system, the epidermis, and overlying structures in the head. The endoderm develops into the lining of the digestive tract, lungs, liver, and pancreas. The mesoderm develops into the parenchyma of the internal organs.

23. C

Osmosis is a special type of diffusion involving water and is a form of passive transport. Hypertonic means high solute and low solvent. Hypotonic means high solvent and low solute. A group of particles moves spontaneously from compact arrangement to diffuse arrangement. Therefore, water will flow from a hypotonic environment to a hypertonic environment.

24. C

Disruptive selection occurs when conditions act to eliminate the intermediate phenotypes and favor the extremes. A stabilizing selection eliminates both extremes and increases the occurrence of the intermediate type. A directional selection eliminates one of the extremes and increases the occurrence of the other extreme. Genetic drift is a random change in the gene pool that occurs over time. Gene flow occurs when groups migrate from place to place, carrying new alleles to a previously isolated population.

25. A

The snake is a secondary consumer because it eats the mouse, a primary consumer. Primary consumers feed directly on plants, which are the primary producers in the ecosystem. An aphid is a primary consumer because it feeds directly on wheat. The fungus in choice (C) is a detrivore or decomposer that feeds on dead matter. It can also be viewed as a primary consumer that feeds directly on the green plant. Photosynthetic bacteria are primary producers. The hawk in choice (E) is a tertiary consumer.

26. A

The main respiratory control center lies in the medulla. Choice (B) is wrong because the hypothalamus controls such things as hunger, thirst, sex drive, water balance, blood pressure, and temperature regulation. It also plays an integral role in controlling the endocrine system. Choice (C) is wrong because the cerebrum processes and integrates sensory input and motor responses and is important for memory and creative thought. Choice (D) is wrong because the cerebellum is important in coordinating muscles. It aids in balance (it receives input from the inner ear), hand-eye coordination, and the timing of rapid movements. Choice (E) is wrong because the pituitary gland, along with the hypothalamus, plays an integral role in controlling the endocrine system.

27. E

Once a virus has injected its genetic material into the cytoplasm of a host cell, it can enter either the lytic cycle or the lysogenic cycle. In the lysogenic cycle, the viral genome integrates into the host genome (if it is an RNA virus, the RNA is first transcribed into DNA using reverse transcriptase) and lies dormant. At this stage, the virus is referred to as a provirus, so choice (C) is correct. The viral genome can remain dormant indefinitely, making choice (A) correct, as it replicates along with the host, making choice (B) correct. At some later time, the viral genome will be activated, and the bacteria will enter the lytic cycle in which the bacteria takes control of the host's genetic machinery and makes numerous progeny. In the last stage, the virus produces an enzyme that causes the cell to burst, releasing all the new viruses.

28. A

The posterior pituitary releases two hormones, the oxytocin hormone and the antidiuretic hormone (ADH, also called vasopressin). Choice (B), FSH, is released by the anterior pituitary. Choice (C), glucagon, is released by the alpha cell of the islets of Langerhans in the pancreas. Choice (D), estrogen, is released by the graafian follicle within the ovary during the menstrual cycle. Choice (E), calcitonin, is released by the thyroid gland.

29. D

When a symbiotic relationship between two organisms benefits both species involved, it is referred to as mutualism. Parasitism, choice (A), is a symbiotic relationship wherein one species benefits at the expense of the other. An example is heartworm in dogs. The worm parasites nourish themselves on the blood of the dog host, while being potentially fatal to the dog. Commensalism, choice (B), is a relationship in which one organism benefits and the other is unaffected. An example is barnacles and whales. Barnacles attach themselves to whales, thereby obtaining more feeding opportunities, while the whale is unaffected by the barnacles' presence. Predation, choice (C), is free-living organisms feeding on other living organisms. Unlike the other relationships above, predation is not a symbiotic relationship.

30. E

In the modern system of classification, all organisms are named as follows: kingdom, phylum, subphylum, class, order, family, genus, species. In the Linnaen classification system, all organisms are assigned a scientific name consisting of the genus followed by the species name. This scheme was originated by the biologist Carl Linn. Therefore *Homo* refers to the genus, and *sapiens* refers to the species.

31. C

Luteinizing hormone (LH) is first released as a surge midway through the menstrual cycle. This surge causes the mature follicle to burst, releasing the ovum from the ovary. Following ovulation, LH induces the ruptured follicle to develop into the corpus luteum, which secretes estrogen and progesterone. Choice (A) is incorrect because progesterone and estrogen inhibit GnRH release in a negative feedback pathway (thereby inhibiting FSH and LH release, thus preventing additional follicles from maturing). Choice (B) is incorrect because LH is secreted by the anterior pituitary. The ovary secretes estrogen and progesterone. Choice (D) is describing the function of progesterone, not LH. Choice (E) is describing the function of prolactin, not LH.

32. D

Choice (A) is incorrect because cardiac muscle is innervated by the autonomic nervous system. Cardiac muscle is striated, eliminating choice (B), and has only one or two centrally located nuclei, eliminating choice (C). Choice (E) is incorrect because cardiac muscle, like skeletal muscle and smooth muscle, requires Ca^{2+} for contraction.

33. D

Fixed action patterns are complex, coordinated, innate behavioral responses to specific patterns of stimulation in the environment. These responses are controlled from all levels of the central nervous system. The characteristic movement of herd animals is an example of a fixed action pattern. The startle response, choice (A), is an example of a complex reflex pattern. These responses are controlled from the brainstem or cerebrum. Choice (B) is an example of a simple reflex. These responses are controlled at the spinal cord. Circadian rhythms, choice (C), are an example of a behavior cycle. These behaviors are a response to both internal and external stimuli and control such behaviors as sleep and wakefulness and eating and satiation.

34. D

The female organ of the flower consists of the stigma (choice E), the site of pollen deposition; the style (choice A), a tubelike structure that connects the stigma to the ovary; and the ovary, which contains ovules and is the site of fertilization and seed development. The petal, choice (B), is a specialized leaf that serves to protect the female organs of the plant and to attract insects to aid in fertilization.

35. A

Pioneer organisms are the first species that inhabit an area that was previously devoid of life. Typically, these organisms have to be able to survive in harsh conditions, such as living on rocky surfaces. Lichens, which are a symbiotic relationship between alga and fungi, are capable of living on rocky surfaces. The acid produced by lichens aids in soil formation, which allows other organisms to colonize the area. Mosses (choice B) usually follow lichens in colonization, but cannot serve as a pioneer organism. Grasses are typically the next succeeding organism, followed by ferns, then birches.

36. B

The area in the kidney with the lowest solute concentration is the cortex. Filtrate that the enters the nephron travels through the proximal convoluted tubule, then through the loop of Henle, followed by the distal convoluted tubule, collecting duct, and renal pelvis, and then out of the kidney to the bladder. The convoluted tubules are within the cortex, and the collecting duct and pelvis are in the medulla. As filtrate travels from the cortex to the medulla, it constantly experiences an increasing concentration gradient, the purpose of which is to reabsorb water so that the urine is concentrated. Choice (A) is incorrect because the solute concentration within the nephron varies according to the region of the kidney through which filtrate is traveling. Choice (C) is incorrect because the medulla has a very high concentration gradient, which is necessary in order for an organism to produce concentrated urine. Choice (D) is incorrect because the pelvis, which is in the medulla, has a very high concentration gradient so that water can be reabsorbed. Choice (E) is incorrect because epithelia does not refer to a region within the kidney.

37. D

A niche defines the functional role of an organism in its ecosystem. A niche describes what the organism eats, where and how it obtains its food, the nature of its parasites and predators, how it reproduces, etc. Organisms occupying the same niche compete for the same limited resources, such as food, water, light, oxygen, and space. This competition will either cause one species to be driven to extinction (eliminating choice A) or cause the species to evolve in divergent directions, changing the niche they occupy and eliminating competition. Choice (B) is wrong because the two species involved may or may not be nocturnal (since they occupy the same niche, they are either both nocturnal or not). Choice (C) is wrong because the species will evolve so that they are more distinct from the other (divergent), not more similar (convergent). Choice (E) is incorrect because two species may indeed occupy two niches, and it is the ensuing competition that drives evolution.

38. E

The resting membrane potential across a nerve cell membrane mainly depends on the physiology of two ions: Na^+ and K^+. The Na^+/K^+ pump is an active transport protein that maintains an electrochemical gradient across the membrane. The membrane is more permeable to K^+ than Na^+, and it is the balance between the pump and the "leaky" membrane that determines the cell's resting potential.

39. E

The cerebellum is involved in balance, hand-eye coordination, and the timing of rapid movements. If a tumor were located in the cerebellum, you would expect loss of hand-eye coordination. Choices (A) and (D) are incorrect because the hypothalamus is responsible for temperature regulation and hunger and thirst drives. Choice (B) is incorrect because the medulla is responsible for controlling heart rate. Choice (C) is incorrect because the cerebrum is responsible for processing sensory input, such as vision, smell, and taste.

40. D

Chlorophyll, the green pigment that participates in the light reactions of photosynthesis, has a magnesium atom in its center. Zinc, copper, and manganese are involved in a variety of cellular functions, none of which needs to be memorized. Iron is found in hemoglobin and provides the ability to bind and release oxygen.

41. A

With the exception of the noble gases, which occupy the last column of the periodic table, the electronegativity of elements increases as one goes toward the upper right-hand corner. The five elements listed in choice (A) are in the same column (or group) but occupy positions that are farther and farther down. The electronegativity thus decreases and is what we are looking for. Choice (B) is incorrect because it contains elements in the same row (or period) in the order of increasing atomic number (moving to the right). The electronegativity increases. Choice (C) is incorrect because the elements move toward the upper right-hand corner (i.e., in the direction of increasing electronegativity). Choice (D) is incorrect because the elements are moving up a group, so electronegativity is increasing. Choice (E) is incorrect because the elements are all noble (or inert) gases and all have very low electronegativity.

42. D

The second ionization energy is the energy needed to remove a second electron from an already positively charged ion. In other words, for the process

$$X^+ \rightarrow X^{2+} + e^- \qquad \Delta E = ?$$

ΔE is the second ionization energy of the element *X*. An element with a high second ionization energy, then, would have a cation with a very stable electron configuration. In particular, if X^+ has an electronic configuration similar to that of a noble gas, then *X* will have a high second ionization energy. Choices (D) and (E), Rb and Cs, are both in the first column of the periodic table. A first ionization would form Rb^+ and Cs^+, both of which will have a noble gas configuration. (Rb^+ will have the configuration of Kr, while Cs^+ will have the configuration of Xe.) Kr has a higher ionization energy than Xe, since its valence orbital has a lower principal quantum number. Rb^+ therefore has a higher ionization energy than Cs^+, which in turn means that Rb has a higher second ionization energy than Cs. Choices (A), (B), and (C) are incorrect because they are Group II elements. A first ionization would cause each of them to be isoelectronic to a Group I element, which has a low ionization energy, since another ionization would bring them to a stable octet of a noble gas configuration.

43. E

Phosphorus has 5 valence electrons. It thus needs 3 more to complete its octet. It can do this by forming three covalent bonds: two to hydrogen and one to chlorine. The Lewis structure is as follows:

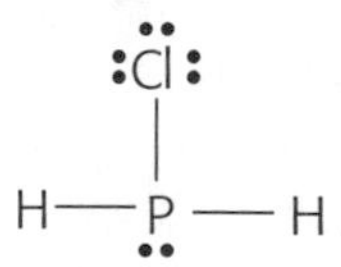

The Lewis structure, however, does not necessarily give an accurate representation of the three-dimensional appearance of the molecule. For that, we have to use VSEPR theory. There are four regions of electron density around the central P atom—three bonding electron pairs and one nonbonding pair. These will want to be as far apart as possible, resulting in a tetrahedral electronic geometry. In describing the actual molecular geometry, however, we ignore the nonbonding pair, and would thus describe the molecule as trigonal pyramidal. It is similar to the structure of NH_3:

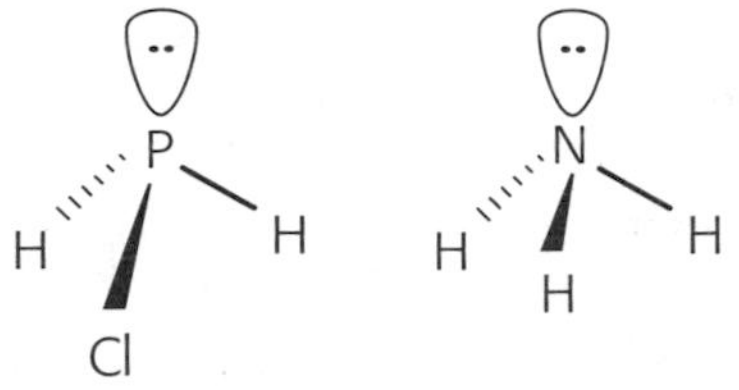

44. D

The pressure has slightly less than doubled on going from 1.00 atm to 1.80 atm. Since temperature and volume are not changing, the number of moles of gas needs to increase proportionally (i.e., it needs to increase to slightly less than the double, 6.00 moles). The only choice that fits this requirement is D: An extra 2.4 moles would bring the total number of moles of gas to 5.4 moles.

For completeness, the setup is as follows. From rearranging the ideal gas law:

$$\frac{P_1}{n_1} = \frac{P_2}{n_2} = \frac{RT}{V} = \text{constant}$$

$$n_2 = \frac{n_1}{P_1} \times P_2 = \frac{3.00}{1.00} \times 1.80 = 5.40 \text{ moles}$$

The extra number of moles needed is therefore

$$5.4 - 3.0 = 2.4$$

Note: Be careful when applying this approach to questions dealing with changes in temperature. Make sure you are using absolute temperature, in Kelvin. An increase from 20°C to 40°C is not a doubling of temperature!

45. E

First we must determine the order of the reaction. On going from experiment 1 to experiment 2, the concentration of B has increased, but the rate of reaction remains the same. The reaction therefore appears to be independent of the concentration of B, or, in other words, it is zero order with respect to B. Comparing experiments 1 and 3, we see that the concentration of A has tripled, while the rate of reaction has increased by about a factor of 9. The reaction is second-order in A. We can therefore write

$$\text{rate} = k[A]^2$$

To determine the rate constant, we need only to arrange the above equation and substitute in values for [A] and the rate for any one experiment:

$$k = \frac{\text{rate}}{[A]^2} = \frac{1.87}{(0.181)^2}$$

46. E

The spontaneity of a reaction is determined by the free energy change, ΔG. A reaction goes from being spontaneous to nonspontaneous (or vice versa) when the value of ΔG crosses the value of 0. $\Delta G = \Delta H - T\Delta S$. Thus $\Delta H = T\Delta S$ or solving for T, $T = \Delta H/\Delta S$. We are given the values $\Delta H = 131$ kJ/mol = 131,000 J/mol and $\Delta S = 134$ J/mol. Plugging these values into the equation yields T, which is approximately 1,000K which equals 700 degrees Celsius. Make sure you do all the calculations in the same units and express the temperature answer in terms of degrees Celsius.

$$\Delta H = 131{,}000 \text{ J/mol}$$

$$0 = 131{,}000 - T(134)$$

$$T = \frac{131{,}000}{134}$$

To convert from Kelvin to degrees Celsius, we need to subtract about 300. This brings the value to about 700, which is choice (E).

The ΔH and ΔS values are reported in different energy units not just to trap you. The magnitude of the enthalpy change is usually much greater than the magnitude of the entropy change for a given reaction, so expressing one with kJ and the other with J (or kcal and cal) is a common practice. Choice (C) may have been tempting if you had forgotten to convert from K to °C.

47. E

A mole of ideal gas occupies 22.4 L at STP, 1 atm pressure, 0°C. The conditions specified in the question stem are thus STP conditions. The mixture occupies a volume of 44.8 L, which means there are 2 moles of gas present. If the mixture contains 1.5 moles of argon, then there must be $2 - 1.5 = 0.5$ mol Ne present.

48. B

Halogens are group VII elements, occupying the second-to-last column on the periodic table. It includes F, Cl, Br, I, and At. Alkaline earth metals are the Group II elements, the ones in the second column. It includes Be, Mg, Ca, etc. Transition metals are the block of elements in the middle columns of the periodic table: from Sc to Hg. Cr, in group VIB, is a transition metal. Choice (A)—Cl, Na, Sr—is incorrect because it lists a halogen, an alkali metal (a Group I element) and an alkaline earth metal. Choice (C) is incorrect because Se is not a halogen and Sn is not a transition metal. Choices (D) and (E) are incorrect because Rb is an alkali metal, not a halogen or an alkaline earth metal.

49. E

The percentage of oxygen by mass is the mass of oxygen divided by the total mass of the compound, multiplied by 100%. Even though we are told that the sample weighs 200 g, we actually don't need this to get the answer. Any sample of $CuSO_4{\bullet}5H_2O$, regardless of its weight, will have the same percentage of O by mass, since this is dictated by the stoichiometric relationships in the chemical formula. We can work with the convenient quantity of 1 mole. The weight of a 1-mole sample is just the molecular weight of the compound: $63.55 + 32.06 + 4 \times 16 + 5 \times (2 \times 1 + 16) = 63.55 + 32.06 + 64 + 90 = 250$ g. The mass of oxygen in this 1-mole sample is $4 \times 16 + 5 \times 16 = 144$, where the first four come from the sulfate and the other five come from the five water molecules hydrated to the compound. The percentage by mass of oxygen is therefore

$$\frac{144}{250} \times 100\%$$

Since 144 is more than half of 250, the percentage is more than 50%, making (E) the correct choice. Note, again, that nowhere did we use the fact that the sample weighs 200 g. Failure to realize that there are five water molecules (each of which contains an oxygen atom) may have led you to choice (C).

50. D

Nonmetallic elements are found in the right of the periodic table, and, if neutral, will always have valence electrons in the *p* subshell, which can hold a maximum of 6 electrons. The requirement that it be in its ground state means that the orbitals are filled in accordance with the Aufbau principle. Only choice (D) satisfies these criteria. Choice (A) is incorrect because its valence electrons are in the *s* subshell. If it is a neutral species, this would be Mg, which is a metal. If it is a nonmetal, it must have had electrons removed or added, making it not neutral (e.g., Al^+.) Choice (B) is incorrect because it has 3 electrons in an *s* subshell, which can accommodate a maximum of only 2 electrons (since it contains only one orbital). Choice (C) is incorrect because the 4*s* orbital should not have filled before the 3*p* orbitals: It does not represent a ground state species. Choice (E) is incorrect because the *p* subshell, with three orbitals, can only have a maximum of 6 electrons.

51. C

Nitrogen is in the second period and hence its valence shell does not have a *d* subshell. It cannot expand its octet and can form no more than four bonds. Choice (C) is the only structure in which neither nitrogen forms more than four bonds. All the other choices contain at least one nitrogen forming five bonds.

52. D

For a molecule to be polar, it must contain a net molecular dipole. Choices (A), (B), and (C) are incorrect because even though they all contain polar bonds, these bonds are arranged spatially so that they cancel one another:

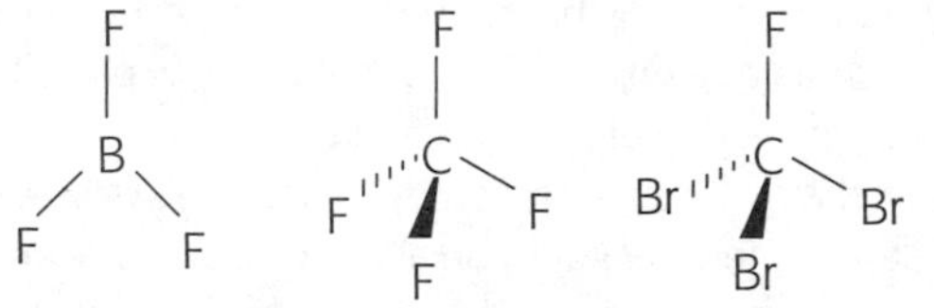

BF_3 has a trigonal planar geometry, and the dipole moments of the polar B–F bonds, when added together vectorially, yield no net dipole moment. The same goes for the tetrahedral CF_4 and CBr_4. Choice (D) is correct because the two polar C–Cl bonds do not completely cancel each other. Compared to choice (E), a C–Cl bond is more polar than a C–Br bond, since Cl is more electronegative than Br. The C–Cl bonds thus have a greater dipole moment.

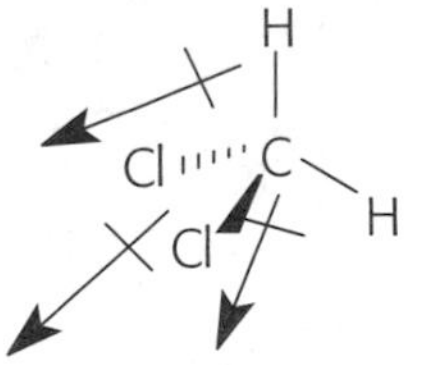

net dipole moment

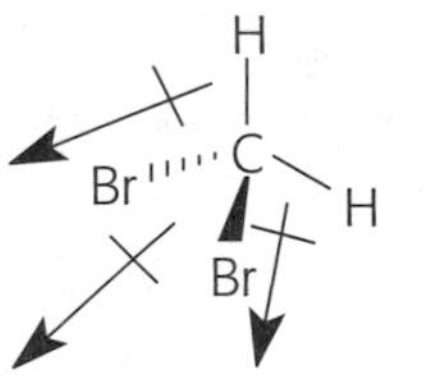

net dipole moment

53. A

First, we need to determine how many moles of hydrogen gas are generated from the reaction and then calculate the volume of the gas under the conditions described. For the first part, the dimensional setup is as follows:

number of moles of H_2 produced =

$$5.05 \text{ g Zn} \times \frac{1 \text{ mol Zn}}{65.4 \text{ g}} \times \frac{1 \text{ mol hydrogen}}{1 \text{ mol Zn}} = \frac{5.05}{65.4}$$

where the atomic weight of Zn of 65.4 g/mol is read from the periodic table and the stoichiometric relationship between Zn and H_2 is read from the balanced equation given in the question stem. For the second part of calculating the volume, we need to use the ideal gas law. We need to be careful about units because we are using the value of R as given in the question stem to determine the volume in liters, but that means that we need our temperature to be in Kelvin and our pressure to be in atmospheres: 40°C = 313 K, and since 1 atm = 760 torr, 763 torr = $\frac{763}{760}$ atm.

$$PV = nRT$$

$$V = \frac{nRT}{P} = \text{number of moles of } H_2 \times \frac{(0.0821 \text{ L•atm/mol•K})(313 \text{ K})}{763/760 \text{ atm}}$$

$$= \text{number of moles of } H_2 \times \frac{760}{763} \times 0.0821 \times 313$$

$$= \frac{5.05}{65.4} \times \frac{760}{763} \times 0.0821 \times 313$$

which is choice (A).

54. A

Isotopes of an element have the same atomic number but different mass numbers. The atomic number is the same as the number of protons, and the mass number is the sum of protons and neutrons. The isotope given in the question has a mass number of 208 and an atomic number of 82; it therefore has 82 protons and 208 – 82 = 126 neutrons. Another isotope of the same element must therefore also have 82 protons (an atomic number of 82) but a different number of neutrons. Choice (A) is correct. Choices (B) and (C) are incorrect because each would imply that the two isotopes are the same. Choices (D) and (E) are incorrect because isotopes of the same element must have the same atomic number.

55. B

The empirical formula gives the simplest whole-number ratio of the different elements in a compound. Since in this question the number of moles of each element in the compound has been given to us already, all we need to do is to find the simplest whole-number ratio among them. Because1.074 is twice the value of 0.537, N:H:Cl = 0.537:1.074:0.537 = 1:2:1. The empirical formula is thus NH_2Cl. Note that in most questions involving empirical formulas, we would probably just be given the mass of each element in the sample, and we would first have to first determine the number of moles of each by dividing by the atomic mass of the elements.

56. D

The standard change in enthalpy of a reaction, $\Delta H°$, is equal to the sum of the standard enthalpies of formation of the products minus the sum of the standard enthalpies of formation of the reactants. Therefore, for the first reaction in the table, we can write:

$$\Delta H° = 729.8 \text{ kcal} = 6 \times \Delta H°_f\,(CO_2) +$$

$$3 \times \Delta H°_f\,(H_2O) - \Delta H°_f\,(C_6H_5OH) - 7 \times \Delta H°_f\,(O_2)$$

O_2 is already in its standard state, so its enthalpy of formation is zero. The last term in the equation thus vanishes. The enthalpy of formation of carbon dioxide is the enthalpy change of the second reaction in the table (i.e., 94.4 kcal/mol). The enthalpy of formation of one mole of H_2O is *one-half* the enthalpy change of the third reaction (i.e., 68.4 kcal/mol). (The reaction leads to the formation of *two* moles of H_2O.) We can now substitute in these values and solve for the unknown, the enthalpy of formation of C_6H_5OH:

$$729.8 = 6 \times 94.4 + 3 \times 68.4 - \Delta H°_f\,(C_6H_5OH)$$

$$\Delta H°_f\,(C_6H_5OH) = 6 \times 94.4 + 3 \times 68.4 - 729.8$$

$$\approx 600 + 210 - 730$$

With this approximation, we can see that only choice (D) is close enough to be correct.

57. D

The percent yield is the actual yield divided by the theoretical yield, multiplied by 100 percent. The theoretical yield is the amount of product expected based purely on stoichiometry. In this question, the theoretical yield is determined as follows:

Amount of $C_6H_5NO_2$ expected

$$= \frac{78 \text{ g } C_6H_6}{78 \text{ g/mol } C_6H_6} \times \frac{1 \text{ mol } C_6H_6}{1 \text{ mol } C_6H_5NO_2}$$

$$\times\ 123 \text{ g/mol } C_6H_5NO_2$$

$$= 123 \text{ g } C_6H_5NO_2$$

The actual yield is 82 g. The percent yield is therefore $\frac{82}{123} \times 100$ percent. Without actually performing the division, we note that 82 is certainly more than half of 123, so the percentage is greater than 50 percent. Choice (D) is the only possible response.

58. C

Hydrogen bonds are a specific type of dipole-dipole interaction. When hydrogen is bound to a highly electronegative atom, such as oxygen, nitrogen, or fluorine, this partially positively charged hydrogen atom interacts with the partial negative charge located on nearby molecules. Water is a liquid at room temperature partially because each molecule can form two hydrogen bonds with neighboring molecules. Hydrogen fluoride can form only one intermolecular hydrogen bond. Choice (A) is incorrect because H_2O and HF differ by only 2 amu; this difference is insignificant relative to boiling point determination. Choice (B) is incorrect because the H–F bond is more polar than the H–O bond (fluorine is more electronegative than oxygen), so the H–F dipole-dipole attraction is stronger than that of O–H. Choice (D) is incorrect because dispersion forces only exist between nonpolar atoms or molecules. So the dispersion forces between H–F and H–O are insignificant. Choice (E) is incorrect because intermolecular forces are measured with pure samples only.

59. D

The easiest way to answer this question is to eliminate wrong answer choices. Choices (A) and (B) can be eliminated because the unknown compound resulted in an acidic solution, so it cannot be a base. We can eliminate choice (C) as follows. We are given a pH of 4.56. Since $pH = -\log[H^+]$, then the $[H^+] = 1 \times 10^{-pH}$. The $[H^+]$ must then be between 1×10^{-5} M and 1×10^{-4} M. Since the volume is 1L, then there are between 1×10^{-5}, and 1×10^{-4} mol H^+. Looking at choice (C), if the acid had a formula weight of 50 g/mol and 100 g was added to the water, then 2 mol of H^+ would form if it were a strong acid. From the previous calculation, we know that is impossible. The unknown must be a weak acid. Choice (E) is incorrect because no acid (weak or strong) has a formula weight of less than 10 g/mol. We can confirm choice (D) as the correct answer as follows. The formula for $K_a = \frac{[H^+][A^-]}{[HA]}$. Since the unknown compound must be a weak acid, there will be more undissociated acid in solution than dissociated, making the $[HA] > [H^+][A^-]$, so then $K_a < 1$. If the $K_a < 1$, then the $pK_a > 1$.

60. D

The molarity of the acid solution can be calculated using the neutralization formula $M_AV_A = M_BV_B$. Since we are given that both the acid and base are monoprotic, the normalities equal the molarities. Solving for the acid molarity and plugging in, we get $M_A = \frac{M_BV_B}{V_A} = \frac{(0.1)(35)}{50}$, choice (D).

61. B

Freezing point depression is a colligative property—one that depends only on the amount of the substance present. Since the compound in the question is ionic, the formula for the freezing point depression has to be multiplied by the number of particles formed upon dissolving. The formula for freezing point depression is $\Delta T_f = k_f m \bullet x$, where x is the number of particles formed, and m is the molarity.

$$\Delta T_f = K_f \frac{\text{mass/MW}}{\text{kg}} = K_f \frac{22.2/111}{1} \approx (2)(0.2) = 0.4°\text{C}.$$

The observed freezing point is −1.12°C, which is 3 times as much as the calculated value. The unknown ionic compound must therefore dissociate into 3 particles, making (B) the correct choice.

62. C

(A)

$2 + x = 0$	$x - 2 - 2 = 0$
↑ ↑	↑ ↑ ↑
+1 x	x −2 −1
H_2S	$SOCl_2$
S = −2	S = +4

(B)

$2 + x - 8 = 0$	$x - 2 - 2 = 0$
↑ ↑ ↑	↑ ↑ ↑
+1 x −2	x −2 −1
H_2SO_4	$SOCl_2$
S = +6	S = +4

(C)

$2 + x - 6 = 0$	$x - 2 - 2 = 0$
↑ ↑ ↑	↑ ↑ ↑
+1 x −2	x −2 −1
H_2SO_3	$SOCl_2$
S = +4	S = +4

(D)

$2 + x = 0$	$2 + x - 8 = 0$
↑ ↑	↑ ↑ ↑
+1 x	+1 x −2
H_2S	H_2SO_4
S = −2	S = +6

(E)

$2 + x - 6 = 0$	$2 + x - 8 = 0$
↑ ↑ ↑	↑ ↑ ↑
+1 x −2	+1 x −2
H_2SO_3	H_2SO_4
S = +4	S = +6

63. C

In beta decay, a neutron decays into a proton and an electron: ${}^1_0n \rightarrow {}^1_1p + {}^0_{-1}e$. The generic formula for beta decay is ${}^A_ZX \rightarrow {}^{A}_{Z+1}Y + {}^0_{-1}e$. In this example, the formula is ${}^{14}_6C \rightarrow X + {}^0_{-1}e$. X must be ${}^{14}_7N$.

64. B

The oxidizing agent is the reduced species. The oxidation state of nitrogen goes from +5 in NO_3^- to −3 in NH_3, getting reduced and serving as an oxidizing agent. Choice (A) is wrong because aluminum goes from 0 in Al(s) to +3 in $Al(OH)_4^-$. Choices (C) and (D) are wrong because they represent products of the reaction. Choice (E) is wrong because neither the oxygen nor hydrogen in OH^- are changed in the reaction.

65. B

This question requires no calculation. Since we are dealing with a base, choices (C), (D), and (E) can all be eliminated. Choice (A) is impossible because the pH can never exceed 14. That leaves only (B) as a possibility.

66. A

The point on the pressure-temperature curve where all three phases exist together in equilibrium is the triple point. The triple point is at point D, answer choice (A).

67. E

Condensation, the conversion of a gas to a liquid, occurs along the gas-liquid boundary, which includes point Z and point D, the triple point.

68. D

Vapor pressure is the amount of pressure the gas phase of a substance exerts over the liquid phase. The vapor pressure of a liquid is affected by temperature and pressure, as well as by the amount of any solute dissolved in the liquid, as determined by Raoult's Law. In this question, the only thing that changes is the amount of liquid in the container. This will have no effect on the ability of liquid molecules to become gas molecules. Therefore, the vapor pressure will remain the same.

69. B

The heat of vaporization is the amount of energy required to turn a liquid into a gas and is represented by the top plateau on the graph. The heat of fusion is the amount of energy required to turn a solid into a liquid and is represented by the bottom plateau on the graph. Since vaporization requires a greater Q than that of fusion, choice (B) is correct. Stated simply, it requires less energy to allow particles to move past one another (solid → liquid) than it does to separate them from one another completely (liquid → gas). Heat capacity is the amount of heat required to raise the temperature of an object by 1 K (or 1°C). The heat capacity of the different phases can be compared by examining the slope of the T versus Q curve. The steeper the slope, the less heat (Q) was required to increase the temperature and, therefore, the lower the heat capacity. The slope for each of the phases is too close to draw any accurate conclusions of their relative values. Choice (A) is incorrect because the graph does not give absolute values for the boiling point and melting point, so you cannot tell if one is more than double the other.

70. B

Oxidation occurs at the anode and reduction at the cathode (mnemonic: An Ox–Red Cat). Only in the reaction shown in choice (B) is chromium being oxidized.

(A) $2x - 14 = -2$ (x ↑, −2 ↑) $Cr_2O_7^{2-}$, Cr = +6 ⟶ $x - 8 = -2$ (x ↑, −2 ↑) CrO_4^{2-}, Cr = +6

(B) Cr^{2+} ⟶ $x - 8 = -2$ (x ↑, −2 ↑) CrO_4^{2-}, Cr = +6

(C) $2x - 14 = -2$ (x ↑, −2 ↑) $Cr_2O_7^{2-}$, Cr = +6 ⟶ Cr^{2+}

(D) $x - 8 = -2$ (x ↑, −2 ↑) CrO_4^{2-}, Cr = +6 ⟶ Cr^{3+}

(E) Cr^{3+} ⟶ Cr^{2+}

71. D

Recall that the convention of Fischer projections is that horizontal lines are bonds projecting toward the front, while vertical lines are bonds toward the back. The Fischer projection given in choice (D) is thus equivalent to

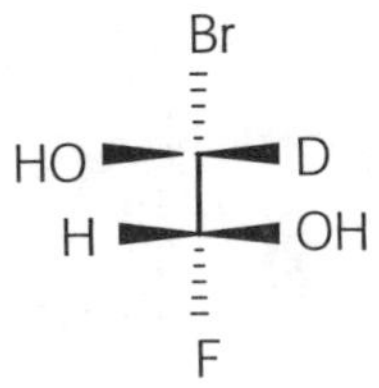

If we then mentally rotate about the C–C single bond (the vertical solid line above), we can verify that indeed it is similar to the first structure shown in choice (D).

A correct Fischer projection that should be drawn for each of the other choices is shown below:

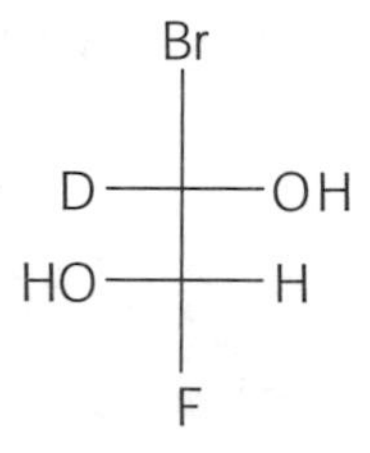

(A)

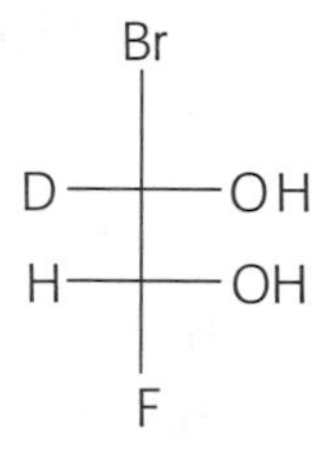

(B)

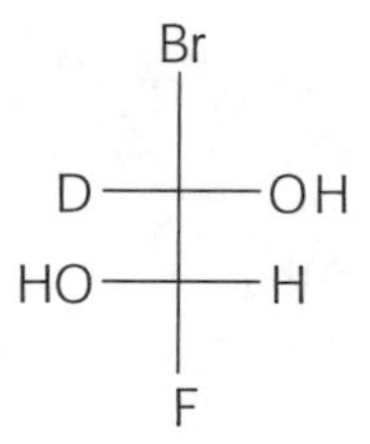

(C)

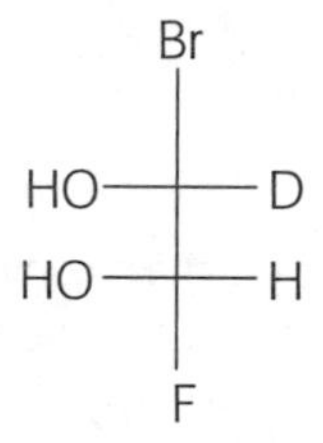

(E)

72. E

Since the –OH group is polar and is capable of hydrogen bonding, alcohols whose alkyl portions are not too big will dissolve in water. (Alkyl groups are nonpolar and thus do not dissolve readily in polar solvents: "Like dissolves like!") Among the answer choices, 3-pentanol has the longest alkyl chain and thus will be the least soluble in water.

73. A

The longest carbon chain containing the double bond (the principal functional group in this case) is made up of 5 carbon atoms. We can therefore eliminate all choices except (A) and (D). We want the position of the double bond to be designated by as low a number as possible, and so we number the carbon atoms from right to left. The alkene functionality thus occurs at carbon number 1, and there are methyl groups attached to carbons #2 and #4, making the molecule 2,4-dimethyl-1-pentene.

74. A

The oxacyclohexane with the least amount of nonbonded strain will have the least steric hindrance by virtue of equatorial positioning of the ring substituents. Methyl groups (or other relatively bulky substituents) in the axial position will experience repulsion from the electron clouds of other substituents (H atoms) occupying axial positions. For example, there are repulsive interactions between the methyl group and each of the pictured H atoms below:

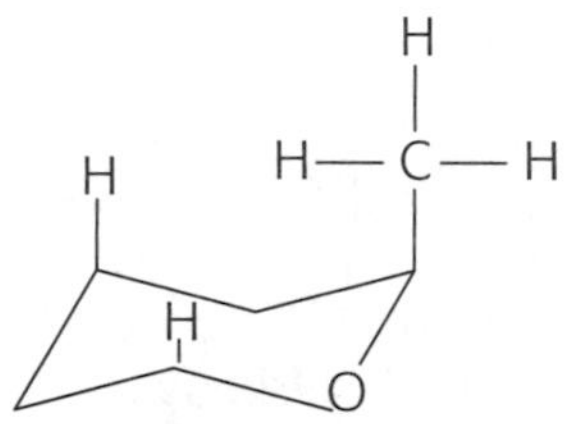

Choice (A) does not have a methyl group in the axial position, and so it has the least nonbonded strain.

75. D

Ethers have the generic formula ROR′, and asymmetric ethers are ones where R ≠ R′. However, we do not even need to know this to answer the question correctly. As indicated in the question, the Williamson ether synthesis is an S_N2 reaction, so we want first of all to identify compounds that will participate in an S_N2 reaction. Choice (D) contains the only pair that satisfies the criteria: the alkoxide ion $CH_3CH_2O^-$ in CH_3CH_2ONa is a strong base, and $CH_3CH_2CH_2CH_2Cl$ possesses a good leaving group (the chloride ion) and is not sterically hindered (it is a primary alkyl halide). The two will therefore readily react via the S_N2 mechanism:

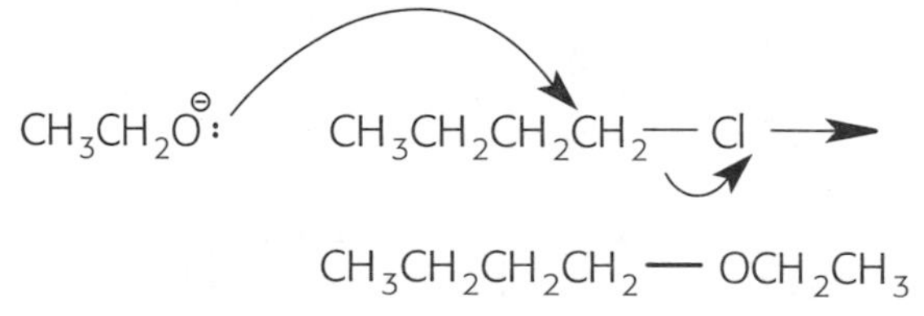

The product is an asymmetric ether (R = butyl group, R′ = ethyl group).

Choice (A) is incorrect because $CH_3CH_2CH_2COONa$ is the salt of a carboxylic acid and is thus not a particularly strong base. The ketone on the left also does not have a good leaving group. Choice (B) is incorrect because even though we have a strong base in $CH_3CH_2CH_2CH_2CH_2O^-$, the alkyl halide is tertiary and thus will not react readily via S_N2. Choice (C) is incorrect because the phenoxide ion ($C_6H_5O^-$) is not as strong a base as an alkoxide ion, and benzaldehyde (C_6H_5CHO) does not have a good leaving group. Choice (E) is incorrect because the substrate is already an ether, which does not have a good leaving group.

76. D

The connectivity of the atoms is different between the two compounds. Note that the compound on the top has a vinylic hydrogen (attached directly to an sp^2 hybridized carbon), but the compound on the bottom does not; both carbon atoms of the double bond are substituted. They are thus constitutional or structural isomers.

77. D

Structural isomers have the same molecular formula same number of each kind of atoms). Only choice (D) satisfies this requirement. Their molecular formula is both C_3H_6O. (Each has three carbon atoms, six hydrogen atoms, and one oxygen atom.) The connections between the atoms, however, are different:

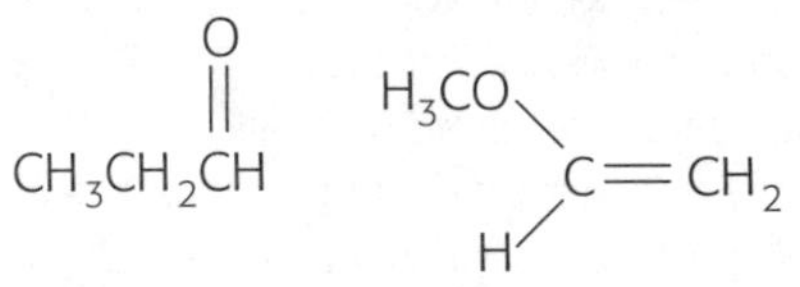

The other choices are incorrect because they do not have the same molecular formula. They are not isomers of any kind.

78. A

The reaction is an S_N2 reaction: DMSO is a polar aprotic solvent, CN^- is a strong nucleophile, and the leaving group is Y^-, which acts as the counter-ion to Na^+ in the product. We thus expect Y^- to be a reasonable leaving group. If Y were I, this would indeed be the case: I^- is a weak base and is a good leaving group. The other choices are incorrect because CH_3^-, SH^-, PH_2^-, and OCH_3^- are not good leaving groups.

79. B

Hydrogen bonding can occur when there is a hydrogen atom bonded to a highly electronegative atom. In such a case, the hydrogen atom may interact with the electronegative atom from another molecule (i.e., other than the one to which it is covalently bonded). This question asks about *intra*molecular hydrogen bonding, which is a more unusual phenomenon. Even if we were not familiar with intramolecular hydrogen bonding, we can still pick the correct answer as choice (B), because it is the only structure where we have a hydrogen atom bonded to an oxygen atom (in the carboxylic acid functional group). The intramolecular part comes in because the hydrogen can also interact with the carbonyl oxygen on the ketone group:

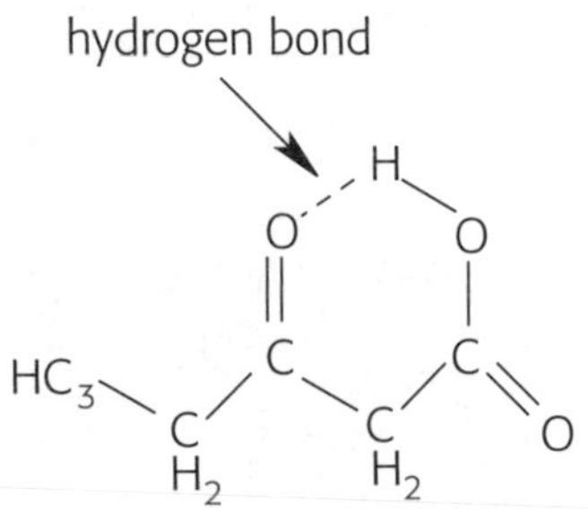

80. E

The longest carbon chain contains 8 carbon atoms. Do not be misled by the way the structure is drawn!

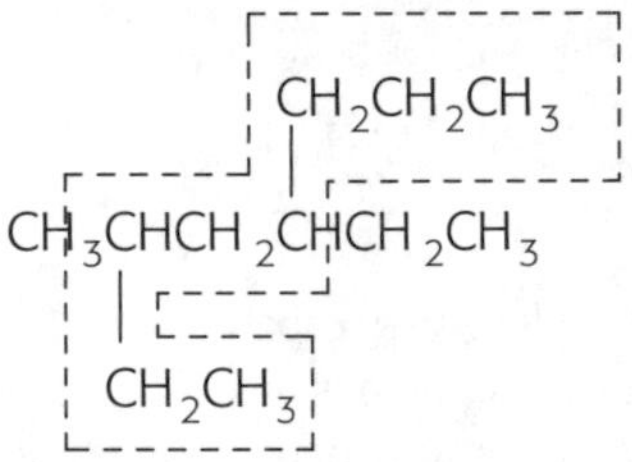

The molecule is thus an octane. This alone is enough for us to pick choice (E) as the correct answer. To verify, we notice that a methyl group and an ethyl group fall outside the octane chain. If we started numbering the carbon from the bottom up, we would get 5-ethyl, 3-methyl; if we numbered the carbon starting from the top, we would get 4-ethyl, 6-methyl. As usual, we go for the option with the lowest number (in this case the lowest sum). Because $5 + 3 < 4 + 6$, the name of the compound is 5-ethyl, 3-methyloctane.

81. C

The first (and rate-determining) step in an S_N1 reaction is the departure of the leaving group, leaving behind a carbocation intermediate. The more stable the carbocation intermediate, the more rapidly this step, and the reaction overall, proceeds. Carbocations are stabilized by the presence of electron-donating alkyl groups, so the more substituted the carbon bearing the positive charge, the more stable the carbocation. Among the answer choices, choice (C), being a tertiary halide, is the most substituted and will form the most stable tertiary carbocation. Choice (A) is a methyl halide, which, having no alkyl group attached to the carbon atom, will not react via an S_N1 reaction. Choices (B) and (D) are both secondary alkyl halides. They will undergo S_N1 reactions but not as readily as a tertiary alkyl halide. Choice (E) is a primary alkyl halide, and the carbocation it forms is not stable.

82. E

The structure shown is a meso compound. It possesses two chiral carbon atoms (indicated by asterisks in the figure below) but also has an internal plane of symmetry and thus is achiral (optically inactive).

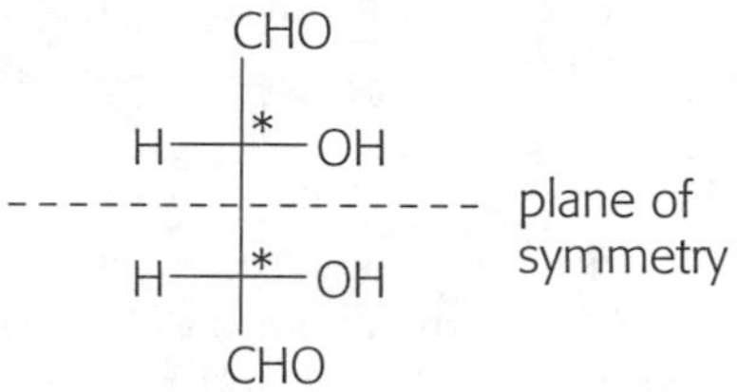

83. B

Aromatic compounds are cyclic and planar and contain ($4n + 2$) π electrons that can be delocalized. All the choices contain a nitrogen atom in the ring, making these all heterocyclic compounds. (Nitrogen, as a "noncarbon," is known as a heteroatom.) The nitrogen atom contains a lone pair of electrons, which may or may not be part of the π system, depending on the orientation of the orbital holding these nonbonding electrons. For the nonbonding electrons to be part of the π system (and thus be counted among the $4n + 2$), the orbital must be perpendicular to the plane of the ring, parallel to the π orbitals of the double bond. Choice (B) satisfies all the criteria for aromaticity. All the carbon atoms in the ring are sp^2 hybridized, forming a delocalized π system with their 4 π electrons. The nitrogen atom in the ring forms three bonds that are in a plane. It is thus also sp^2 hybridized, and the nonbonding electrons are in an unhybridized p orbital that is perpendicular to the plane. These nonbonding electrons can thus be conjugated with the π electrons of the double bond, giving a total of 6 ($= 4 \times 1 + 2$) π electrons.

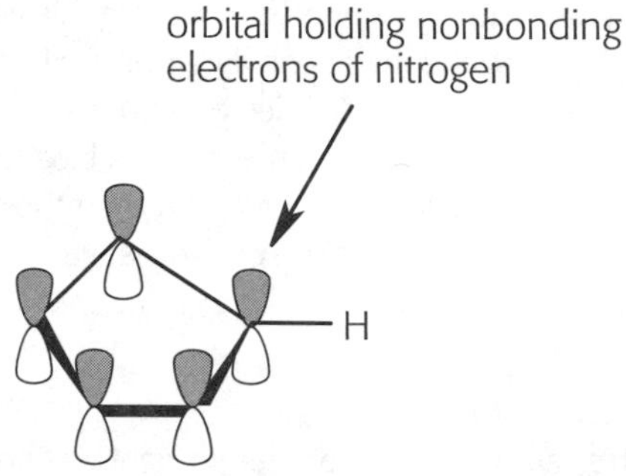

Choice (A) is incorrect because the nonbonding electrons of nitrogen are in an orbital lying in the plane of the ring. They thus do not form part of the π system, and the compound only has the 4 π electrons, one from each atom in the ring. It does not satisfy Hückel's rule.

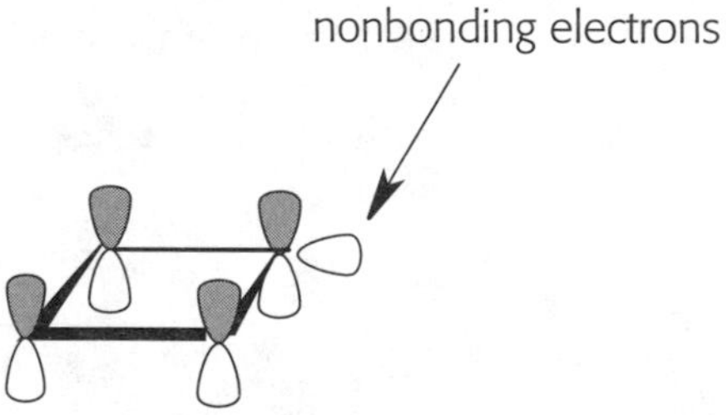

Choice (C) is not aromatic because the carbon opposite to the nitrogen is a saturated sp^3 hybridized carbon. Because the C–C–C bond angle is 109.5° for saturated carbons, the molecule is actually not planar. Choice (D) is not correct for the same reason as choice (C). Choice (E) is not aromatic because it has 8 π electrons, and thus does not satisfy Hückel's rule.

84. D

An E isomer is one in which the higher-priority group on each end of the double bond faces opposite sides (E = "epposite"). Priority is assigned based on atomic weight. In choice (D), the higher-priority group is F on both ends, and these two F atoms are on opposite sides. It is thus an E isomer. Choice (A) is incorrect because the molecule does not have geometric isomers: the carbon atom on one end of the double bond is bonded to the same group (F). Choice (B) is a Z isomer because the higher priority groups (again, F's on each end) are on the same side. Choice (C) is incorrect because the higher-priority group on one end is F, while it is a methyl group on the other. These two are on the same side, making this also a Z isomer. In fact, since the lower-priority group is H on both ends, we can forego the Z/E designation and refer to the compound as the *cis* isomer. Choice (E) is incorrect because the higher-priority methyl groups are on the same side. Again, we can refer to it as the *cis* isomer (*cis*-2-butene).

85. E

Numbering the carbon atoms from left to right, we notice that carbon 2 and carbon 3 form a triple bond and a single bond each. They are thus both sp hybridized, and the bond angles *a* and *b* must be 180° (i.e., carbons 1–4 are linear). Carbon 4 forms a double bond and a single bond (with presumably another single bond, not shown, to a hydrogen atom or something else). It is thus sp^2 hybridized with a bond angle of 120°. A more accurate representation of the structure of the molecule may be as follows:

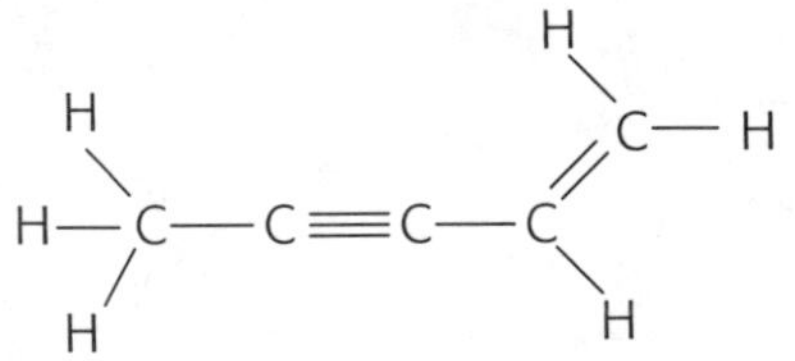

86. D

A more-substituted alkyl halide is less likely to undergo an S_N2 reaction, because the incoming nucleophile is sterically hindered from approaching the substrate. Choice (D) is a tertiary alkyl halide and is thus the most sterically hindered.

87. C

The compound in choice (C) is an alkyl halide, which is a very reactive species formed from a carboxylic acid and a chlorinating group, such as PCl_3 or $SOCl_2$. Acyl chlorides react with amines to form amides (carboxylic acids and amines can also form amides, but the acyl chloride form is much more reactive). Answer choices (A) and (D) are ethers, which are very stable and do not react with amines. Answer choice (B) is pyridine, which is even more stable than benzene. Considering that benzene will not react with amines, pyridine certainly will not. Answer choice (E) is a ketone. It resembles the acyl chloride of choice (C), but here instead of Cl^- as the leaving group, a primary cabanion (CH_3^-), would have to serve as the leaving group, a very unstable compound. Therefore the amine will not react with choice (E).

88. A

In this reaction, a carboxylic acid is being reduced to an alcohol. The correct answer must therefore be a strong reducing agent. $LiAlH_4$ is a strong reducing agent (THF is just a solvent—reactions involving $LiAlH_4$ must be anhydrous) that can donate H^- to bring the acid down to the alcohol. Choice (B) is incorrect because organomercury compounds are unreactive and cannot be used to yield the given product. The reactants in choice (C) would produce an ester. The reactants in choice (D) are used to convert an alkene to an alcohol. They will not convert a carboxylic acid to an alcohol. The reactants in choice (E) promote oxidation, not reduction.

89. E

When 1,3-cyclopentadiene reacts with sodium, it goes from a nonaromatic to an aromatic compound. A cyclic compound is aromatic if it satisfies Hückel's rule, that is it has $4n+2$ π electrons, where n is any integer. The product of the reaction has 6 π electrons, so it is therefore aromatic. An aromatic compound is very stable because the π electrons are delocalized throughout ring. In this reaction, the products are much more stable, so the reaction will have a very negative ΔH, and the reaction will still be spontaneous ($-\Delta G$), even under low temperatures (as determined by the formula $\Delta G = \Delta H - T\Delta S$).

90. C

The reactants used to produce compound X, an alkyl halide and Lewis acid, promote Friedel-Crafts alkylation. The alkyl group attached to the chlorine will add to the benzene ring, and the product will be isopropyl benzene. In the next step, the reactants promote halogenation of the benzene ring. The chlorine will add para to the isopropyl group of product X (R groups are ortho or para directing). Notice this eliminates choices (A) and (B). In the final step, a free radical halogenation reaction, bromine will add to the most substituted carbon atom (since it is the most stable free radical intermediate). The most substituted carbon is the tertiary carbon attaching the isopropyl group to the ring. This leaves only choice (C) as the correct answer.

91. E

The compound pictured is ethyl propionate—the ester formed from the dehydration reaction of ethanol and propionic acid. If water is added to an ester, the parent acid and alcohol are formed. Choices (A) and (D) are incorrect because there are no chiral carbons in the molecule. Choices (B) and (C) are incorrect because propionic acid would be formed, not acetic acid.

92. E

When *p*-aminobenzioc acid dissociates, it assumes a −1 charge. Any resonance structure that can be drawn must have the same charge. This eliminates choice (A) as a possible answer. Answer choices (B) and (D) are not even benzene derivatives; rather they are pyridine derivatives. Choice (C) can be eliminated because the carbonyl carbon has only three bonds and no formal charge. This leaves only choice (E) as the correct answer.

93. C

This question is nearly the same as the final reaction in question 90. The halide in free radical halogenation reactions always adds to the most-substituted carbon. The most-substituted carbon is the tertiary carbon connecting the isopropyl group to the benzene ring, making choice (C) the only possibility. Choices (A), (B), and (D) are incorrect because the free radical reaction will not involve the benzene ring (don't confuse this with a halogenation reaction, which requires a Lewis acid catalyst). Choice (E) is incorrect because the bromination will not cause the benzene ring to open up.

94. A

IR spectroscopy is useful in distinguishing different functional groups of a molecule. Only in choice (A) do the two molecules pictured have different functional groups.

95. A

There are three steps in a radical reaction: initiation, propagation, and termination. Termination is when two radicals combine, forming a compound with an even number of electrons. Since termination reactions decrease the number of free radicals, terminations decrease the reaction rate and eventually cause the reaction to stop. Only choice (A) depicts two free radicals combining to form a compound with an even number of electrons. Choices (B) and (D) depict propagation steps. Choice (C) is not a radical reaction, and choice (D) does not even occur during the course of a radical reaction.

96. E

Elimination reactions involve the removal of inorganic acid (hydrogen and a halide) from an alkane to form an alkene. This bit of information eliminates all the incorrect answer choices: Choices (A), (C), and (D) still have the chlorine attached, and choice (B) is an alkyne. This leaves only choice (E).

97. B

We can recognize this reaction as a Friedel-Crafts acylation—we are reacting a benzene ring with an acyl halide and a Lewis acid. The $CH_3C{=}O$ will add to the ring with the aid of the $AlCl_3$ Lewis acid catalyst, either ortho or para to the alkoxide group, because O–R groups are activating ortho or para directors. Choice (B) is the only answer that assigns the correct placement of the $CH_3C{=}O$ group. Choices (A) and (C) are incorrect because the ether functional group will not react with the acyl halide. Choice (D) is incorrect because the acyl group is meta to the alkoxide group. It must be either ortho or para, since that is where O–R groups direct addition reactions. Choice (E) would be formed if Cl_2 and $FeCl_3$ were being added.

98. D

When diethylamine, $(CH_3CH_2)_2NH$, acts as a Brønstead-Lowry base and binds an H^+, it forms the conjugate acid $(CH_3CH_2)_2NH_2^+$, answer choice (D).

99. C

When an ester is reduced, the alcohol function of the ester is first liberated, then the carboxylic acid is converted into a primary alcohol. The reduction of methyl propanoate would thus yield methanol and propanol.

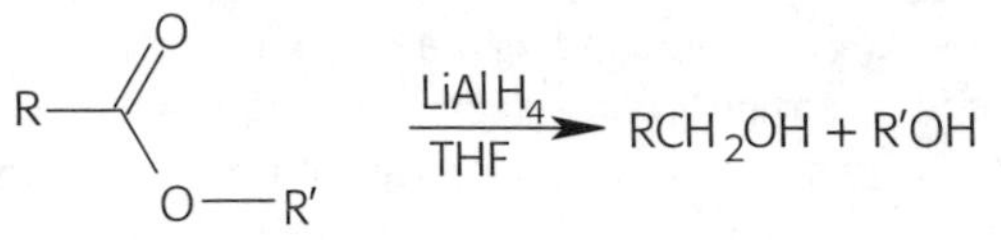

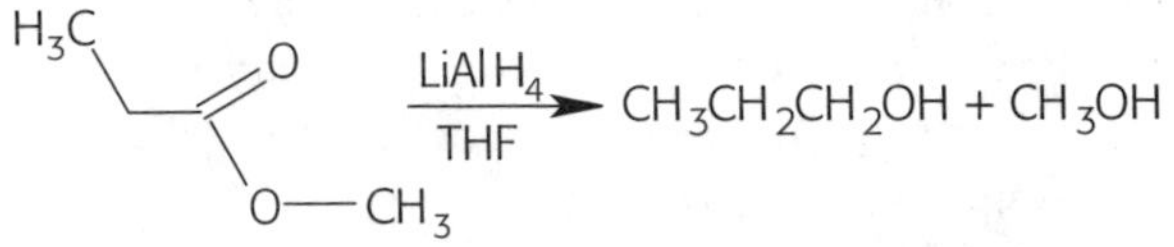

The addition of acid to the alcohol mixture will have no effect, so the correct answer is (C).

100. D

The first step of the reaction will lead to the addition of a nitro group to the ring through a diazonium intermediate. The nitro group will add either ortho or para, as R groups are ortho or para directors. This leaves only choices (D) and (E) as possibilities. In the second step of the reaction, the potassium permanganate will oxidize the toluene to benzoic acid. Therefore, the answer must be (D).

Answers and Explanations

1. C	11. D	21. C	31. C	41. C
2. D	12. E	22. D	32. A	42. B
3. D	13. B	23. E	33. D	43. E
4. E	14. B	24. B	34. D	44. C
5. B	15. A	25. C	35. B	45. B
6. E	16. E	26. B	36. D	46. A
7. B	17. A	27. E	37. E	47. E
8. C	18. D	28. B	38. D	48. D
9. A	19. E	29. C	39. C	49. D
10. B	20. D	30. E	40. B	50. B

1. C

The different types of spectroscopy are discussed in lines 60–94, which tell us that HREEL was used under vacuum conditions. Starting on line 83, the author states that infrared (IR) spectroscopy has an advantage over HREEL because it can be used under both vacuum and high-pressure conditions. We can infer from this that HREEL cannot be used under high-pressure conditions, making answer choice (C) correct. Choice (A) is wrong, given the above discussion. Choice (B) is wrong based on further information provided on lines 81–83—that is, HREEL uses electrons to cause vibrations. The context of choices (D) and (E) are out of the scope of the passage and can be eliminated.

2. D

The difficulties applying the results of surface chemistry to commercial catalysts are discussed starting on line 14. Choice (C) is a valid reason and is the reason why choices (A) and (B) are also valid reasons. The surface chemistry experiments were done under vacuum (no pressure) conditions, while commercial catalysts operate under high pressure, resulting in more molecules impacting the surface. This alters the kinetics of the reaction. Choice (E) is also valid and is derived from the lines 26–28. Choice (D), the availability of catalysts, was never discussed in the passage and so is the correct answer.

3. D

The correct answer to this question can be found in paragraph 3, specifically from the sentence that begins with, "The primary function of converters . . ." (lines 32–35) Choice (A) is incorrect because nitric oxide reacts with air, not water. Choice (B) does not describe the function of catalytic converters but rather why they have a certain shape (honeycomb). Choice (C) is fundamentally incorrect—catalysts need not be regenerated. Choice (E) is incorrect because catalytic converters serve to minimize further pollution of the environment; they do not clean the environment.

4. E

The experiments conducted in the mid-1980s are discussed in lines 50–94. On lines 67–68, the author states that the GM workers studied the reduction of NO. Choice (E) states that oxidation of NO was studied, which is incorrect, making (E) the correct answer choice.

5. B

The question stem is quoting from the sentence starting on line 135. At the end of the same paragraph, we are told that catalysts should promote the production of useful hydrocarbons, remove sulfur, and not promote the production of carbon and hydrogen. We can then measure the performance based any of these three measures. Choices (A), (C), (D), and (E) address the rate of the reactions, while choice (B) addresses yield. The measure of performance is determine by the amount produced (or not produced), not how fast it does so. Therefore, (B) is the correct choice.

6. E

The desulfurization process is discussed in lines 161–175. The second sentence (line 165) reads, "The first step is the cleavage of the sulfur-hydrogen bond." This leaves only choice (E) as the correct choice.

7. B

The rate of formation of carbon and hydrogen is addressed in the last paragraph. Carbon and hydrogen will be formed if a C–H bond is broken before a C–S bond. This is stated accurately in choice (B).

8. C

The effects sulfur has on the environment are briefly addressed in lines 98–104. The author states that sulfur-oxygen compounds contribute to acid rain, as also stated in choice (C). Choices (A) and (D) do not involve the environment, so are incorrect. Choice (B) could be applied to carbon emissions (CO is toxic), not sulfur emissions. Choice (E) is a true statement but is never addressed by the author, so is also incorrect.

9. A

This question addresses the same concepts as in question 7. At the end of the last paragraph, we are told that thiols with low carbon-sulfur bond strengths will yield a large fraction of hydrocarbons. So if a compound has high bond strengths, it would yield a small fraction of hydrocarbons—choice (A).

10. B

The correct statements in this question are taken directly from the first paragraph. The technology (choice A), synthesis (choice C), and development (choice D) of catalysts are all stated, as well as the removal of pollutants (choice E). The study of decomposition mechanisms is never mentioned, making (B) the correct answer choice.

11. D

The answer to this question can be found in lines 112–114. The question stem is lifted directly from the passage, and the correct answer merely fills in the blank, "[At the time of writing], the best catalyst for desulfurization is … "

12. E

The role of Pt and Rh in catalytic converters is discussed in lines 42–45. The metals function to remove NO, CO, and uncombusted hydrocarbons, choice (E). Choice (A) is incorrect because the metals are catalysts, not coenzymes. The metals do not serve any role in heat and friction, making choice (B) incorrect. Choices (C) and (D) are incorrect because it is the ceramic honeycomb surface to which the metals are deposited that influences the surface area, not the metals themselves.

13. B

The correct answer to this question can be found in lines 105–112. The desulfurization process encourages sulfur removal without breaking down pure hydrocarbons. Choice (B) is the only one that properly addresses this.

14. B

The nature of thiols is described in lines 118–124. The passage states that thiols are hydrocarbons that have attached a sulfur atom with an adjoining hydrogen atom, as described in choice (D).

15. A

The construction of a catalytic converter is decribed in lines 40–49. The amount of metals used in a catalyst is minimized because they are very expensive. None of the other choices is mentioned. Again, don't be tempted by a true statement if it is not addressed in the passage, such as choice (B).

16. E

The environmental dangers of nitric oxide, nitrogen-oxygen compounds, and carbon monoxide are addressed in lines 35–39. The danger of sulfur-oxygen compounds is addressed in lines 97–104. The dangers of thiols are never addressed. The passage states that sulfur compounds have to be burned before they become harmful but never addresses the dangers of thiols released directly into the atmosphere.

17. A

The series of events involved in an inflammation reaction is described in lines 37–55. The initial event in inflammation is vasoconstriction of the arterioles near the area of injury. Choice (E) is tempting but can be eliminated based on the fact that ischemia develops as a result of vasoconstriction so cannot occur first.

18. D

The definition of inflammation is provided in lines 10–12. Choices (A) and (B) are incorrect because they describe events that would incite an inflammatory response. Choice (C) is too specific—it describes only one part of the inflammatory response. Choice (E) is incorrect because inflammation is a local response, not a generalized one as described.

19. E

The findings of 19th-century scientists, specifically those of Cohnheim and Metchnikoff, are discussed in lines 28–36. The advent of the microscope allowed scientists to learn about the vascular and cellular changes that are responsible for the signs of inflammation. Choice (A) is incorrect because the outward signs of inflammation were described as early as the 1st century AD (lines 21–24). Choice (B) misrepresents the work of Metchnikoff. It was not pinocytosis that was studied but rather the process of phagocytosis. Choice (C) is an incorrect statement, for reasons addressed in the previous question. Choice (D), although a correct statement, was not described in relation to 19th-century studies and was understood well before that.

20. D

A local deficiency of blood in tissues is the definition of ischemia. The definition is provided in lines 46–47.

21. C

The opening of precapillary sphincters is one of the vascular events that occurs during inflammation, as discussed in lines 52–55. Going to the passage to paraphrase our answer before looking at the choices, we know that the answer must involve hyperemia, described as a local excess of blood. Only choice (C) involves hyperemia.

22. D

Neutrophils are discussed in lines 113-121. We can eliminate choice (A), as neutrophils can engulf particles up to half their size, not twice their size. Choice (B) can be eliminated: the relative effectiveness of leukocytes is never addressed. Choice (C) in also incorrect. Lines 67–69 inform us that macrophages are the first line of cellular defense. Choice (E) can also be eliminated—lines 124–125 state that eosinophils are not nearly as efficient as neutrophils in phagocytosis. Only choice (D) is correct.

23. E

We can go back to lines 113–121 to answer this question. Phagocytosed particles are digested in free-flowing vesicles in the cytoplasm. Since vesicle is not an answer choice, choice (E), the cytoplasm, must be the correct answer. The only other tempting choice is (B), lysosomes. We can eliminate this by looking at the last sentence of the paragraph—lysosomes are the source of the digestive enzymes but are not where digestion occurs.

24. B

To get this question correct, we have to combine two pieces of information provided for us in lines 83-88. We are told that neutrophils constitute about 60 percent of circulating leukocytes and that the number of leukocytes can reach a high of 30,000 cells/mm^3. So the number of neutrophils can reach a high of $0.60 \times 30{,}000$ or 18,000 cells/mm^3.

25. C

On lines 62–65, we are told that a key event in inflammation is the walling off of the affected area by fibrin clots. The fibrin was able to enter the area from the blood because of the increased permeability of the blood vessels. This makes choice (C) the only possibility.

26. B

The effects of enzymes, toxins, etc., are described in lines 98–112. The effects include stimulating inflammatory cells to migrate to the area, marginate, and then pass through the vessel wall. The cells can pass through because the products also increase the permeability of the capillaries and damage their walls. Answer choice (B) is the opposite of what happens—cells are induced to leave the circulatory system, not stay within.

27. E

In the last paragraph of the passage, the author attaches modern definitions to the 1st-century Latin terms used to describe inflammation. *Tumor* is caused by the accumulation of fluid leaking from blood vessels to the damaged tissue.

28. B

Leukocytosis-inducing factor is discussed in lines 89–97. The chemical is released from inflamed tissue and travels in the blood to the bone marrow, where it activates neutrophils. The factor is not stored in the bone marrow, making choice (B) the correct response to this EXCEPT question.

29. C

The four cardinal signs of inflammation are *tumor*, *calor*, *rubor*, and *dolor* (lines 21–24).

Answers and Explanations

1. A	11. B	21. B	31. E
2. A	12. A	22. C	32. A
3. E	13. E	23. C	33. B
4. B	14. B	24. D	34. E
5. E	15. D	25. B	35. D
6. D	16. E	26. B	36. C
7. C	17. C	27. B	37. A
8. B	18. E	28. D	38. E
9. B	19. B	29. B	39. B
10. C	20. A	30. D	40. D

1. A

The simplest way to solve this problem is to use conservation of energy. In other words, (potential energy at top of incline) = (kinetic energy at bottom of incline). Potential energy is mgh and kinetic energy is $\frac{1}{2}mv^2$, so we have $mgh = \frac{1}{2}mv^2 \Rightarrow v^2 = 2gh$, where v is the velocity at the bottom of the incline. Therefore, the velocity only depends on h and g. Given that both inclines have equal heights, we conclude both masses have the same velocity at the bottom.

2. A

Constant velocity means zero acceleration, which means there's no net force on the air bubble. Physically, there are two equal and opposite forces on the bubble: the force of gravity downward and the buoyant force upward. Applying an additional force, so that there is now a net downward force on the bubble, will result in acceleration downward. The bubble will accelerate in the downward direction.

3. E

Recall that the equations for two-dimensional projectile motion only require the acceleration of gravity and the initial velocity as inputs. Of course by initial velocity we mean the initial velocity vector, which tells us the initial horizontal and initial vertical velocities. Once initial velocity and acceleration of gravity are given, the equations are complete and every aspect of the motion can then be determined.

4. B

We're given a system of three masses attached by springs. We're also given a force on mass A of 8 lb to the right and a force on mass C of 3 lb to the right. Because the masses are connected by springs, they will move together with a common acceleration. Thus, the acceleration of mass B is the same as the acceleration of the system of masses. The net force on the system of masses is 11 lb to the right. From Newton's 2nd law, we have $11 = (m_A + m_B + m_C)a$, where a is the acceleration of the system. Solving for a, we have $a = 11/(m_A + m_B + m_C)$ ft/s^2. From the above remarks, this is also the acceleration of mass B.

5. E

As a spring oscillates back and forth it undergoes periodic motion, i.e., the displacement from the center repeats its trajectory at regular intervals. The only periodic function mentioned in the answer choices is the sinusoidal function. So if we didn't know that the displacement was indeed sinusoidal, we should know it's periodic and then choose (E).

6. D

We're given that A and B have the same kinetic energy. Thus, $\frac{1}{2}m_Av_A{}^2 = \frac{1}{2}m_Bv_B{}^2$. If the velocity of A is tripled, its kinetic energy becomes $\frac{1}{2}m_A(3v_A)^2 = 9\left(\frac{1}{2}m_Av_A{}^2\right)$. Clearly the ratio of the kinetic energy of A to that of B will be 9:1.

7. C

The mechanical energy of a body is defined as the sum of the kinetic energy and the potential energy, and is conserved when no friction or other dissipative forces are present.

8. B

The simplest way to solve this problem is with the principle of conservation of energy. The initial energy of the cart, at the top of the track, is mgh_0 because the cart is at rest. The energy at any other time is also equal to this energy. In particular, numerically when the cart has a speed of 8 ft/s, its total energy will be $\frac{1}{2}m\ (8)^2 + mg(h_0 - y)$, where y is the vertical distance of the cart from the point at which it started its descent. When the cart is moving at 8 ft/s it will have a potential energy of $mg(h_0 - y)$, $mgh_0 = \frac{1}{2}mv^2 + mg(h_0 - y)$

$mgh_0 = \frac{1}{2}mv^2 + mgh_0 - mgy$

$\frac{1}{2}mv^2 = mgy;\ \frac{1}{2}v^2 = gy$

$hy = v^2/2g$

Notice that mgh_0 on both sides cancels, as does the mass, so we didn't have to know h_0 or m. The equation then simplifies to $gy = \frac{1}{2}(8)^2$ ($g = 32$ ft/s^2 in British units). Thus, $y = \frac{1}{2}\left(\frac{64}{32}\right) = 1$ ft.

9. B

$$\text{Efficiency} = \frac{\text{Energy out}}{\text{Energy in}}$$

So we'll have to calculate energy expended by the engine and actual work done. Consider the energy expended by the engine. Recall power = energy/time, so energy = power × time. Given power = 4 horsepower = 4 (550) ft·lb/s, we have power = 2,200 ft·lb/s. Given a duration of 4 s, we have energy expended = (2,200)(4) = 8,800 ft·lb. The actual work done is the change in potential energy of the 200-lb object. The change in potential energy is mgh = (200)(11) = 2,200 ft·lb (i.e., we're already given mg = 200 lb). So efficiency $= \frac{2{,}200}{8{,}800} = \frac{1}{4} = 25\%$.

10. C

Because an ideal pendulum conserves energy, its mechanical energy is constant. The potential energy (mgh) is the smallest at point C because it's closest to the ground. So point C is the point of maximum kinetic energy. The point of maximum kinetic energy is also the point of maximum velocity.

11. B

Because the car is slowing down, its kinetic energy is decreasing. We can then rule out (C). The other choices involve the time dependence of the kinetic energy (i.e., $v = v_o + at$). So we have $v^2 = v_o^2 + 2v_o at + a^2t^2$. Thus, the square of the velocity depends nonlinearly on time, so the kinetic energy also depends nonlinearly on time.

12. A

The braking force decelerates the car, resulting in a decrease in its velocity. Because momentum is mass times velocity, we know that momentum is also decreasing with time. Thus, we can rule out (C). Momentum is given by mv, so to determine the time dependence of momentum, we'll need the time dependence of the velocity. Because the force is constant, we know the acceleration is also constant. Thus, the velocity is described by $v = v_o + at$, which means the momentum is given by $m(v_o + at)$. The momentum depends linearly on time.

13. E

The temperature of the brake shoes will increase due to the heat produced by the frictional force between the brake shoes and the wheels of the car. Recall that the change in temperature of an object is related to the heat it absorbs by $\Delta Q = mc\Delta T$. Thus, the change in temperature is given by $\Delta T = \Delta Q/[mc]$. To determine how the temperature changes with time, we need to know how the heat absorbed by the brake shoes changes with time. From conservation of energy, this heat is produced by the loss of kinetic energy of the car, which depends on time nonlinearly. Thus, the heat absorbed by the brake shoes will change nonlinearly with time. The above equation for ΔT says that the time dependence of ΔT is given by the time dependence of ΔQ. Given that ΔQ changes nonlinearly with time, we know the temperature changes nonlinearly with time.

14. B

We're told that two objects have the same mass and velocity. As p = mv, just as mv is the same for both objects, so too is p .

15. D

Weight is the force of Earth's gravity on an object and is given generally by $F = GMm/r^2$, where M is the mass of the Earth, m is the mass of the object, and r is the distance from the object to the center of the Earth. The weight of the object at an altitude of 32,000 miles is $F_1 = GMm/(36{,}000)^2$. The weight of the object at an altitude of 5,000 miles is given by $F_2 = GMm/(9{,}000)^2$. Notice that the distance from the object to the center of the Earth is the altitude of the object plus the radius of the Earth.

$\frac{F_2}{F_1} = (36{,}000)^2/(9{,}000)^2 = \left(\frac{36{,}000}{9{,}000}\right)^2 = 16.$

The percent increase is therefore $\frac{16F_1 - F_1}{F_1} \times 100\%$

$= \frac{16-1}{1} \times 100\% = 15 \times 100\% = 1{,}500\%.$

16. E

Choice (A) suggests the sliding body reaches the ground first. The falling body has the acceleration g. The sliding body has an acceleration down the incline given by a = F/m, where F is the force down the incline. If the angle of the incline is θ, then $F = mg\sin\theta$, so that $a = g\sin\theta$. As $g\sin\theta < 1$, so the falling mass has a larger acceleration than does the sliding mass. This implies that the falling mass reaches the ground sooner. We can then eliminate (A) and (B). (C) suggests the sliding body has a lower speed at the ground. Both masses start from the same height so both have initial energy mgh (h is the height). Both have zero potential energy at the bottom so their energy at the bottom is $\frac{1}{2}mv^2$. Conservation of energy says $mgh = \frac{1}{2}mv^2$. Thus, both masses strike the ground with the same speed. We then eliminate (C). Choice (D) says the sliding mass has a lower kinetic energy at the bottom. From our conservation of energy equation, we see that given equal masses, both objects have the same kinetic energy at the bottom. Thus, we eliminate (D), which leaves (E) as the correct choice. For completeness, consider (E). From conservation of energy we have $mgh = \frac{1}{2}mv^2 + mgy$, where h is the initial height, y is some intermediate height, and v is the velocity at that height. Given identical initial heights, this says the speed at any intermediate height is the same. So indeed (E) is correct.

17. C

We're told that a certain chain of decays starts from the nucleus $^{238}_{92}U$ and eventually ends up with $^{234}_{92}U$. In addition, we're told that the decay process takes us to both $^{234}_{91}Pa$ and $^{234}_{90}Th$. Recall that in alpha decay, the atomic number decreases by 2, and the mass number decreases by 4. In beta-minus decay the atomic number increases by one (neutron into a proton), and the mass number stays the same. To reach either of the intermediate nuclei we have to decrease the atomic number, which means the first decay has to be an alpha decay. An alpha decay from $^{238}_{92}U$ will produce a nucleus with atomic number 90 and mass number 234 (i.e., precisely $^{234}_{90}Th$). Thus, we can eliminate answer choices (A), (B), and (E). To get from $^{234}_{90}Th$ to $^{234}_{91}Pa$ requires a beta-emission. The atomic number increases by one and the mass number remains the same. Thus, we know choice (C) is correct. For completeness, consider the final decay from $^{238}_{91}Pa$ to $^{234}_{92}U$. Clearly this will also be a beta decay.

18. E

Let's consider the answer choices. Choice (A) suggests light doesn't carry energy. This is false. The energy of a photon of light of frequency f is E = hf. Choice (B) suggests that the speed of light isn't equal to the product of wavelength and frequency. Like any wave phenomena, the speed of a light wave is related to the frequency and wavelength by $v = \lambda f$. For the propagation of light in a vacuum, the speed is always equal to $c = 3 \times 10^8$ m/s. Choice (C) suggests that sound and light are different in that sound requires a medium through which to travel. This is certainly the case. Sound cannot travel in a vacuum, since it requires the existence of molecules to propagate. So choice (C) is a true statement. Choice (D) suggests that the modes of travel for sound and light are different in that sound travels by the transfer of energy between molecules. This is certainly true. The energy in a light wave travels through empty space, requiring no molecular processes for transmission. Thus, (C) and (D) are both correct, so choice (E) is the correct answer.

19. B

The bubble of air can be treated as a volume of an ideal gas, where the pressure of the gas will be equal to the pressure of its surroundings. Let's denote P1, v1 to be the pressure and volume, respectively, of the gas at a depth of 30 meters and P2, v2 to denote the pressure and volume of the gas at the surface. Recall the ideal gas law pv = nRT, where n is the number of moles of gas and T is the temperature. In this case, both n and T are constant and therefore we can apply Boyle's Law: P1v1 = P2v2. Now recall that the pressure at a depth of h below the surface of a liquid is P = Po + ρgh, where Po is the pressure at the surface (atmospheric pressure in the present case, measured in Pascals) and ρ is the density of the liquid. We then have P1 = Po + 30ρg and P2 = Po. We are also told that v1 = 0.25 L and v2 = 1.0 L. Inserting these values into our above equation relating pressures and volumes we have $[(1.01\times10^5) + (10)(30)(\rho)](0.25) = [(1.01\times10^5)(1.0)]$. Simplifying and solving for density, ρ, we find that the average density of the lake water is 1,000 kg/m^3.

20. A

The equation you need to answer this question was derived by Neils Bohr. It predicts the frequency of light produced when an electron falls from one quantum level to another in a hydrogen atom, though it doesn't work for other kinds of atoms, since those have more complex subshells. The equation states that E equals –A times the quantity $(1/n_i^2 - 1/n_f^2)$, where n_i is the principle quantum number of the electron in its initial state and n_f is the first quantum number of the electron in its final state. A is the complete dissociation energy, which is constant for a given action. The negative sign indicates the electron's emission of energy as it transitions to a lower energy state. So we have to multiply –A by $\frac{1}{3^2} - \frac{1}{2^2}$. This comes to $-A = -\frac{5}{36}$, which is equal to 0.14 A, choice (A).

21. B

We're told that an airplane with a mass of 150,000 kilograms produces a thrust of 200,000 newtons to go from rest to a cruising speed of 720 kilometers per hour. So we're given a mass, force, and speed, and we're asked to find the time it takes to reach that speed.

An equation that accomplishes this is the familiar kinematic equation $v = v_0 + a\,t$, where v is the final speed, v_0 is the initial speed, a is the acceleration (which is equal to the force over the mass), and t is the time. The plane starts from rest, so $v_0 = 0$. Solving for t, we find that t = v/a. We know v = 720 kilometers per hour, but what is the acceleration? As noted earlier, we can calculate the acceleration from Newton's second law, F = m a, where F is the force and m is the mass. We know that F = 200,000 newtons and m = 150,000 kilograms. So we can calculate a by dividing F by m. We get a = 200,000 over 150,000, or four-thirds. Now that we have a, we can calculate t from the equation t = v/a. But before we can substitute our numbers in, we must first convert the speed of the aircraft from kilometers per hour to meters per second. Multiply the speed by the number of meters in a kilometer and divide it by the number of seconds in an hour; we get that the speed equals (720 × 1,000)/3,600, or 200 meters per second. Plugging that number into our equation, we find that the time t equals v over a or 200 over $\frac{4}{3}$ or 150 seconds, which is answer choice (B).

You could also use the formula for impulse to answer this question. Impulse, J, is the product of the force, F, and the time over which the force acts, t. It also equals the change in momentum, Δp, which equals the final momentum minus the initial momentum. Therefore, we can say that J = Δp = Ft. Since momentum is the product of mass and speed and the aircraft is initially at rest, the initial momentum of the aircraft is zero. So the change in momentum Δp is simply the final momentum of the aircraft. Thus, our equation becomes mv = Ft, where m is the mass of the aircraft and v is the final speed of the aircraft. We are trying to find the time, so rearranging to get an equation in terms of the time t, we get that t = mv over F. Plugging in the values for m and v, we get that $t = \frac{(150{,}000 \times 200)}{200{,}000}$, or 150 seconds.

22. C

There are two ways you could do this problem: an easy way if you have the Henderson-Hasselbach equation memorized and a longer way based on the definition of the acid dissociation constant, K_a, if you don't remember that equation. If you don't, you'll have to decide if it's worth trying to memorize. It can potentially save you time on the exam, but on the other hand, if you try to memorize it, that's one more equation you could forget or get mixed up. If you understand how to figure out questions like this one based on pK_a, it may take longer but you'll be less likely to forget how to do it. By definition, the pK_a of an acid solution is –log of the acid dissociation constant, or K_a. The acid dissocation constant, in turn, is equal to (the concentration of the hydrogen ion) × (the concentration of the anion, X^-) divided by (the concentration of the undissociated acid, HX). If the concentration of X^- and the concentration of HX are equal, they'll cancel each other out. This means that the concentration of hydrogen ion will be equal to the value of the acid constant. In that case, the pH, which is the *negative log* of the hydrogen ion concentration, will be equal to the negative log of the acid constant—that is, equal to the pK_a.

So any time the pH is equal to the pK_a, the concentration of X^- must also be equal to the concentration of HX. In this example, the pH is not equal to the pK_a, so the concentrations of X^- and of HX will not be equal. But you can figure out what they will be just by remembering that the pK_a is the negative log of the acid constant. Since the pH is 6, the hydrogen ion concentration will be 1×10^{-6}. Since the pK_a is 5, the acid constant must be 1×10^{-5}. If you plug these values into the equation for the acid constant, and then divide both sides of the equation by the hydrogen ion concentration, you find that the concentration of X^- divided by the concentration of HX is equal to 1×10^{-5} divided by 1×10^{-6}. This comes to 10^1, or 10. So the concentration of X^- must be 10 times the concentration of HX, and choice (C) is correct.

The Henderson-Hasselbach equation says that for a weak acid solution, the pH equals the pK_a plus the log of the ratio of the concentration of conjugate base to the concentration of acid. For an acid HX, the conjugate base is the X^- ion that's formed when the acid dissociates. Now, if the pK_a of an acid is 5, then for its pH to be 6, the log of that concentration ratio must be 1, or in other words, the ratio must be 10. This means that the concentration of conjugate base, and therefore of dissociated acid, must be 10 times the concentration of acid.

23. C

We are told that a metal plate is completely illuminated by a monochromatic light source, and we are asked which of the Roman numeral statements would increase the number of electrons ejected from the surface of the metal. Statement I suggests that increasing the intensity of the light source would increase the number of electrons ejected. Light may be thought of as being made of particles. These light particles are more commonly known as photons and have an energy given by the equation $E = hf$, where E is the energy, h is Planck's constant, and f is the frequency of the light. The intensity of a light source is the number of photons produced per unit time. Therefore, when we increase the intensity of the light source, we increase the number of photons striking the metal plate, resulting in more electrons being ejected from the metal. Thus Statement I is true, so we can eliminate answer choice (D). Statement II suggests that increasing the frequency of the light source would increase the number of electrons ejected. From the equation $E = hf$, we see that by increasing the frequency of the light, we increase the energy of the incident photons. This means that a photon that strikes the metal will eject an electron with a higher kinetic energy. However, it will not increase the number of electrons ejected, since the number of electrons ejected is proportional to the number of incident photons. Therefore, Statement II is false, and we can eliminate answer choices (B) and (E). This leaves us with answer choices (A) and (C). The final statement suggests that increasing the surface area of the metal plate would increase the number of electrons ejected. The key point to remember here is that the metal plate is completely illuminated by the light source. Therefore, by increasing the area of the metal plate, we increase the area on which the light source is incident. This implies that more photons will strike the plate, resulting in an increase in the number of electrons ejected. Since Statements I and III are true, the correct answer must be choice (C).

24. D

The time required for a ball to fall to the ground from a height h is found from using the equation $h = 1/2gt^2$, where g is the acceleration of gravity on the planet. So $t = \sqrt{2h/g}$. The acceleration of gravity near the surface of a planet depends on the mass of the planet and the radius of the planet. The equation is derived noting that the gravitational force on a mass m is given by $F = GMm/r^2$, where M is the planet's mass and r is the radius. Newton's second law says $F = ma$, and in this case the acceleration is g. Therefore $GMm/r^2 = mg \Rightarrow g = GM/r^2$, and doubling the mass of the planet and keeping its radius the same means doubling g. The new time to fall the height h is then given by $t_1 = \sqrt{2h/2g} = t/\sqrt{2} = 10/\sqrt{2} = 5\sqrt{2}$ seconds.

25. B

Recall that the magnitude of torque is given by $rF\sin\theta$, where r is the distance from the fulcrum, F is the force, and θ is the angle between the force and the lever arm. In the present case, the force is the weight W and is equal for both children. The distance r is simply D and is equal for both. Because the children must balance, their weight force will be perpendicular to the lever arm, so $\sin\theta = \sin 90° = 1$. Thus, the magnitude of torque due to each child is the same. Torques also have direction in the sense of giving rise to either clockwise or counterclockwise rotation. Clearly, one of the children will tend to give rise to a clockwise torque and the other to a counterclockwise torque. The torques are thus equal in magnitude and opposite in direction.

26. B

For the monkey to climb upward with an acceleration of 2.5 m/s^2, there must be an upward force on the monkey of magnitude F = ma, where a is the upward acceleration of the monkey and m is the mass of the monkey. This upward force must be supplied by tension in the rope. In addition to providing this upward force, the rope must also support the weight of the monkey. The total tension in the rope must therefore be the sum of the weight of the monkey and the force necessary to accelerate the monkey upward. However, we are told that the rope can support a maximum weight of 530 Newtons. In other words, the maximum tension in the rope before it will snap is 530 N. So, we need to determine if the combined weight of the monkey and the upward force accelerating the monkey is greater or less than 530 N. Since the mass of the monkey is 45 kg, the weight of the monkey, w = mg, is (45 kg)(9.8 m/s^2) = 441 N. The tension in the rope necessary to accelerate the monkey can not exceed 89 N. The force required to accelerate the monkey at 2.5 m/s^2 is (45 kg)(2.5 m/s^2) = 112.5 N. To support this acceleration, the total tension in the rope would have to be 112.5 N + 441 N = 553.5 N, which is greater than the maximum tension than can be sustained by this particular rope. Thus, the rope will snap.

27. B

Consider a rocket at rest in empty space. The initial momentum of the rocket with its fuel contents is zero. When the engines are fired, exhaust gases move at high speed out the back of the rocket. Thus, the exhaust gases have momentum in the backward direction. For momentum to be conserved, the rocket must acquire an equal momentum in the opposite direction. The total momentum of rocket plus exhaust gases is still zero, and the rocket moves forward. Thus, conservation of momentum provides the explanation.

28. D

Consider the given function $a = 0.34Bt^{-1/2} + A$. This is the same as $a = \frac{0.34B}{\sqrt{t}} + A$. Clearly, as time increases, the acceleration decreases. Because time is raised to a negative exponent (and as a square root), we know the time variation is nonlinear.

29. B

Let's determine both kinetic and potential energies for the given spring length of 3 m. The equilibrium length of the spring is 2 m, and the maximum length is 4 m. Thus, the maximum displacement from equilibrium is 2 m. Note that at maximum displacement, all the energy is potential because the mass is momentarily at rest. Given that energy is conserved, we then know that the total energy of the system is simply the potential energy at maximum displacement. Potential energy of a spring is $\frac{1}{2}kx^2$. Using the given values, we have $\frac{1}{2}kx^2 = \frac{1}{2}(5)(2)^2 = 10$ J, so the total energy of the system is 10 J. When the spring length is 3 m, the total energy is still 10 J, but the displacement from equilibrium is 1 m. The potential energy is then $\frac{1}{2}kx^2 = \frac{1}{2}(5)(1) = 2.5$ J. The total energy is $\frac{1}{2}kx^2 + \frac{1}{2}mv^2 = 2.5 + \frac{1}{2}mv^2 = 10$, so $\frac{1}{2}mv^2 = 10 - 2.5 = 7.5$ J, so the kinetic energy is greater than the potential energy.

30. D

The maximum velocity occurs when the block has maximum kinetic energy. As total energy is conserved, maximum kinetic energy occurs at minimum potential energy, and minimum potential energy is when the block is at the equilibrium position, when the velocity and so kinetic energy is zero. From the last problem, we know that the total energy is 10 J. When the block is at the equilibrium position, its potential energy is zero so its total energy is kinetic energy. We then have $1/2mv^2 = 10 \Rightarrow v^2 = (10)(2)/10 = 2 \Rightarrow v = \sqrt{2}$ m/s.

31. E

This question describes the essence of Newton's third law: action equals reaction. Object A exerts a force on object B, and object B exerts an equal and opposite force on object A. The point, though, is that the only force on object B is the force due to A. The reaction force is not on B but on A.

32. A

To determine the units of x, we simply solve for x using the given equation. We then have $x = \frac{Fd}{V\eta}$. Substituting in the units of all the quantities, $x = \frac{(N)(m)}{(m/s)(N\text{–}s/m^2)} = m^2$. Thus, x has the units of area.

33. B

The equation describing the travel distance of the train is $d = 1/2at^2$. Given a distance of D and a time of T, we have $a = 2D/T^2$. To determine the time to travel half this distance, use

$(D/2) = 1/2at^2 = 1/2[2D/T^2]t^2 \Rightarrow t^2 = T^2/2 \Rightarrow t = T/\sqrt{2}$.

34. E

Given is constant deceleration, $v^2 = v_o^2 + 2ad$, where v is the velocity after a distance d. The initial velocity is v_o, and the acceleration is a. In this case the acceleration is negative, the initial velocity is v, and the velocity after a distance d is 0. Thus the equation becomes $0 = v^2 - 2ad$, where a is the magnitude of the deceleration. Solving for d, we have $d = v^2/2a$. If we keep a constant but double the speed, the stopping distance increases by a factor of 4.

35. D

The weight of something is simply the force that is exerted on it by gravity: $W = F_{grav} = mg$, where m is the mass and g the gravitational acceleration. Because we are given the weight, we do not need to do any calculation: A weight of 800 N means that the Earth exerts a force of 800 N on the person. According to Newton's third law, the person exerts an equal and opposite force on the Earth.
Thus, the person exerts a force of 800 N on the Earth.

36. C

A scale measures as a force equal in magnitude but opposite in direction to the normal force. The normal force and gravity are the two opposing forces and provide for the 1m/s^2 downward acceleration the person is undergoing: mg – scale reading = ma ⇒ 800 – scale reading = m (1). The mass m can be determined using the person's weight when at rest: m(10) = 800. Hence m = 80 kg. Thus, 800 – scale reading = 80 ⇒ scale reading = 800 – 80 = 720.

37. A

The gravitational force on an object is $F = GMm/r^2$, where M is the Earth's mass, m the mass of the object, G the gravitational constant, and r the distance from the object to the center of the Earth. First notice that r is equal to the radius of Earth when the object is at the surface. Then we have r equal to twice the radius of the Earth when the object is at a distance of one Earth radius above the surface. From the equation for the gravitational force, we see that doubling the distance r results in a force one-quarter as large as the original. Thus, the force at the height of one Earth radius above the surface is 100/4 = 25 N.

38. E

Let us examine each of the three quantities. The magnitude of torque is rFsinθ, where F is the magnitude of the force exerted, r is the distance between the axis of rotation and the point where the force is exerted, and θ is the angle between the two previous quantities. As a trigonometric function, sinθ is dimensionless, r has the units of length, and F has the units of force, which in the SI system would be N, or kg•m/s^2 (i.e., mass•length/time^2). Multiplying the quantities, we can determine that torque has units of length × (mass•length/time^2) = mass•length^2/time^2. Item I must therefore be among the items in our answer choice. Work is force × distance. Distance is the same as length, and so we see that work can be expressed in the same units as torque. Item II is also correct. Work and energy have the same units (because work is a way of changing the energy of a system), and so the two quantities have to be dimensionally equivalent. Item III has to be correct also. In other words, all three quantities, torque, work, and energy, can be expressed dimensionally as $M \cdot L^2/T^2$.

39. B

There are two forces on the mass as it executes its motion: the centripetal force and the friction force. In the direction of vector A is the centripetal force, provided by the tension in the rope connecting to the mass. The friction force acts in the direction opposite to the motion of the object. At the given position, the direction of motion is in the direction of vector C. Thus, the frictional force will be parallel to vector D. The net force on the mass is the vector sum of these two forces and is thus in the general direction of vector B.

40. D

To find power, let's recall that power = $\frac{\text{work}}{\text{time}}$ = $\frac{\text{(force)(distance)}}{\text{time}}$. Because $\frac{\text{distance}}{\text{time}}$ = speed, we have power = (force)(speed). Given that the force is the frictional force, the above equation is the rate at which energy is being drained from the system. To keep the mass moving with the same speed, this same power must be supplied to the mass. The frictional force is given by $\mu N = \mu mg = (0.2)(10)(10) = 20$ N. Therefore, power = $(20)(2) = 40$ watts.

Answers and Explanations

1. C	11. B	21. B	31. A	41. D
2. E	12. E	22. C	32. D	42. B
3. A	13. D	23. D	33. E	43. A
4. A	14. B	24. E	34. A	44. E
5. E	15. D	25. A	35. C	45. C
6. C	16. E	26. B	36. E	46. B
7. D	17. D	27. D	37. C	47. B
8. D	18. D	28. A	38. E	48. A
9. C	19. A	29. D	39. B	49. D
10. C	20. C	30. B	40. A	50. B

1. C

The question stem states that the ratio of boys to girls is $\frac{5}{3}$, so for every 8 students, there are 3 girls. We can express this as the fraction $\frac{3 \text{ girls}}{8 \text{ students}}$.

If there are 120 students, then the number of girls $= 120 \text{ students} \times \frac{3 \text{ girls}}{8 \text{ students}} = 45$ girls.

2. E

In order to solve verbal math problems, you have to change the words into math:

What percent	of	$\sqrt{0.005}$	is	$\sqrt{2}$?
↓	↓	↓	=	↓
y%	×	$\sqrt{0.005}$	=	$\sqrt{2}$?

$$y = \frac{\sqrt{2}}{\sqrt{0.005}} \times 100\%$$

When we divide two radicals, we can divide the numbers under one radical sign.

$$x = \sqrt{\frac{2}{0.005}} \times 100\% = \sqrt{\frac{2{,}000}{5}} \times 100\% =$$

$$\sqrt{400} \times 100\% = 20 \times 100\%$$

$y = 2{,}000\%$, choice (E).

3. A

We can solve for the length of the side of the room in inches as it would appear on the blueprint by using the conversion given in the question stem:

$$\frac{3\frac{1}{8} \text{ blueprint in.}}{125 \text{ feet}} = \frac{\frac{25}{8} \text{ in.}}{125 \text{ feet}} = \frac{\frac{1}{8}}{5} = \frac{1 \text{ in.}}{40 \text{ feet}}.$$

Converting the length of the room, we get

$$\frac{20 \text{ ft} \times 1 \text{ in.}}{40 \text{ feet}} = \frac{1}{2} \text{ in.}$$

The area is then $\frac{1}{2} \times \frac{1}{2} = \frac{1}{4} \text{ in}^2$.

4. A

Since the dimensions of the floor are given in feet, we'll change all the costs to dollars per square foot. The area of the floor $= 10 \times 15 = 150 \text{ ft}^2$.

One firm:

$$\text{Cost} = 150 \text{ ft}^2 \times \$0.80/\text{ft}^2 = 150 \times \frac{4}{5}$$
$$= 30 \times 4 = \$120$$

Another firm:

$$\text{Cost} = \frac{\$7.50}{\text{yd}^2} \times \frac{1 \text{ yd}^2}{9 \text{ ft}^2} \times 150 \text{ ft}^2 = \frac{7.50}{3} \times 50$$
$$= 2.50 \times 50 = \$125$$

The possible savings is $\$125 - \$120 = \$5$.

5. E

We can solve this question using dimensional analysis. We take the expression we are given and multiply it by conversion fractions to cancel out units until we are left with the units we are looking for:

$$\frac{60 \text{ miles}}{\text{hour}} \times \frac{5{,}280 \text{ feet}}{1 \text{ mile}} \times \frac{1 \text{ hour}}{60 \text{ min}} \times \frac{1 \text{ min}}{60 \text{ sec}}$$
$$= \frac{(60)(5{,}280)}{3{,}600} = \frac{88 \text{ ft}}{\text{sec}}$$

21. B

Since the circumference and the radius of a circle are directly proportional ($C = 2\pi r$), the percent increase will be the same for both. If the circumference increases by 20%, then the radius increases by 20%. If we let the radius of the original circle be 5, the radius of the new circle is $5 + (20\% \text{ of } 5) = 5 + 1 = 6$.

The area of a circle is proportional to the square of the radius ($A = \pi r^2$). The area of the original circle $= \pi 5^2 = 25\pi$. The area of the new circle $= \pi 6^2 = 36\pi$.

Therefore,

$$\text{the \% increase} = \frac{\text{amount of increase}}{\text{original amount}} \times 100\%$$

$$= \frac{36\pi - 25\pi}{25\pi} \times 100\% = \frac{11}{25} \times 100\% = 44\%$$

22. C

Pick numbers since you are given percents and asked for percents.

Volume of cylinder = area of base × height

Let radius of the first cylinder = 5.

It is increased by 20%. New radius $= 5 + \frac{1}{5}(5) = 6$

Let the height of the first cylinder = 6.

It is decreased by $16\frac{2}{3}\%$. New height $= 6 - \frac{1}{6}(6) = 5$

A cylinder has a circular base. Therefore,

Volume of first cylinder $= \pi(5)^2 \times 6 = 25\pi \times 6 = 150\pi$

Volume of new cylinder $= \pi(6)^2 \times 5 = 36\pi \times 5 = 180\pi$

$$\text{\% increase in volume} = \frac{\text{increase in volume}}{\text{original volume}}$$

$$= \frac{30\pi}{150\pi} = \frac{1}{5} = 20\%$$

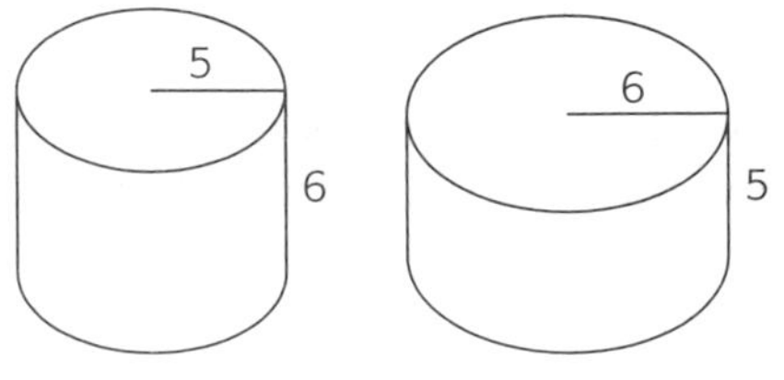

23. D

When the numerator is doubled, the value of the fraction is doubled. When the denominator is halved, the value of the fraction is again doubled. The net result is quadrupling (multiplying by 4), choice (D).

24. E

Let the width be 10 (for the rectangle). Therefore, the length is 20 and the perimeter is $2(10 + 20) = 60$. The perimeter of the square is also 60, which gives a side of 15. The area of the rectangle is $(10)(20) = 200$. The area of the square is $(15)(15) = 225$. The ratio = 200:225 = 40:45 = 8:9

25. A

No tax is paid on the first $50,000. A tax of 6% is paid on the remaining $100,000. The amount of tax = 6% Δ $100,000 = $6,000, choice (A).

26. B

In a 60-foot fence, there are forty $1\frac{1}{2}$ foot sections (distance between pickets). Forty sections are made by 41 pickets. If the fence is extended to 80 feet without adding any pickets, there are still 41 pickets and 40 sections formed. Each section is $\frac{80}{40}$ or 2 ft.

27. D

No matter the shape of the pool, a given amount of water will take up the same volume. The volume of a swimming pool in the shape of a rectangular solid equals length × width × height.

Let h = the height the water would reach in the second pool.

$$(24 \text{ feet})(16 \text{ feet})(1 \text{ foot}) = (20 \text{ feet})(8 \text{ feet})(h \text{ feet})$$

After canceling like factors:

$$12 \text{ feet}^2 = 5h \text{ feet}^2;\ h = 2\frac{2}{5} \text{ feet}$$

28. A

$x + y + 3z = 7;\ 3x + 6y + 6z = 8$

We want to solve for $(y - z)$, so we first have to eliminate x. Multiply the first equation by 3 and subtract it from the second equation.

$$\begin{aligned} 3x + 6y + 6z &= 8 \\ -(3x + 3y + 9z) &= -21 \\ 3y - 3z &= -13 \\ \hline 3(y - z) &= -13 \\ 3(y - z) &= -13 \\ y - z &= -\frac{13}{3} \end{aligned}$$

29. D

B will have his maximum number of marbles when the others (A and C) have their minimum number according to the constraints. Since C has fewer than both A and B, his minimum is 0. Therefore, A and B have 24 together. If A is to have more than B and B is to have a maximum, A will have 13 and B will have 11.

30. B

The graph of a line has to satisfy the equation $y = mx + b$, where m is the slope and b is the y-intercept. If two lines are perpendicular to each other, then the slope of one line is the negative inverse of the other. We are told that line ℓ is perpendicular to the line $y = -\frac{1}{5}x$, so the slope of ℓ must equal 5. In $y = mx + b$, we know that m must equal 5. To find b, we substitute the point (3, −10) into the equation. We are given that the point (3, −10) is on the line, so $x = 3$ and $y = -10$ must satisfy the equation $y = 5x + b$. By substituting $x = 3$ and $y = -10$, we get

$$\begin{aligned} y &= mx + b \\ y &= 5x + b \\ -10 &= 5\,(3) + b \\ -10 &= 15 + b \\ -10 - 15 &= b \\ -25 &= b \end{aligned}$$

Now we know that $m = 5$ and $b = -25$, so our equation is $y = 5x - 25$, which is choice (B).

31. A

Using a simple mnemonic and some common sense, this question can be answered quickly. Recalling the mnemonic SOH CAH TOA, the $\sin\theta = \frac{\text{opposite}}{\text{hypotenuse}}$ and $\cos\theta = \frac{\text{adjecent}}{\text{hypotenuse}}$. From this, it is easy to see that the functions sine and cosine are not inversely related.
The true relationship is $\cos\theta = \sin(90 - \theta)$.
Therefore the $\cos 59° = \sin 31°$.

If you were not sure of the relationship between the sine and cosine functions, you can still get this question correct by eliminating answer choices. Answer choices (B) and (D) can easily be eliminated—the only cosine function that can equal the cos 59° is the cos 59°. Answer choice (C) can also be eliminated—since the functions of sine and cosine are different, the cosine of an angle cannot equal the sine of the same angle.

32. D

Choice (D) happens to be a rearrangement of the trigonometric identity:

$$\sin^2 x + \cos^2 x = 1$$

This is true for all values of x. If you didn't know this identity—and you aren't required to memorize identities for the OAT—you could easily solve this problem by picking values for x, plugging them in, and seeing which choice works. We'll pick a value between 0 and $\frac{\pi}{2}$. How about $\frac{\pi}{4}$? Remember that $\frac{\pi}{4} = 45°$.

(A)
$$\begin{aligned} \sin\frac{\pi}{4} &= \cos^2\frac{\pi}{4} + 1 \\ \frac{\sqrt{2}}{2} &= \left(\frac{\sqrt{2}}{2}\right)^2 + 1 \\ \frac{\sqrt{2}}{2} &= \frac{2}{4} + 1 \\ \frac{\sqrt{2}}{2} &= 1.5 \qquad \text{No.} \end{aligned}$$

(B)
$$\begin{aligned} \tan\frac{\pi}{4} &= \left(\sin\frac{\pi}{4}\right)\left(\cos\frac{\pi}{4}\right) \\ 1 &= \left(\frac{\sqrt{2}}{2}\right)\left(\frac{\sqrt{2}}{2}\right) \\ 1 &= \frac{2}{4} \\ 1 &= 0.5 \qquad \text{No.} \end{aligned}$$

(C) $\tan\frac{\pi}{4} = \dfrac{\cos\frac{\pi}{4}}{\sin\frac{\pi}{4}}$

$1 = \dfrac{\frac{\sqrt{2}}{2}}{\frac{\sqrt{2}}{2}}$

$1 = 1$ Possible . . .

(D) $\sin^2\frac{\pi}{4} = 1 - \cos^2\frac{\pi}{4}$

$\left(\frac{\sqrt{2}}{2}\right)^2 = 1 - \left(\frac{\sqrt{2}}{2}\right)^2$

$\frac{2}{4} = 1 - \frac{2}{4}$

$0.5 = 0.5$ Possible . . .

(E) $\sin\frac{\pi}{4} = \dfrac{1}{\cos\frac{\pi}{4}}$

$\frac{\sqrt{2}}{2} = \dfrac{1}{\frac{\sqrt{2}}{2}}$

$\frac{\sqrt{2}}{2} = \frac{2}{\sqrt{2}}$ No.

So now let's check (C) and (D) with another value. We'll use $\frac{\pi}{6}$ or 30°.

(C) $\tan\frac{\pi}{6} = \dfrac{\cos\frac{\pi}{6}}{\sin\frac{\pi}{6}}$

$\frac{1}{\sqrt{3}} = \dfrac{\frac{\sqrt{3}}{2}}{\frac{1}{2}}$

$\frac{1}{\sqrt{3}} = \sqrt{3}$ No.

Therefore, (D) must be the correct answer.

33. E

Let's look at each term of the expression $(x^2 - 6)(y + 7)$ separately. In evaluating the term $x^2 - 6$, notice that x is being squared, so the term is largest when the absolute value for x is largest. Since x ranges from –4 to 2, the largest value will be when $x = -4$. In evaluating the value for y, the term $y + 7$ will be greatest when y is greatest. Since y ranges from 3 to 5, the largest value will be when $y = 5$.

34. A

We are given that ΔABC is equilateral, which means that each leg of the triangle is equal. The altitude of an equilateral triangle bisects the base, so $BD = CD = \frac{1}{2}AB$. Labeling the legs as shown, we can use the Pythagorean theorem to solve for the length of AB.

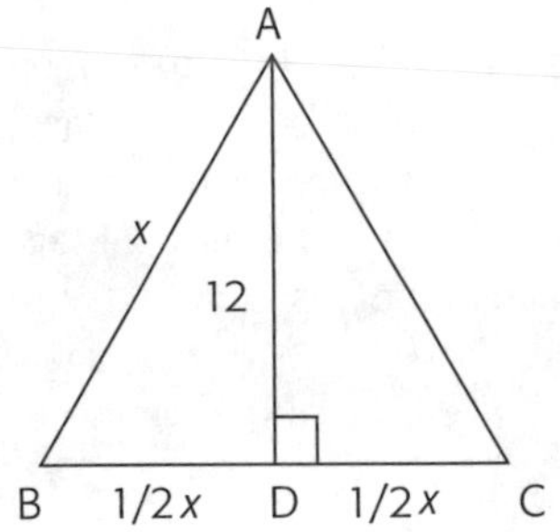

$\left(\frac{1}{2}x\right)^2 + 12^2 = x^2$

$\frac{1}{4}x^2 + 144 = x^2$

$x^2 - \frac{1}{4}x^2 = 144$

$\frac{3}{4}x^2 = 144$

$x^2 = 144 \times \frac{4}{3}$

$x^2 = 48 \times 4$

$x = \sqrt{192} = 8\sqrt{3}$

35. C

This is a simple arithmetic problem, as long as you remember the rules for handling exponents and scientific notation;

$$\frac{6 \times 10^{-4}}{30 \times 10^{5}} = \frac{6}{30} \times 10^{-9}$$
$$= \frac{1}{5} \times 10^{-9}$$
$$= 0.2 \times 10^{-9}$$
$$= 2 \times 10^{-10}$$

36. E

The number of different ways to arrange x number of objects, given no repeats, is $x!$, the factorial of x.
The number of ways to arrange 5 students equals $5! = 5 \times 4 \times 3 \times 2 \times 1 = 120$.

37. C

The probability of two independent events occurring together is the product of their individual probabilities. The probability of selecting the first marble is $\frac{5}{11}$, and the probability of selecting the second marble is $\frac{4}{10}$ (don't forget to subtract 1 since you are not putting the second one back!). The probability of drawing two purple marbles is then $\frac{5}{11} \times \frac{4}{10} = \frac{20}{110} = \frac{2}{11}$.

38. E

To solve verbal math problems, you have to convert words into equations:

(A) "$34 in nickels, dimes, and quarters" is expressed as $\$34 = (n)\left(\frac{1}{20}\right) + (d)\left(\frac{1}{10}\right) + (q)\left(\frac{1}{4}\right)$

where

n = # of nickels, which is one-twentieth of a dollar

d = # of dimes, which is one-tenth of a dollar

q = # of quarters, which is one-fourth of a dollar

(B) "3 times as many dimes as quarters" is expressed as $3q = d$.

(C) "2 times as many nickels as dimes" is expressed as $n = 2d$.

Substituting the equations for q and n (from B and C above) into the equation from A, and then solving for d, we get

$$\$34 = (n)\left(\frac{1}{20}\right) + (d)\left(\frac{1}{10}\right) + (q)\left(\frac{1}{4}\right)$$
$$\$34 = (2d)\left(\frac{1}{20}\right) + (d)\left(\frac{1}{10}\right) + \left(\frac{d}{3}\right)\left(\frac{1}{4}\right)$$
$$= \frac{d}{10} + \frac{d}{10} + \frac{d}{12}$$
$$= \frac{2d}{10} + \frac{d}{12}$$
$$= \frac{24d}{120} + \frac{10d}{120}$$
$$34 = \frac{34d}{120}$$
$$d = 120$$

39. B

To find the distance between two points on an x-y axis, plot the points and construct a right triangle. The distance between the points is measured by the hypotenuse of the right triangle (see figure). The length of legs are measured using the graph, and the hypotenuse is calculated using the Pythagorean theorem ($a^2 + b^2 = c^2$). Plugging in the lengths of the legs of the triangle in this example yields $9^2 + 12^2 = c^2$. Notice that these values are the 3-4-5 triple multiplied by 3, so the hypotenuse = 15.

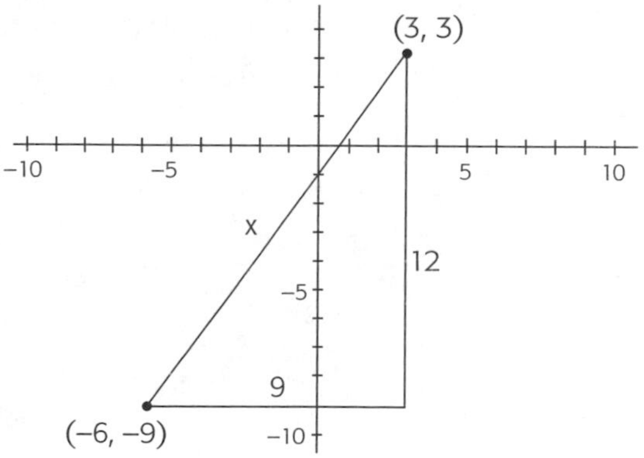

40. A

The average of a set of numbers equals $\frac{\text{sum of the numbers}}{\text{number of items}}$.
The average of the given set of numbers

$= \frac{3 + 5 + 5 + 11 + 13}{5} = \frac{37}{5} = 7\frac{2}{5}$.

41. D

Given the numerical coefficients, for all the terms to be equivalent, the variables would have to be in the following order: *y* is the smallest (because it has the highest numerical coefficient), *z* is larger than *y*, and finally *x* is the largest (because its numerical coefficient is the smallest).

42. B

$\cos 45° = \sin 45° = \frac{\sqrt{2}}{2}$

43. A

1, 2, 5, 10, 13, 26, 65, and 130 are the integers that can replace *x* in the given equation and still give an integer.

44. E

The best option here would be to backsolve. Let's take (A). If the wire is 24 m, then each part would have to 8 m. Given that the question says the resulting segments of 4, 6, and 8 parts from the three parts of 8 have to be of integral length (as in the number has to be an integer), we can see that (A) is wrong (because $\frac{8}{6}$ is not an integer).

Going through all the choices gives us (E) as the answer. A 72-m wire can be divided into three equal parts of 24 m, each of which can give us integral lengths when further divided into 4, 6, and 8 parts each ($\frac{24}{2}$, $\frac{24}{6}$, and $\frac{24}{8}$ are all integers).

45. C

Average = sum/total number of parts.
The sum = (n) + (n + 1) + (n + 2) + (n + 3) =
4n + 6. The total number of parts here = 4.

Therefore, the average $= \frac{(4n + 6)}{4} = n + 1.5$.

46. B

For every 1 pound of tin, we need 3 pounds of copper to make the alloy. The simplest way to get the right answer would be to go through all the choices. (A) says 25 pounds of tin, which means we need 75 pounds of copper. Together, that only makes 100 pounds of the alloy, one-half the required amount. Therefore, the answer is (B).

47. B

The amount of alcohol in the 25-ounce solution =

$\left(\frac{20}{100}\right) \times 25 = 5$ ounces.

When the 50 ounces of water are added, the total volume now becomes 25 ounces (original) + 50 ounces = 75 ounces. Basically, the question is asking what % of this 75 ounces is alcohol (5 ounces)?

$\left(\frac{X}{100}\right) \times 75 = 5$

Solving for X gives us 6.67%, which is (B).

48. A

Using FOIL (firsts, outers, inners, and lasts), we get
$5 + \sqrt{20} \times \sqrt{20} - 4 = 1$.

49. D

(A), (B), (C), and (E) give 0.0675. Only (D) gives us 0.675.

50. B

Basically, we are asked to solve for *b* given the equation
$\frac{2}{3b} = 12c$.

Cross multiplying it out gives us $b = \frac{2}{36c}$, which can be simplified further to $\frac{1}{18c}$.

ANSWER SHEET

MARK ONE AND ONLY ONE ANSWER TO EACH QUESTION. BE SURE TO FILL IN COMPLETELY THE SPACE FOR YOUR INTENDED ANSWER CHOICE. IF YOU ERASE, DO SO COMPLETELY. MAKE NO STRAY MARKS.

RIGHT MARK: ● WRONG MARKS:

Survey of the Natural Sciences

1. A B C D E	11. A B C D E	21. A B C D E	31. A B C D E	41. A B C D E
2. A B C D E	12. A B C D E	22. A B C D E	32. A B C D E	42. A B C D E
3. A B C D E	13. A B C D E	23. A B C D E	33. A B C D E	43. A B C D E
4. A B C D E	14. A B C D E	24. A B C D E	34. A B C D E	44. A B C D E
5. A B C D E	15. A B C D E	25. A B C D E	35. A B C D E	45. A B C D E
6. A B C D E	16. A B C D E	26. A B C D E	36. A B C D E	46. A B C D E
7. A B C D E	17. A B C D E	27. A B C D E	37. A B C D E	47. A B C D E
8. A B C D E	18. A B C D E	28. A B C D E	38. A B C D E	48. A B C D E
9. A B C D E	19. A B C D E	29. A B C D E	39. A B C D E	49. A B C D E
10. A B C D E	20. A B C D E	30. A B C D E	40. A B C D E	50. A B C D E

51. A B C D E	61. A B C D E	71. A B C D E	81. A B C D E	91. A B C D E
52. A B C D E	62. A B C D E	72. A B C D E	82. A B C D E	92. A B C D E
53. A B C D E	63. A B C D E	73. A B C D E	83. A B C D E	93. A B C D E
54. A B C D E	64. A B C D E	74. A B C D E	84. A B C D E	94. A B C D E
55. A B C D E	65. A B C D E	75. A B C D E	85. A B C D E	95. A B C D E
56. A B C D E	66. A B C D E	76. A B C D E	86. A B C D E	96. A B C D E
57. A B C D E	67. A B C D E	77. A B C D E	87. A B C D E	97. A B C D E
58. A B C D E	68. A B C D E	78. A B C D E	88. A B C D E	98. A B C D E
59. A B C D E	69. A B C D E	79. A B C D E	89. A B C D E	99. A B C D E
60. A B C D E	70. A B C D E	80. A B C D E	90. A B C D E	100. A B C D E

Reading Comprehension

1. A B C D E	11. A B C D E	21. A B C D E	31. A B C D E	41. A B C D E
2. A B C D E	12. A B C D E	22. A B C D E	32. A B C D E	42. A B C D E
3. A B C D E	13. A B C D E	23. A B C D E	33. A B C D E	43. A B C D E
4. A B C D E	14. A B C D E	24. A B C D E	34. A B C D E	44. A B C D E
5. A B C D E	15. A B C D E	25. A B C D E	35. A B C D E	45. A B C D E
6. A B C D E	16. A B C D E	26. A B C D E	36. A B C D E	46. A B C D E
7. A B C D E	17. A B C D E	27. A B C D E	37. A B C D E	47. A B C D E
8. A B C D E	18. A B C D E	28. A B C D E	38. A B C D E	48. A B C D E
9. A B C D E	19. A B C D E	29. A B C D E	39. A B C D E	49. A B C D E
10. A B C D E	20. A B C D E	30. A B C D E	40. A B C D E	50. A B C D E

MARK ONE AND ONLY ONE ANSWER TO EACH QUESTION. BE SURE TO FILL IN COMPLETELY THE SPACE FOR YOUR INTENDED ANSWER CHOICE. IF YOU ERASE, DO SO COMPLETELY. MAKE NO STRAY MARKS.

RIGHT MARK: ⬬ WRONG MARKS: ⊘ ⊗ ⊙

Physics

1. Ⓐ Ⓑ Ⓒ Ⓓ Ⓔ	11. Ⓐ Ⓑ Ⓒ Ⓓ Ⓔ	21. Ⓐ Ⓑ Ⓒ Ⓓ Ⓔ	31. Ⓐ Ⓑ Ⓒ Ⓓ Ⓔ
2. Ⓐ Ⓑ Ⓒ Ⓓ Ⓔ	12. Ⓐ Ⓑ Ⓒ Ⓓ Ⓔ	22. Ⓐ Ⓑ Ⓒ Ⓓ Ⓔ	32. Ⓐ Ⓑ Ⓒ Ⓓ Ⓔ
3. Ⓐ Ⓑ Ⓒ Ⓓ Ⓔ	13. Ⓐ Ⓑ Ⓒ Ⓓ Ⓔ	23. Ⓐ Ⓑ Ⓒ Ⓓ Ⓔ	33. Ⓐ Ⓑ Ⓒ Ⓓ Ⓔ
4. Ⓐ Ⓑ Ⓒ Ⓓ Ⓔ	14. Ⓐ Ⓑ Ⓒ Ⓓ Ⓔ	24. Ⓐ Ⓑ Ⓒ Ⓓ Ⓔ	34. Ⓐ Ⓑ Ⓒ Ⓓ Ⓔ
5. Ⓐ Ⓑ Ⓒ Ⓓ Ⓔ	15. Ⓐ Ⓑ Ⓒ Ⓓ Ⓔ	25. Ⓐ Ⓑ Ⓒ Ⓓ Ⓔ	35. Ⓐ Ⓑ Ⓒ Ⓓ Ⓔ
6. Ⓐ Ⓑ Ⓒ Ⓓ Ⓔ	16. Ⓐ Ⓑ Ⓒ Ⓓ Ⓔ	26. Ⓐ Ⓑ Ⓒ Ⓓ Ⓔ	36. Ⓐ Ⓑ Ⓒ Ⓓ Ⓔ
7. Ⓐ Ⓑ Ⓒ Ⓓ Ⓔ	17. Ⓐ Ⓑ Ⓒ Ⓓ Ⓔ	27. Ⓐ Ⓑ Ⓒ Ⓓ Ⓔ	37. Ⓐ Ⓑ Ⓒ Ⓓ Ⓔ
8. Ⓐ Ⓑ Ⓒ Ⓓ Ⓔ	18. Ⓐ Ⓑ Ⓒ Ⓓ Ⓔ	28. Ⓐ Ⓑ Ⓒ Ⓓ Ⓔ	38. Ⓐ Ⓑ Ⓒ Ⓓ Ⓔ
9. Ⓐ Ⓑ Ⓒ Ⓓ Ⓔ	19. Ⓐ Ⓑ Ⓒ Ⓓ Ⓔ	29. Ⓐ Ⓑ Ⓒ Ⓓ Ⓔ	39. Ⓐ Ⓑ Ⓒ Ⓓ Ⓔ
10. Ⓐ Ⓑ Ⓒ Ⓓ Ⓔ	20. Ⓐ Ⓑ Ⓒ Ⓓ Ⓔ	30. Ⓐ Ⓑ Ⓒ Ⓓ Ⓔ	40. Ⓐ Ⓑ Ⓒ Ⓓ Ⓔ

Quantitative Reasoning

1. Ⓐ Ⓑ Ⓒ Ⓓ Ⓔ	11. Ⓐ Ⓑ Ⓒ Ⓓ Ⓔ	21. Ⓐ Ⓑ Ⓒ Ⓓ Ⓔ	31. Ⓐ Ⓑ Ⓒ Ⓓ Ⓔ	41. Ⓐ Ⓑ Ⓒ Ⓓ Ⓔ
2. Ⓐ Ⓑ Ⓒ Ⓓ Ⓔ	12. Ⓐ Ⓑ Ⓒ Ⓓ Ⓔ	22. Ⓐ Ⓑ Ⓒ Ⓓ Ⓔ	32. Ⓐ Ⓑ Ⓒ Ⓓ Ⓔ	42. Ⓐ Ⓑ Ⓒ Ⓓ Ⓔ
3. Ⓐ Ⓑ Ⓒ Ⓓ Ⓔ	13. Ⓐ Ⓑ Ⓒ Ⓓ Ⓔ	23. Ⓐ Ⓑ Ⓒ Ⓓ Ⓔ	33. Ⓐ Ⓑ Ⓒ Ⓓ Ⓔ	43. Ⓐ Ⓑ Ⓒ Ⓓ Ⓔ
4. Ⓐ Ⓑ Ⓒ Ⓓ Ⓔ	14. Ⓐ Ⓑ Ⓒ Ⓓ Ⓔ	24. Ⓐ Ⓑ Ⓒ Ⓓ Ⓔ	34. Ⓐ Ⓑ Ⓒ Ⓓ Ⓔ	44. Ⓐ Ⓑ Ⓒ Ⓓ Ⓔ
5. Ⓐ Ⓑ Ⓒ Ⓓ Ⓔ	15. Ⓐ Ⓑ Ⓒ Ⓓ Ⓔ	25. Ⓐ Ⓑ Ⓒ Ⓓ Ⓔ	35. Ⓐ Ⓑ Ⓒ Ⓓ Ⓔ	45. Ⓐ Ⓑ Ⓒ Ⓓ Ⓔ
6. Ⓐ Ⓑ Ⓒ Ⓓ Ⓔ	16. Ⓐ Ⓑ Ⓒ Ⓓ Ⓔ	26. Ⓐ Ⓑ Ⓒ Ⓓ Ⓔ	36. Ⓐ Ⓑ Ⓒ Ⓓ Ⓔ	46. Ⓐ Ⓑ Ⓒ Ⓓ Ⓔ
7. Ⓐ Ⓑ Ⓒ Ⓓ Ⓔ	17. Ⓐ Ⓑ Ⓒ Ⓓ Ⓔ	27. Ⓐ Ⓑ Ⓒ Ⓓ Ⓔ	37. Ⓐ Ⓑ Ⓒ Ⓓ Ⓔ	47. Ⓐ Ⓑ Ⓒ Ⓓ Ⓔ
8. Ⓐ Ⓑ Ⓒ Ⓓ Ⓔ	18. Ⓐ Ⓑ Ⓒ Ⓓ Ⓔ	28. Ⓐ Ⓑ Ⓒ Ⓓ Ⓔ	38. Ⓐ Ⓑ Ⓒ Ⓓ Ⓔ	48. Ⓐ Ⓑ Ⓒ Ⓓ Ⓔ
9. Ⓐ Ⓑ Ⓒ Ⓓ Ⓔ	19. Ⓐ Ⓑ Ⓒ Ⓓ Ⓔ	29. Ⓐ Ⓑ Ⓒ Ⓓ Ⓔ	39. Ⓐ Ⓑ Ⓒ Ⓓ Ⓔ	49. Ⓐ Ⓑ Ⓒ Ⓓ Ⓔ
10. Ⓐ Ⓑ Ⓒ Ⓓ Ⓔ	20. Ⓐ Ⓑ Ⓒ Ⓓ Ⓔ	30. Ⓐ Ⓑ Ⓒ Ⓓ Ⓔ	40. Ⓐ Ⓑ Ⓒ Ⓓ Ⓔ	50. Ⓐ Ⓑ Ⓒ Ⓓ Ⓔ

INSTRUCTIONS FOR TAKING THE PRACTICE TEST

Before taking the practice test, find a quiet place where you can work uninterrupted. Make sure you have a comfortable desk and several No. 2 pencils.

Use the answer grid provided to record your answers. You'll find the answer key and score conversion chart following the test.

The test consists of four sections: Survey of the Natural Sciences (90 minutes), Reading Comprehension (60 minutes), Physics (50 minutes), and Quantitative Reasoning (45 minutes). Remember, if you finish a section early, you may review any questions within that section, but you may not go back or forward a section.

Good luck.

PERIODIC TABLE OF THE ELEMENTS

1 **H** 1.0																	2 **He** 4.0
3 **Li** 6.9	4 **Be** 9.0											5 **B** 10.8	6 **C** 12.0	7 **N** 14.0	8 **O** 16.0	9 **F** 19.0	10 **Ne** 20.2
11 **Na** 23.0	12 **Mg** 24.3											13 **Al** 27.0	14 **Si** 28.1	15 **P** 31.0	16 **S** 32.1	17 **Cl** 35.5	18 **Ar** 39.9
19 **K** 39.1	20 **Ca** 40.1	21 **Sc** 45.0	22 **Ti** 47.9	23 **V** 50.9	24 **Cr** 52.0	25 **Mn** 54.9	26 **Fe** 55.8	27 **Co** 58.9	28 **Ni** 58.7	29 **Cu** 63.5	30 **Zn** 65.4	31 **Ga** 69.7	32 **Ge** 72.6	33 **As** 74.9	34 **Se** 79.0	35 **Br** 79.9	36 **Kr** 83.8
37 **Rb** 85.5	38 **Sr** 87.6	39 **Y** 88.9	40 **Zr** 91.2	41 **Nb** 92.9	42 **Mo** 95.9	43 **Tc** (98)	44 **Ru** 101.1	45 **Rh** 102.9	46 **Pd** 106.4	47 **Ag** 107.9	48 **Cd** 112.4	49 **In** 114.8	50 **Sn** 118.7	51 **Sb** 121.8	52 **Te** 127.6	53 **I** 126.9	54 **Xe** 131.3
55 **Cs** 132.9	56 **Ba** 137.3	57 **La** * 138.9	72 **Hf** 178.5	73 **Ta** 180.9	74 **W** 183.9	75 **Re** 186.2	76 **Os** 190.2	77 **Ir** 192.2	78 **Pt** 195.1	79 **Au** 197.0	80 **Hg** 200.6	81 **Tl** 204.4	82 **Pb** 207.2	83 **Bi** 209.0	84 **Po** (209)	85 **At** (210)	86 **Rn** (222)
87 **Fr** (223)	88 **Ra** 226.0	89 **Ac** † 227.0	104 **Rf** (261)	105 **Db** (262)	106 **Sg** (263)	107 **Bh** (264)	108 **Hs** (269)	109 **Mt** (268)	110 **Ds** (269)	111 **Rg** (272)	112 **Uub** (277)	113 **Uut** (284)	114 **Uug** (289)	115 **Uup** (288)	116 **Uuh** (292)	117 **Uus** (291)	118 **Uuo** (293)

*	58 **Ce** 140.1	59 **Pr** 140.9	60 **Nd** 144.2	61 **Pm** (145)	62 **Sm** 150.4	63 **Eu** 152.0	64 **Gd** 157.3	65 **Tb** 158.9	66 **Dy** 162.5	67 **Ho** 164.9	68 **Er** 167.3	69 **Tm** 168.9	70 **Yb** 173.0	71 **Lu** 175.0
†	90 **Th** 232.0	91 **Pa** (231)	92 **U** 238.0	93 **Np** (237)	94 **Pu** (244)	95 **Am** (243)	96 **Cm** (247)	97 **Bk** (247)	98 **Cf** (251)	99 **Es** (252)	100 **Fm** (257)	101 **Md** (258)	102 **No** (259)	103 **Lr** (260)

Full-Length Practice Test II

SURVEY OF THE NATURAL SCIENCES

100 questions–90 minutes

Directions: This examination is composed of 100 items: Biology (1–40), General Chemistry (41–70), and Organic Chemistry (71–100). Choose the best answer for each question from the five choices provided

1. Which of the following might appear in an F_2 generation but could not appear in an F_1 generation if one parent is homozygous dominant and the other is homozygous recessive?

   (A) Heterozygous genotype
   (B) Dominant phenotype
   (C) Recessive phenotype
   (D) All of the above
   (E) None of the above

2. Which of the following is not a distinction between plants and animals?

   (A) Plants contain cell walls made of cellulose.
   (B) Plants have intermediate larval stages.
   (C) Plants are extensively branched.
   (D) Animals are generally heterotrophic and motile.
   (E) All of the above

3. Ectoderm : endoderm:

   (A) Heart : stomach
   (B) Retina : lungs
   (C) Skeletal muscles : liver
   (D) Skin : stomach muscle
   (E) Taste buds : uterus

4. An organism is heterozygous with respect to three pairs of genes, namely Aa, Bb, and Cc. How many different types of gametes can be formed?

   (A) 2
   (B) 4
   (C) 6
   (D) 8
   (E) 9

5. Breeding animals of close genotypes or phenotypes is known as

   (A) inbreeding.
   (B) hybridization.
   (C) cross-breeding.
   (D) selective breeding.
   (E) test breeding.

6. $CO_2 + H_2O \rightarrow C_6H_{12}O_6 + O_2$
   The above reaction is catalyzed by

   (A) light.
   (B) ADP.
   (C) CO_2.
   (D) chlorophyll.
   (E) None of the above

GO ON TO THE NEXT PAGE

7. The membrane that functions in respiration in the embryo is the
   (A) amnion.
   (B) allantois.
   (C) chorion.
   (D) umbilical cord.
   (E) yolk sac.

8. A process that CANNOT take place in haploid cells is
   (A) mitosis.
   (B) meiosis.
   (C) cell division.
   (D) growth.
   (E) digestion.

9. The Krebs cycle involves
   (A) formation of NAD.
   (B) regeneration of oxaloacetic acid.
   (C) transamination.
   (D) breaking of peptide bonds.
   (E) glycogen formation.

10. Which is CORRECTLY associated?
   (A) RNA : thymine
   (B) DNA : uracil
   (C) RNA : replication
   (D) mRNA : picks up amino acids
   (E) RNA : ribose sugar

11. Enzymes
   (A) are carbohydrates.
   (B) work best at pH greater than 8.
   (C) always require a coenzyme.
   (D) are necessary in respiration.
   (E) are changed during a reaction.

12. A B C D

   If the diagram above represents genes on a chromosome, which genes would have the highest frequency of crossover?
   (A) A and B
   (B) A and D
   (C) B and C
   (D) B and D
   (E) The frequencies are the same for all crossovers.

13. What is the best evidence that genes control synthesis of proteins?
   (A) Proteins are macromolecules.
   (B) RNA directs amino acid synthesis.
   (C) Amino acid sequence of polypeptides is changed by gene mutation.
   (D) DNA serves as a template for RNA.
   (E) mRNA is found in the ribosome.

14. The different appearance of the rough endoplasmic reticulum compared to the smooth endoplasmic reticulum is due to the presence of
   (A) lysosomes.
   (B) ribosomes.
   (C) mitochondria.
   (D) Golgi apparati.
   (E) histones.

15. In humans, the site of fertilization is the
   (A) ovary.
   (B) fallopian tube.
   (C) uterus.
   (D) cervix.
   (E) vagina.

GO ON TO THE NEXT PAGE

16. Which of the following is found in eukaryotes but not prokaryotes?
    (A) Ribosomal RNA
    (B) Plasma membrane
    (C) Nuclear membrane
    (D) Ribosomes
    (E) None of the above

17. A totipotent cell
    (A) has 100% of its developmental potential.
    (B) has limited developmental potential.
    (C) has reached complete development.
    (D) can develop into any organism.
    (E) always forms a unicellular organism.

18. The hypothesis that chloroplasts and mitochondria were originally prokaryotic organisms living within eukaryotic hosts is supported by the fact that mitochondria and chloroplasts
    (A) possess protein synthetic capability.
    (B) possess genetic material.
    (C) possess plasma membrane.
    (D) possess characteristic ribosomes.
    (E) All of the above

19. The site of storage and maturation of sperm is the
    (A) seminiferous tubule.
    (B) seminal vesicle.
    (C) vas deferens.
    (D) epididymis.
    (E) prostate.

20. During the process of oxidative phosphorylation, oxygen serves as
    (A) the initial acceptor of H electrons.
    (B) the final acceptor of H electrons.
    (C) a high-energy intermediate.
    (D) a phosphorylating agent.
    (E) a reducing agent.

21. From which germ layer do the kidneys form?
    (A) Ectoderm
    (B) Mesoderm
    (C) Endoderm
    (D) Ectoderm and mesoderm
    (E) Mesoderm and endoderm

22. As a consequence of gastrulation, the embryo possesses
    (A) an archenteron.
    (B) a blastopore.
    (C) a blastocoel.
    (D) Two of the above
    (E) All of the above

23. Neurulation is induced by cells of the
    (A) archenteron.
    (B) notochord.
    (C) endodermal layer.
    (D) neural ectoderm.
    (E) neural crest.

24. Which of the following statements regarding photosynthesis is NOT true?
    (A) The light cycle occurs only during exposure to light.
    (B) The dark cycle occurs only in the absence of light.
    (C) During the light cycle, ATP is produced.
    (D) During the dark cycle, sugars are produced.
    (E) Red and blue light are optimal for photosynthetic function.

GO ON TO THE NEXT PAGE

25. Which statement about the blastula stage of embryonic development is FALSE?

(A) It consists of a solid ball of cells.
(B) It contains a fluid-filled center called the blastocoel.
(C) It is the stage of development that precedes the gastrula.
(D) It is a more advanced stage than a morula.
(E) It is a less advanced stage than a neurula.

26. Which of the following foods contains the greatest amount of energy/gram?

(A) Sugar
(B) Starch
(C) Fat
(D) Protein
(E) Vitamins

27. The tRNA code for the amino acid valine is AAC. What is the mRNA code for valine?

(A) TTG
(B) GGU
(C) CCA
(D) CCG
(E) UUG

28. The source of oxygen given off in photosynthesis is

(A) water.
(B) carbon dioxide.
(C) glucose.
(D) starch.
(E) chlorophyll.

29. Laboratory mice are to be classified based on genes A, B, and C. How many genetically distinct offspring can be produced from a cross of an AaBbCc individual with an AaBBCc individual?

(A) 12
(B) 16
(C) 32
(D) 48
(E) 64

30. The BEST description of identical twins is

(A) twins of the same gender.
(B) twins from a single egg.
(C) twins from two eggs that have been fertilized by the same sperm.
(D) twins from two eggs fertilized by two separate sperm.
(E) twins from a single egg fertilized by two separate sperm.

31. The first major part of the photosynthetic process involves

(A) the conversion of water and carbon dioxide into starch and oxygen.
(B) the conversion of sugar into water and CO_2.
(C) the splitting of water into oxygen, hydrogen, and electrons.
(D) the changing of CO_2 into a bicarbonate ion.
(E) the splitting of CO_2 into carbon, oxygen, and an electron.

32. The ABO human blood groups are inherited through a system of

(A) multiple alleles.
(B) dihybrid crosses.
(C) recessive alleles.
(D) independent assortments.
(E) spontaneous mutations.

GO ON TO THE NEXT PAGE

33. Which of the following occurs in the cell nucleus?
    (A) RNA synthesis
    (B) Protein synthesis
    (C) DNA synthesis
    (D) A and C
    (E) A, B, and C

34. The gene for red-green color blindness is recessive and located on the X chromosome. If a man suffering from red-green color blindness had children with an unaffected woman, how would their children be affected?
    (A) 50% of the females would be carriers, 100% of the males would be affected.
    (B) 100% of the females would be normal, 50% of the males would be affected.
    (C) 100% of the females would be carriers, 100% of the males would be normal.
    (D) 50% of the females would be affected, 100% of the males would be affected.
    (E) 100% of the females would be normal, 50% of the males would be carriers.

35. A mutation in a gene in a somatic cell is deleterious because
    (A) it will affect gamete formation.
    (B) it will be dominant.
    (C) it may be passed on to subsequent generations.
    (D) it may lead to a tumor in that tissue.
    (E) None of the above

36. A single nondisjunction may cause all of the following except
    (A) spontaneous miscarriage of the fetus.
    (B) 47 chromosomes.
    (C) 45 chromosomes.
    (D) congenital diseases such as Down syndrome.
    (E) breakage near the centromere.

37. Which of the following is FALSE regarding DNA replication?
    (A) DNA replication is semiconservative.
    (B) DNA replication occurs during prophase.
    (C) Okasaki fragments are formed.
    (D) Purines bind to pyrimidines.
    (E) None of the above

38. Red is dominant over white in a certain flower. To test whether a red offspring is homozygous or heterozygous in this flower
    (A) cross it with a red plant that had a white parent.
    (B) cross it with a red plant that had two red parents.
    (C) cross it with a white plant.
    (D) Two of the above will work.
    (E) None of the above will work.

39. Blood types A and B are dominant over type O. If a male with genotype AO marries a female with genotype AB, which of the following types is impossible for a first-generation child?
    (A) Type B
    (B) Type A
    (C) Type O
    (D) Type AB
    (E) All blood types are possible.

40. If one-twelfth of the males in a population are red-green color blind, what fraction of the females from that population are red-green color blind?
    (A) $\frac{1}{6}$
    (B) $\frac{1}{12}$
    (C) $\frac{1}{48}$
    (D) $\frac{1}{144}$
    (E) No females will have color blindness because it is sex-linked.

GO ON TO THE NEXT PAGE

41. A gaseous compound consists of element X (atomic weight = 12) and element Y (atomic weight = 1). Its empirical formula is XY_2, and its density is 1.25 g/L at STP. Its molecular formula is

(A) XY.

(B) XY_2.

(C) X_2Y_2.

(D) X_2Y_4.

(E) X_4Y_8.

42. How many grams of O_2 are necessary to oxidize 88 g of C_3H_8 to CO_2 and H_2O? (Atomic weights: C = 12, H = 1, O = 16)

(A) 32 g

(B) 64 g

(C) 120 g

(D) 160 g

(E) 320 g

43. What is the approximate mass of 1.204×10^{24} bromine atoms?

(A) 79.9 g

(B) 159.8 g

(C) 160.2 g

(D) 239.7 g

(E) 340.4 g

44. Element X has atomic number 16 and atomic weight 32. How many electrons are present in the ion X^{2-}?

(A) 2

(B) 14

(C) 16

(D) 18

(E) 32

45. Chlorophyll, the green pigment involved in photosynthesis, consists of 2.4312% Mg by mass. If you are given a 100-g sample of chlorophyll, how many Mg atoms will it contain? (Atomic weight of Mg: 24.312 g/mol)

(A) 6.02×10^{22}

(B) 6.02×10^{23}

(C) 6.02×10^{24}

(D) 6.02×10^{25}

(E) None of the above

46. If 88 g of C_3H_8 and 160 g of O_2 are allowed to react maximally to form CO_2 and H_2O, how many grams of CO_2 will be formed? (Atomic weights: C = 12, H = 1, O = 16)

(A) 33 g

(B) 66 g

(C) 132 g

(D) 264 g

(E) None of the above

47. The most important factor in determining the chemical properties of an element is

(A) the number of electrons in *s* orbitals.

(B) the number of protons.

(C) the number of valence electrons.

(D) the total number of electrons.

(E) the atomic mass.

GO ON TO THE NEXT PAGE

48. Which of the following is generally true of atomic radii?

(A) They increase from left to right across a period of the periodic table, and increase down a group.

(B) They decrease across a period from left to right and decrease down a group.

(C) They increase from left to right across a period and decrease down a group.

(D) They decrease from left to right across a period and increase down a group.

(E) Atomic radii do not vary in any regular pattern.

49. According to VSEPR theory, the molecular geometry of NF_3 is

(A) planar.

(B) tetrahedral.

(C) pyramidal.

(D) octahedral.

(E) linear.

50. Which of the following lists the atoms/ions in decreasing order by size?

(A) Te^{2-}, Cs^+, Xe, La^{3+}, I^-, Ba^{2+}

(B) Cs^+, Ba^{2+}, La^{3+}, Te^{2-}, I^-, Xe

(C) La^{3+}, Ba^{2+}, Cs^+, Xe, I^-, Te^{2-}

(D) Te^{2-}, I^-, Xe, Cs^+, Ba^{2+}, La^{3+}

(E) None of the above

51. If an electron on an atom has a principal quantum number of $n = 4$, what possible values of l can it have?

(A) 0

(B) 0, 1

(C) 0, 1, 2

(D) 0, 1, 2, 3

(E) 0, 1, 2, 3, 4

52. $Mg_3N_2 + 6H_2O \rightarrow 3Mg(OH)_2 + 2NH_3$

How many moles of ammonia are liberated when 2 moles of Mg_3N_2 is reacted with 9 moles of H_2O?

(A) 1

(B) 2

(C) 3

(D) 4

(E) 5

53. Which of the following compounds is (are) held together by ionic bonds?

NaH, MgH_2, NH_3

(A) NaH only

(B) MgH_2 only

(C) NaH and MgH_2

(D) All of the three

(E) None of the three

54. Calculate the heat released when 8.0 g of hydrogen react according to the following reaction:

$$2H_2(g) + O_2(g) \rightarrow 2H_2O(g); \Delta H = -115.60 \text{ kcal}$$

(A) 57.80 kcal

(B) 115.60 kcal

(C) 173.4 kcal

(D) 231.2 kcal

(E) 462.4 kcal

55. The electron configuration $1s^22s^22p^63s^23p^63d^2$ represents

(A) an excited, neutral Ca atom.

(B) a ground state, neutral Ca atom.

(C) an excited, neutral Sc atom.

(D) an excited, neutral K atom.

(E) a ground state K^+ ion.

GO ON TO THE NEXT PAGE

56. If ΔH°_f of $CO_2(g)$ is –94.05 kcal/mol and ΔH°_f of $CO(g)$ is –26.41 kcal/mol, calculate ΔH for the following reaction:

$$CO(g) + \frac{1}{2}O_2(g) \rightarrow CO_2(g)$$

(A) –120.46 kcal
(B) –67.64 kcal
(C) 67.64 kcal
(D) 120.46 kcal
(E) None of the above

57. One mole of gas A exerts a pressure of 25 mmHg. How many molecules of gas B are required to exert a pressure of 125 mmHg in an identical container at the same temperature?

(A) 5.00
(B) 6.02×10^{23}
(C) 3.00×10^{23}
(D) 3.00×10^{24}
(E) Cannot be determined

58. If 0.15 mL of oxygen is obtained from analysis of a 1.0 mL sample of whole blood at STP, how many millimoles of oxygen would be obtained from 100.0 mL of the same blood at STP?

(A) $\frac{0.015}{22.4}$
(B) $\frac{15}{16}$
(C) $\frac{1.5}{32}$
(D) $\frac{15}{22.4}$
(E) $\frac{0.15}{32}$

59. The equilibrium

$$4HI(g) + O_2(g) \leftrightarrow 2H_2O(g) + 2I_2(g) + \text{heat}$$

has reached equilibrium at 350°C and 1.0 atm. To increase the yield of I_2, one could

(A) raise the temperature to 500°C.
(B) introduce a catalyst.
(C) add more oxygen.
(D) introduce H_2O into the reaction vessel.
(E) decrease the pressure.

60. Which of the following atoms has the largest electron affinity?

(A) He
(B) Li
(C) Na
(D) Br
(E) Cl

61. In an exothermic reaction, it is always TRUE that

(A) ΔG is positive.
(B) ΔH is positive.
(C) ΔH is negative.
(D) ΔG is negative.
(E) ΔS is positive.

62. When the following equation is balanced, what is the difference between the sum of the coefficients of the products and the sum of the coefficients of the reactants?

$$KMnO_4 + NH_3 \rightarrow KNO_3 + MnO_2 + KOH + H_2O$$

(A) 3
(B) 4
(C) 5
(D) 6
(E) 7

GO ON TO THE NEXT PAGE

63. What could be the empirical formula of a compound that contains 6 g of C for each gram of H? (Atomic weights: C = 12.011, H = 1.008)

(A) CH_3OH
(B) CH_4
(C) C_2H_4
(D) $C_6H_{12}O_6$
(E) CH_2O

64. ΔH°_f of $H_2O(g)$ is –57.798 kcal/mol, and ΔH°_f of $WO_3(s)$ is –200.84 kcal/mol. Calculate ΔH for the reaction

$$3H_2(g) + WO_3(s) \rightarrow W(s) + 3H_2O(g)$$

(A) –258.638 kcal
(B) –143.042 kcal
(C) 27.45 kcal
(D) 143.042 kcal
(E) 258.638 kcal

65. If an electron has a secondary quantum number of $l = 3$, what possible values of m_l can it have?

(A) –3, –2, –1, 0, 1, 2, 3
(B) 1, 2, 3, 4
(C) 0, 1, 2
(D) $-\frac{1}{2}, +\frac{1}{2}$
(E) None of the above

66. Which of the following ions has the smallest ionic radius?

Mg^{2+}, Ca^{2+}, Sr^{2+}, Be^{2+}

(A) Mg^{2+}
(B) Ca^{2+}
(C) Sr^{2+}
(D) Be^{2+}
(E) They all have the same ionic radius.

67. Which of the following will change the numerical value of an equilibrium constant?

(A) An increase in pressure
(B) A decrease in temperature
(C) An increase in the concentration of a reactant
(D) Addition of a catalyst
(E) An increase in the volume of the reaction vessel

68. If the temperature of an endothermic reaction is increased by 10°C, as a rule of thumb, which of the following is approximately doubled?

(A) Rate of reaction
(B) Velocity of molecules
(C) Concentration
(D) Pressure (of gases)
(E) Heat evolved

69. Approximately how many molecules are contained in 16.2 g of quinine, $C_{20}H_{24}N_2O_2$? (Atomic weights: C = 12.011, H = 1, N = 14.0, O = 15.999)

(A) 2.5×10^{21} molecules
(B) 3.0×10^{21} molecules
(C) 2.5×10^{22} molecules
(D) 3.0×10^{22} molecules
(E) 3.0×10^{23} molecules

70. Arrange the following elements in order of increasing metallic character.

Ge, Sn, Pb, Si

(A) Pb, Sn, Ge, Si
(B) Ge, Sn, Pb, Si
(C) Si, Ge, Sn, Pb
(D) Si, Sn, Ge, Pb
(E) All four are equally metallic.

GO ON TO THE NEXT PAGE

71. Acetylene is completely saturated through hydrogenation. The carbon-carbon bond distance in acetylene is 1.20 Å. After saturation, the carbon-carbon bond distance is

(A) 1.07 Å.
(B) 0.60 Å.
(C) 0.40 Å.
(D) 1.20 Å.
(E) 1.54 Å.

72. Which molecule is most likely to react via an S_N1 mechanism?

(A) $CH_3CH_2CH_2Br$
(B) $CH_3CH_2CHBrCH_3$
(C) $CH_3CH_2CBr(CH_3)_2$
(D)

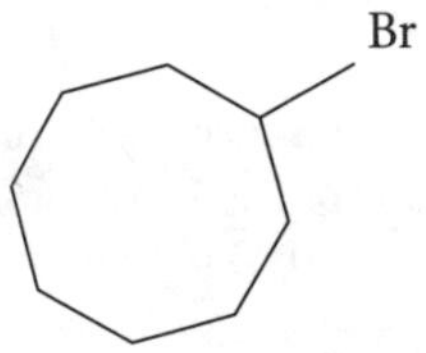

(E)

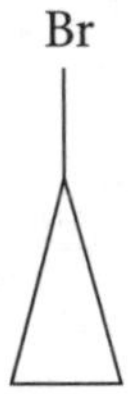

73. The isomerization of 2-butane from configuration A to configuration B requires

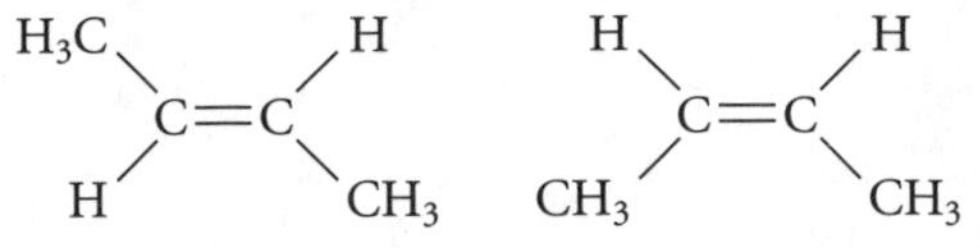

A B

(A) the breakage of one σ bond.
(B) the breakage of both a σ and a π bond.
(C) the breakage of one π bond and rotation about the σ bond.
(D) the breakage of one σ bond and rotation about the π bond.
(E) no breakage of bonds but simple rotation about the carbon-carbon bond.

74. Which of the following carbon atoms is *sp* hybridized?

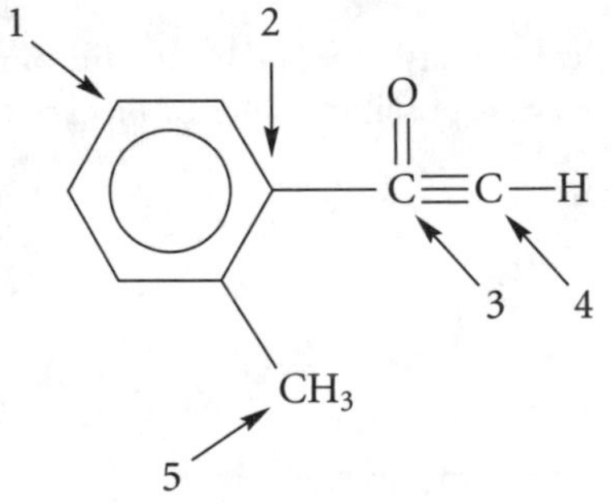

(A) 1
(B) 2
(C) 3
(D) 4
(E) 5

GO ON TO THE NEXT PAGE

75. Which of the following structures has the largest number of stereoisomers?

(A)
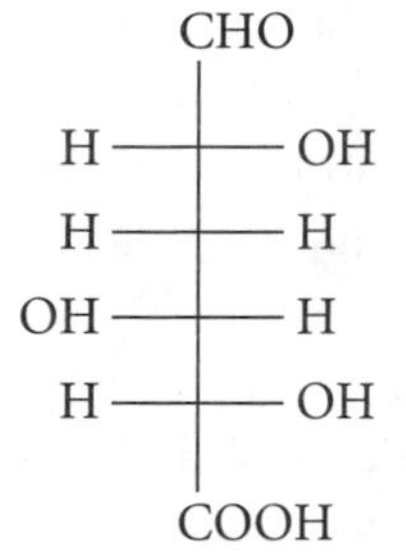

(B)
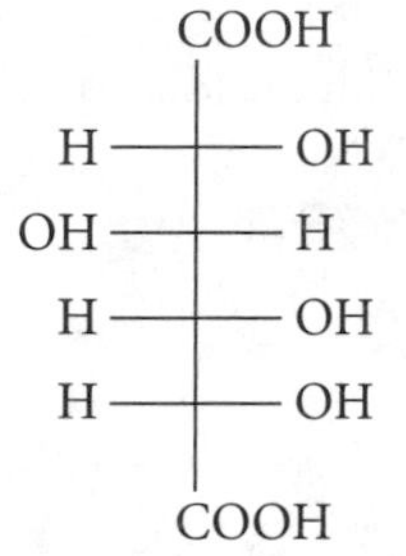

(C)
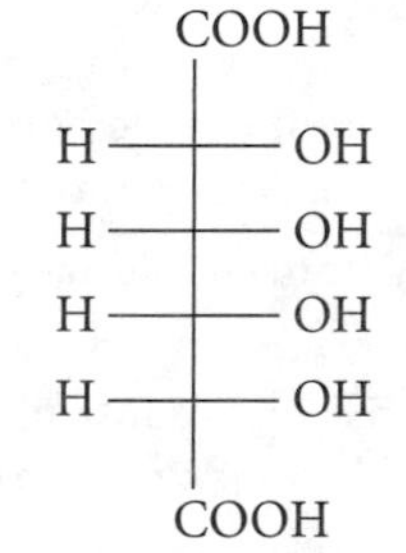

(D)
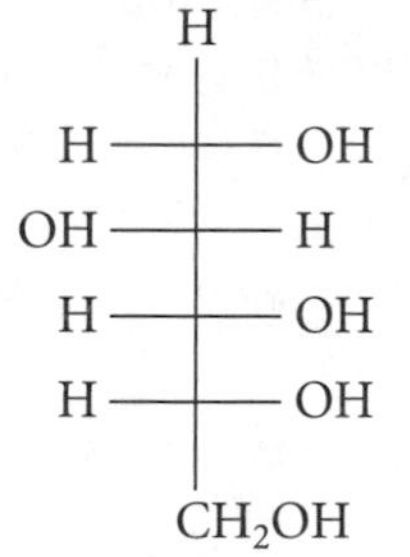

(E)
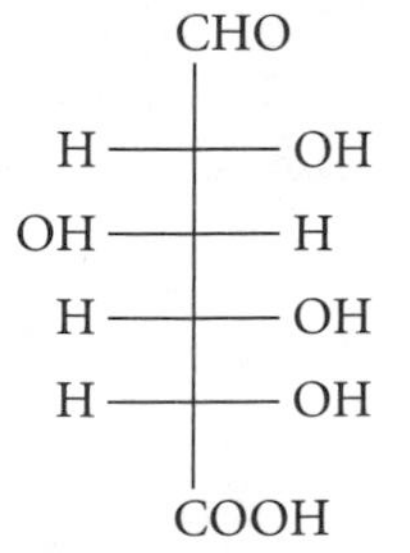

76. Which of the following is methyl acetate?

(A) CH_3COOH
(B) $CH_3COO^-Na^+$
(C) CH_3OCH_3
(D) $CH_3COOCH_2CH_3$
(E) CH_3COOCH_3

77. Which of the following condition(s) favor(s) S_N2 reactions over S_N1 reactions?

(A) Nonpolar solvent
(B) Low temperature
(C) Weak nucleophile
(D) High concentration of nucleophile
(E) All of the above

78. When an atom goes from its ground state to an excited state

(A) the number of core electrons must decrease.
(B) the number of valence electrons must decrease.
(C) the total energy of the electrons must increase.
(D) the total energy of the electrons must decrease.
(E) the nucleus must always obtain a greater positive charge.

79. Dimethylpropylamine (*N*,*N*-dimethyl-1-propanamine) will be LEAST soluble in which of the following?

(A) Dilute KOH(*aq*)
(B) Dilute HCl(*aq*)
(C) Dimethyl ether
(D) Benzene
(E) Concentrated H_2SO_4

GO ON TO THE NEXT PAGE

80. Benzene and cyclohexane are similar in which of the following ways?

(A) Both contain six carbon atoms.

(B) Both exist primarily in the chair conformation.

(C) Both are equally stable.

(D) A and C

(E) A, B, and C

81. The IUPAC name of the following structure is

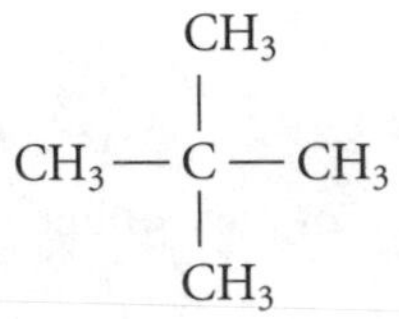

(A) *sec*-butyl methane.

(B) *tert*-butyl methane.

(C) 1,1-dimethyl isopropane.

(D) 2,2-dimethyl propane.

(E) None of the above

82. Which of the following Fischer projections are enantiomers of each other?

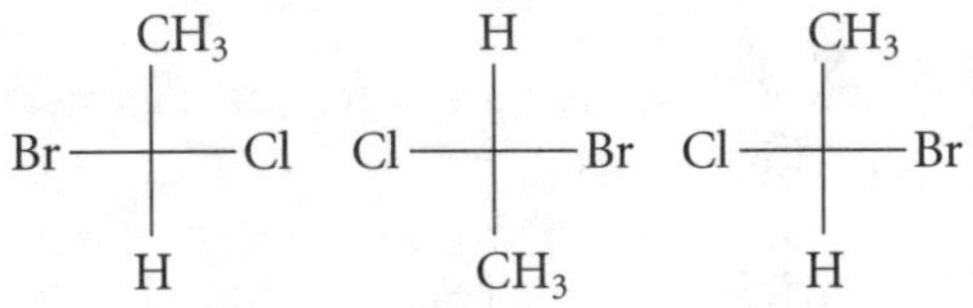

I II III

(A) I and II only

(B) I and III only

(C) II and III only

(D) All are enantiomeric to each other.

(E) I and III and II and III are enantiomers, but I and II are not.

83. Which of the following is TRUE of benzene?

(A) Each pair of consecutive carbon atoms is connected only by a single bond.

(B) Each pair of consecutive carbon atoms is connected only by a double bond.

(C) All of the carbon-carbon bonds in benzene are the same length.

(D) Benzene exists as an equilibrium mixture of two energetically equivalent structures.

(E) Two of the above

84. What is wrong with the following Lewis structure?

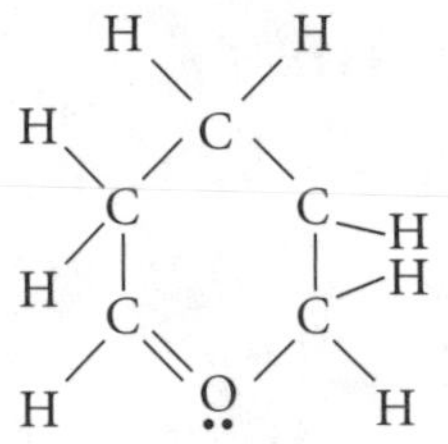

(A) The carbon atom double bonded to oxygen should have a formal positive charge.

(B) The oxygen atom should have a formal positive charge.

(C) Six-membered rings containing carbon-oxygen double bonds never exist.

(D) Both B and C are correct.

(E) This structure is perfectly acceptable as shown.

GO ON TO THE NEXT PAGE

85. The name of the following alkane is

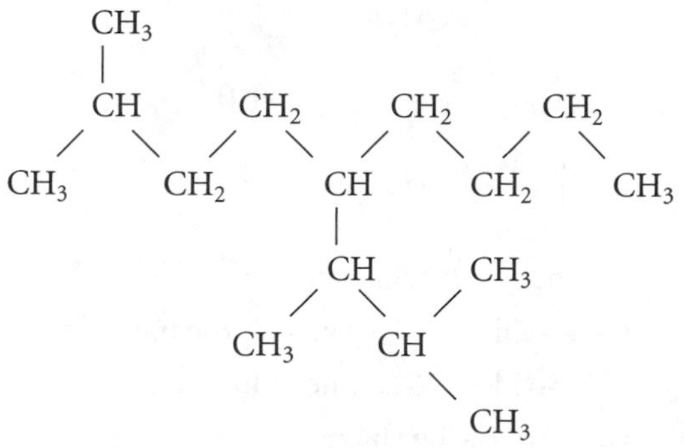

(A) 5-(1,2-dimethylpropyl)-8-methylnonane.
(B) 4-(3-methylbutyl)-2,3-methyloctane.
(C) 5-(1,2-dimethylpropyl)-2-methylnonane.
(D) 5-(1,2-dimethylpropyl)-2-methyldecane.
(E) None of the above

86. Which of the following is/are aromatic?

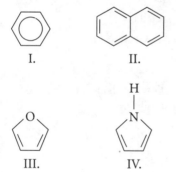

I.

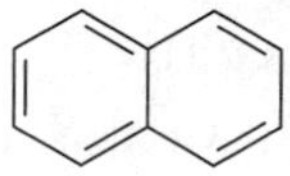

II.

III.

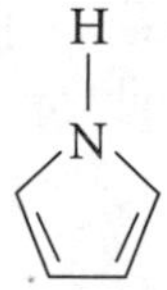

IV.

(A) I only
(B) I and II only
(C) II and IV only
(D) I, II, and IV only
(E) All of the above

87. Arrange the following molecules in order of increasing boiling point.

I. $CH_3(CH_2)_4CO_2H$
II. $CH_3(CH_2)_5CH_3$
III. $CH_3(CH_2)_5CO_2H$
IV. $CH_3(CH_2)_4CH_2OH$
V. $CH_3(CH_2)_4CH_2Br$

(A) II, V, IV, I, III
(B) II, V, IV, III, I
(C) II, IV, V, III, I
(D) V, II, IV, I, III
(E) III, I, IV, II, V

88. Which of the following compounds is an amide?

(A) $CH_3(CH_2)_5OCH_2NH_2$
(B) $CH_3CH_2NHCH_3$
(C)

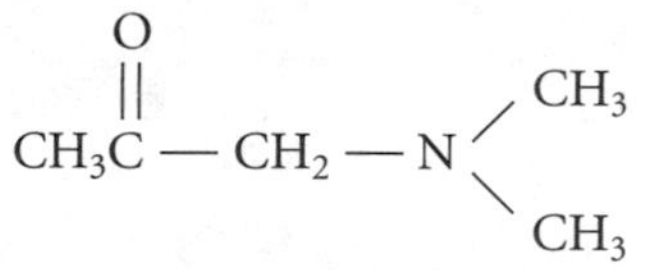

(D)

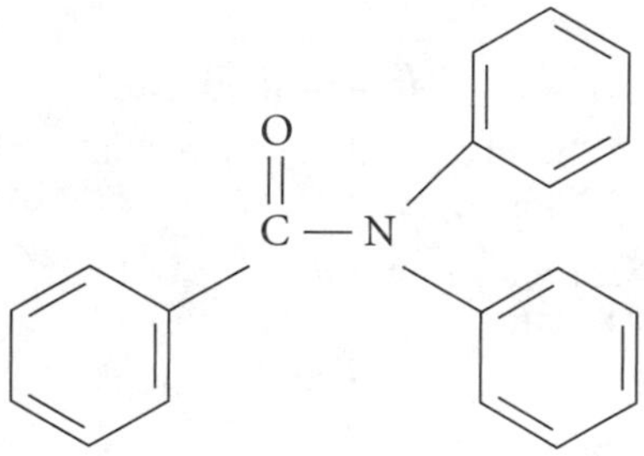

(E) Two of the above

89. How many different stereoisomers of the following molecule exist?

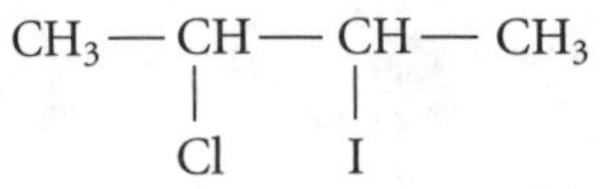

(A) 1
(B) 2
(C) 4
(D) 8
(E) 16

90. The diagram below indicates a pair of *p* orbitals. What kind of bond is formed by overlapping *p* orbitals within a molecule?

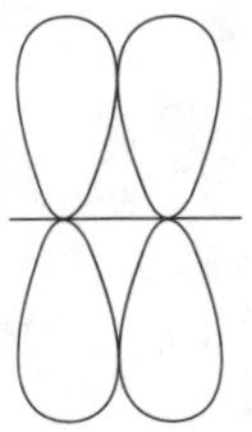

(A) σ bonds found in single bonds
(B) σ bonds found in single, double, and triple bonds
(C) π bonds found in triple but not in double bonds
(D) π bonds found in double but not in triple bonds
(E) π bonds found in double and triple bonds

91. The following compound is called

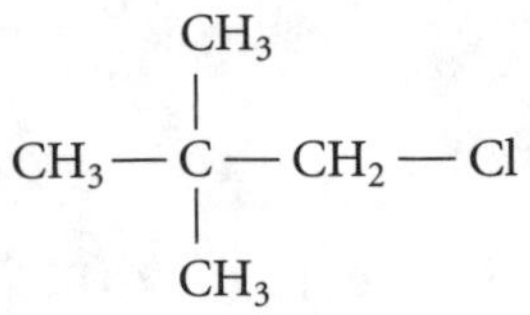

(A) neopentyl chloride.
(B) 1-chloro-2,2-dimethylpropane.
(C) 3-chloro-2,2-dimethylpropane.
(D) Two of the above
(E) All of the above

92. Which of the following is a secondary amine?

(A)
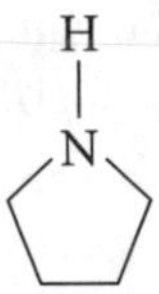

(B) $(CH_3)_3N$
(C) $(CH_3)_3CNH_2$
(D) $[(CH_3)_3CCH_2]_4N^+$
(E) NH_3

93. Rank the following alkenes in order of increasing stability:

I. $CH_3CH{=}CHCH_3$
II. $(CH_3)_2C{=}CHCH_3$
III. $CH_2{=}CH_2$
IV. $(CH_3)_2C{=}C(CH_3)_2$
V. $CH_3CH{=}CH_2$

(A) IV, II, I, V, III
(B) III, V, I, II, IV
(C) V, III, I, II, IV
(D) III, V, I, IV, II
(E) II, IV, I, V, III

GO ON TO THE NEXT PAGE

94. C_nH_{2n+2} + excess $O_2 \rightarrow$ products

The above reaction

(A) is endothermic.
(B) is the oxidation of an alkene.
(C) yields CO_2 and H_2O as products.
(D) yields a mixture of alcohols as products.
(E) yields an alkene and H_2O as products.

95. Which of the following is NOT true of acetylene?

(A) It does not have a permanent dipole moment.
(B) The carbon atoms are sp^2 hybridized.
(C) Its formula is C_2H_2.
(D) It has two π bonds.
(E) It is a linear molecule.

96. Resonance structures do NOT contribute to the stability of which of the following?

(A) Benzene

(B) 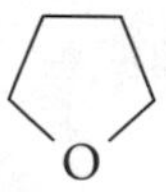

(C) $CH_3-C(=O)-O^{\ominus}$

(D) 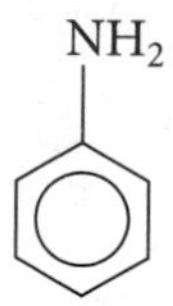

(E) $CH_2=C-\overset{\oplus}{C}H_2$

97. Which is the MOST stable carbocation?

(A) $CH_3-CH=CH-\overset{\oplus}{C}H_2$

(B) $CH_3-CH=CH-CH_2-\overset{\oplus}{C}H_2$

(C) 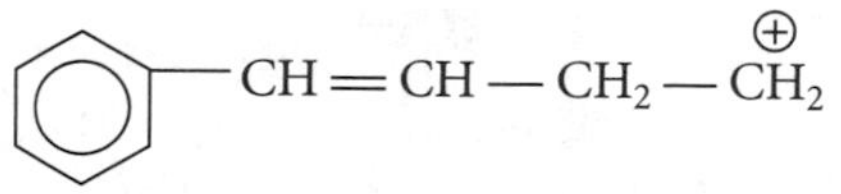

(D) 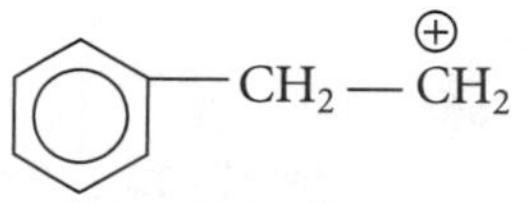

(E) $CH_2=\overset{\oplus}{C}H$

98. Among molecules of similar formula weight, which of the following compound classes will exhibit the highest boiling point?

(A) Alcohol
(B) Ether
(C) Ketone
(D) Cyclic ether
(E) Alkane

GO ON TO THE NEXT PAGE

99. Which is the most stable isomer of di-bromo-di-phenyl ethene?

(A)

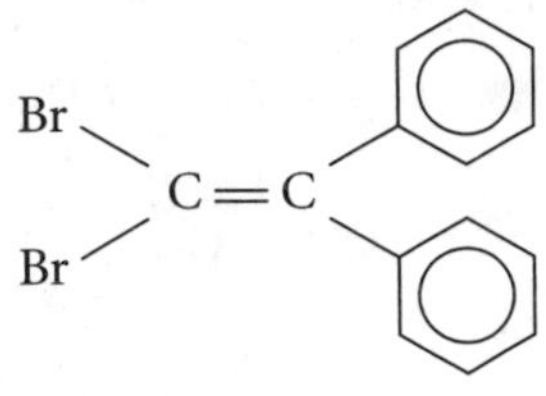

(B)

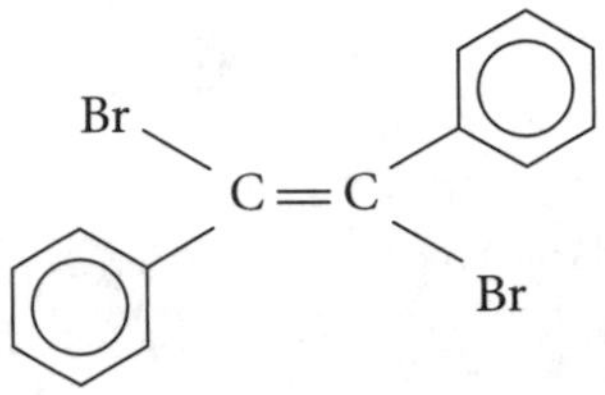

(C)

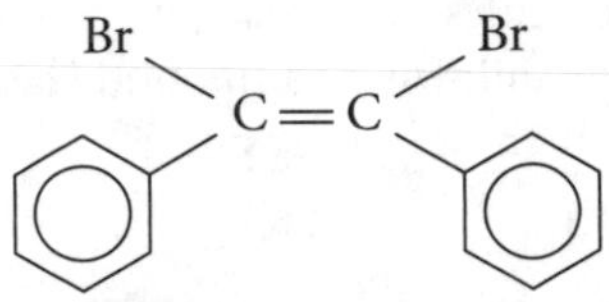

(D) Choices A and C
(E) Choices B and C

100. $C_2H_5ONa + CH_3I \rightarrow$ products

The products of this synthesis are

(A) ethyl methyl ether and sodium iodide.
(B) ethyl iodide and sodium methoxide.
(C) propane, sodium iodide, and nascent oxygen.
(D) propyl alkoxide and sodium iodide.
(E) No reaction occurs.

IF YOU FINISH BEFORE TIME IS CALLED, YOU MAY CHECK YOUR WORK ON THIS SECTION ONLY. DO NOT TURN TO ANY OTHER SECTION IN THE TEST. **STOP**

READING COMPREHENSION

50 questions—60 minutes

Directions: The following test consists of several reading passages and questions that test your comprehension of the passages. Choose the best answer for each question from the five choices provided.

Therapy for speech disorders is the joint concern of orthodontists and speech therapists. However, these two groups of specialists should by no means be thought of as working in an identical manner on identical problems. The contrast between the aims of speech therapy and orthodontics is analogous to the difference between treatment of functional and structural disorders.

The speech pathologist is concerned with a patient's functional disorders, employing therapy aimed simply at correcting the speech difficulty. Cases involving children with problems in sibilant articulation are generally important to the speech therapist, because of the fact that *s* sounds: 1) belong to the most difficult speech groups with regard to articulation, 2) generally appear last in the course of language development, and 3) are most easily disturbed by behavioral and/or pathological factors. Therefore, an examination of the methods employed by speech therapists for treating children with open bite or lisps is instructive.

A cardinal rule of speech therapy is that the patient must learn an entirely new sound to compensate for the one he or she is incapable of articulating. The therapist does not attempt to "improve" the faulty sound or require the child to imitate correct articulation. Either "passive" or "active" methods are used by therapists for correcting the sibilant problem.

Passive methods have as their purpose the direction of the child's articulatory organs into the proper position for making a correct sound. This is accomplished through the use of objects such as mirrors, probes, plates, or tubes, all of which enable the therapist to show the child what he or she is doing, and, where necessary, to manipulate the articulatory organs themselves. For example, illustration of correct tongue position is as follows: the therapist shows the child how to approximate the position of the front teeth, to touch or steady the tongue tip lightly against the lower front teeth, and then blow against the biting edge of the four inner incisor teeth.

Active methods of speech therapy are deductive in nature, beginning with sounds the child can already make and working toward the sound which is to be learned. In the case of sibilants, it is frequently observed that while one or more sounds are affected by lisping, many others in the sibilant series can be properly articulated by the child. In these cases, it is best to develop the desired new sound from the one which is already present. For example: children who are unable to pronounce the *s* may be able to articulate the Greek θ or *th* sound. The *th* corresponds to interdental protrusion of the tongue and is a rather common form of lisping. The therapist induces the child to pull the tongue tip back slightly while articulating a prolonged *th*. A correct *s* will occur spontaneously as soon as the tongue tip disappears behind the teeth. The most important action to avoid here is demonstration by the therapist of perfect pronunciation. Such demonstrations are generally of no use to the patient and may only create tension and nervousness, thus hindering progress.

As a form of preventive dentistry, orthodontics is usually concerned with the correction of dental anomalies for the purpose of heading off future difficulties. With regard to speech disorders, it has been demonstrated that misaligned teeth and tooth loss can cause or contribute to defects in articulation. Therefore, orthodontists are frequently called on to assist in the correction of speech disorders through the realignment or other adjustment of the patient's teeth.

In dealing with malocclusion—a faulty meshing of teeth in the upper and lower jaws when biting—the orthodontist generally places the child into one of three basic categories. The first, class I, includes

GO ON TO THE NEXT PAGE

patients who have irregularities in the front teeth, despite fairly normal relationships between the jaws and proper meshing of the back teeth (though other teeth may also be irregular). This condition can be treated with fixed or removable appliances that help turn or straighten irregular teeth. Fixed appliances work all the time, delivering even and consistent forces to the teeth. Removable appliances may be taken off on occasion, although neglect can bring progress to a halt.

Class II malocclusion involves an underdevelopment of the lower jaw, with upper molars falling in front of the lower ones. Frequently, this is accompanied by protrusion of the upper front teeth, a condition commonly referred to as "buck teeth." An appliance such as an elastic band and night brace may be worn for at least 13 hours each day and serves to push the molars back. If the other teeth do not then follow, they are moved individually into the proper alignment.

Class III children have prominent lower jaws and protruding lower front teeth. They are treated in much the same way as those in class II, through the use of the elastic band and night brace. The child's profile remains the same, with jaw structure correctable only through surgery.

Clearly, the speech pathologist and the orthodontist deal with the problems of improper speech in different contexts, one functional and the other structural. In many cases, the two are permitted to work together, as in the elimination of lisping by removing speech patterns with simultaneous speech correction. However, it has been shown that the problems of sibilant articulations, as well as other speech difficulties, can be treated with considerable success by speech therapy alone. Also, there is abundant evidence that the correction by the orthodontist of dental anomalies such as malocclusion or missing teeth will spontaneously result in formal speech patterns. The conclusion drawn by many parents is that one or another of these types of therapy should suffice or that their effects are interchangeable.

This is a very dangerous assumption to make, however. It has often been the case that a child is taken to a speech pathologist for therapy when very young and achieves some success in overcoming his or her speech disorder. Then, he or she is taken to an orthodontist, who subjects the child to treatments for the correction of structural problems. The result is that the child must return to the speech therapist to begin a new sequence of treatment in order to acquire normal abilities in articulation.

The reason for this is simple. The speech therapist works with the child's existing articulatory organs and, with the help of artificial devices, helps the child to pronounce a particular sound in a particular way. By altering the structural context through orthodontics, the orthodontist has made the child's acquired techniques less effective, and a return to the therapist is necessary. This frequently results in emotional trauma for the child and, in most cases, inflicts a senseless and unnecessary burden.

The recommended attitude is one of isolating the very different approaches to speech improvement practiced by the speech therapist and the orthodontist. Our example of sibilant articulation in children leads to the conclusion that both specialists are able to employ methods and achieve significant results. If they worked together, the results would most probably be faster and more positive. Once the orthodontist has completed the correction of any dental problems, the speech therapist can reeducate the child's tongue and lips to function within the new structural context, thus assisting in maintaining the orthodontic results.

GO ON TO THE NEXT PAGE

1. According to the passage, the major difference between orthodontics and speech therapy is that orthodontics
   - (A) corrects structural anomalies rather than functional disorders.
   - (B) requires much more rigorous medical training than speech pathology.
   - (C) is contraindicated in cases of lisping.
   - (D) works best on adolescents, while speech therapy can begin much earlier.
   - (E) corrects functional disorders rather than structural anomalies.

2. A distinguishing feature of passive methods of speech therapy is that they
   - (A) begin with sounds the child can already articulate and develop gradually toward the correct sound.
   - (B) attempt to induce the child's speech organs to form the proper position for correct articulation.
   - (C) involve less personal contact between therapist and child than do active methods.
   - (D) tend to be effective even in cases of severe malocclusion.
   - (E) involve little manipulation of the articulatory organs.

3. Many of the children treated by speech therapists
   - (A) never achieve their desired results.
   - (B) are better served by orthodontic intervention.
   - (C) do not receive sufficient emotional support from their parents.
   - (D) must also contend with learning disabilities.
   - (E) do not require surgery.

4. Speech therapists in general believe that it is necessary to
   - (A) instruct the child by setting a correct example.
   - (B) treat children before any orthodontic treatment is attempted.
   - (C) employ active methods whenever possible.
   - (D) teach the child an entirely new sound.
   - (E) use passive methods over active methods.

5. The essential characteristic of active methods of speech therapy is that they
   - (A) retrain the child's articulatory organs following orthodontic treatment.
   - (B) use related sounds that the child can already correctly articulate.
   - (C) avoid using mirrors or other external objects to cure speech disorders.
   - (D) eliminate the need for passive therapeutic methods.
   - (E) work with the physical manipulation of the mouth.

GO ON TO THE NEXT PAGE

6. Problems with the articulation of sibilants
   (A) can easily be corrected through speech therapy.
   (B) are difficult to eliminate without surgery.
   (C) are usually structural or anatomical in origin.
   (D) often appear late in the child's language development.
   (E) originate from early Greek alphabets.

7. Class I malocclusions are treated with
   (A) fixed or removable appliances.
   (B) surgery.
   (C) prosthetic teeth.
   (D) passive speech therapy.
   (E) active speech therapy.

8. One error speech therapists must avoid is
   (A) treating children who have class III malocclusions.
   (B) demonstrating to the child correct articulation.
   (C) associating articulative mechanisms with particular sounds.
   (D) attempting to correct lisps without the help of an orthodontist.
   (E) teaching the child new sounds.

9. The author probably believes that, as a general rule, children with speech disorders
   (A) benefit from speech therapy only if orthodontic work is not required.
   (B) should never receive orthodontic treatment after completing speech therapy.
   (C) could benefit from recent advances in dental surgery.
   (D) respond best to a coordinated effort of speech therapist and orthodontist.
   (E) should avoid any professional intervention.

10. The night brace is used for treating
    (A) open bite.
    (B) tongue protrusion.
    (C) problems in sibilant articulation.
    (D) class I malocclusion.
    (E) class II malocclusion.

11. According to the passage, orthodontics is considered a form of
    (A) functional therapy.
    (B) speech pathology.
    (C) preventive dentistry.
    (D) sibilant modification.
    (E) active therapy.

12. Which of the following would strongly indicate a diagnosis of class III malocclusion?
    (A) Open lips
    (B) Pronounced lisp
    (C) Underdeveloped lower jaw
    (D) Overdeveloped lower jaw
    (E) Sibilant misarticulation

13. Active methods of speech therapy are especially effective in cases of lisping where the child
    (A) has already completed orthodontic treatment.
    (B) has not yet begun orthodontic treatment.
    (C) is able to articulate some sibilants correctly.
    (D) is not suffering from severe malocclusion.
    (E) suffers from class III malocclusion.

GO ON TO THE NEXT PAGE

14. The passage indicates that a speech therapist employing passive methods might have the child begin by

    (A) listening to recordings of the sound, articulated first incorrectly and then correctly.
    (B) doing exercises to increase tongue flexibility.
    (C) learning proper alignment of the front teeth.
    (D) recognizing that changing one's speech habits is an emotional process as well as a physical one.
    (E) wearing a night brace.

15. A child whose lower molars stand behind the corresponding upper molars would probably be described as having a

    (A) class I malocclusion.
    (B) class II malocclusion.
    (C) class III malocclusion.
    (D) condition not specified in this article.
    (E) problem with sibilant articulation.

16. Patients receiving removable orthodontic appliances

    (A) sometimes experience irritation of the gums.
    (B) rarely correct their problems with the positioning of their teeth.
    (C) are considered too young for fixed appliances.
    (D) suffer from the condition commonly known as "buck teeth."
    (E) may fail to make progress if they neglect to wear them.

GO ON TO THE NEXT PAGE

The population of the United States is growing older and will continue to do so until well into the next century. As the 1900s began, the median age of the U.S. population had risen from around 28, in the 1950s, to 33. It will be 36 by the beginning of the 21st century and 42 by the year 2050. The elderly—those people 65 and older—now outnumber teenagers for the first time in American history; the population of elders has doubled in just forty years. The U.S. Census Bureau projects that 39 million Americans will be 65 or older by the year 2010, 51 million by 2020, and 65 million by 2030. This demographic trend is due mainly to two factors: increased life expectancy and the occurrence of a "baby boom" in the generation born immediately after World War II.

To begin with, more people than ever before are surviving into old age. In 1900, the average life expectancy for a U.S. citizen was 47.3 years; only about one out of every ten Americans lived to the age of 65. Today, eight out of ten will see their 65th birthday, and the average life expectancy has increased to approximately 75 years. People are living well beyond the average life expectancy in greater numbers than ever before, too. In fact, the number of U.S. citizens 85 years old and older is growing six times as fast as the rest of the population.

Numerous subsidiary factors contribute to Americans' increased life expectancy, including improved methods of food production and public sanitation, the ever growing popularity of physical fitness, and federal and state aid for the poor and the elderly. Another important factor, of course, has been the explosive advancement of medicine in this century, which has helped sustain lives of all ages. Better prenatal and neonatal care, for example, have helped reduce infant mortality. Vaccines, new drugs and surgical techniques, and other technological innovations have vastly increased physicians' ability not only to save lives but also to extend them.

The "graying" of the United States is also due in large measure to the aging of the generation born after World War II, the "baby boomers." With the advent of peace, in an economic climate of unparalleled prosperity, the birth rate of post–World War II America increased dramatically. The baby boom peaked in 1957 with over 4.3 million births that year. More than 75 million Americans were born between 1946 and 1964, the largest generation in U.S. history. Today, millions of "boomers" are already moving into middle age; in less than two decades, they will join the ranks of America's elderly. Those ranks, it must be noted, will be predominantly female. In the United States, as in the rest of the world, the gender ratio at birth is 105 males for every 100 females. By the age of 65, however, there are only 81 men left for every 100 women, and at age 85 and above, only 41 men for every 100 women.

What will be the social, economic, and political consequences of the aging of America? One likely development will involve a gradual restructuring of the family unit, moving away from the traditional nuclear family and toward an extended, multigenerational family dominated by elders, not by their adult children. This restructuring has already begun to occur. With one out of every two U.S. marriages currently ending in divorce, a significant number of today's grandparents are suddenly faced with the task of raising or helping to raise their grandchildren, even as they continue to provide financial assistance to their adult children. Indeed, far from being a financial burden to their children, today's elders often find themselves acting as family bankers. Roughly 75 percent of today's elders already own their own homes, something their offspring are finding increasingly difficult to accomplish without parental assistance.

The aging of the U.S. population is also likely to have far-reaching effects on the nation's workforce. In 1989, there were approximately 3.5 workers for every person 65 and older; by the year 2030, there'll only be 2 workers for every person 65 and older. As the number of available younger workers shrinks, elderly people will become more attractive as prospective employees. Many will simply retain their existing jobs beyond the now-mandatory retirement age of 65. In fact, the phenomenon of

GO ON TO THE NEXT PAGE

early retirement, which has transformed the U.S. workforce over the past four decades, will probably become a thing of the past. In 1950, about 50 percent of all 65-year-old men still worked; today, only 15 percent of them do. The median retirement age is currently 61. Yet recent surveys show that almost half of today's retirees would prefer to be working, and in decades to come, their counterparts will be doing just that.

The housing needs of an aging population will generate further social and economic changes. Over the past 30 years, hundreds of thousands of senior citizens migrated south to Sunbelt states such as Arizona, California, and Florida, where they pioneered retirement communities and other congregate living arrangements that foreshadow some of the possible housing options for future retirees. But many demographic experts and social scientists predict that this southward migration will diminish in the future, since surveys have found that the great majority of people age 55 and older would prefer not to relocate. Tomorrow's elders may well decide to adapt the Sunbelt's retirement village format to the areas in which they have lived for the majority of their adult lives.

Finally, the great proportional increase in older Americans will have significant effects on the nation's economy in the areas of Social Security and health care. A recent government survey showed that 77 percent of elderly Americans have annual incomes of less than $20,000; only 3 percent earn more than $50,000. As their earning power declines and their need for health care increases, most elderly Americans come to depend heavily on federal and state subsidies. With the advent of Social Security in 1935 and Medicaid/Medicare in 1965, the size of those subsidies has grown steadily until by 1990, spending on the elderly accounted for 30 percent of the annual federal budget.

Considering these figures, and the fact that the elderly population will double within the next forty years, it's clear that major government policy decisions lie ahead. In the first 50 years of its existence, for example, the Social Security fund has received $55 billion more in employee/employer contributions than it has paid out in benefits to the elderly. Yet time and again, the federal government has "borrowed" from this surplus—without repaying it—in order to pay interest on the national debt.

Similarly, the Medicaid/Medicare system is threatened by the continuous upward spiral of medical costs. The cost of caring for disabled elderly Americans is expected to double in the next decade alone. Millions of Americans of all ages are currently unable to afford private health insurance. In fact, the United States is practically unique among developed nations in lacking a national health care system. Its advocates say such a system would be far less expensive than the present state of affairs, but the medical establishment and various special interest groups have so far blocked legislation aimed at creating it. Nonetheless, within the next few decades, an aging U.S. population may well demand that such a program be implemented.

17. According to the passage, the segment of the U.S. population currently aged 85 years and older

(A) is predominantly male.

(B) is located primarily in the Sunbelt states.

(C) is growing six times faster than the rest of the population.

(D) is largely responsible for the high cost of medical care.

(E) on average has an annual income between $20,000 and $50,000.

18. The passage states that by the year 2030, there will be

(A) no money left in the Social Security fund.

(B) only 81 men for every 100 women in the United States.

(C) 51 million elderly Americans.

(D) only two workers for every American over the age of 65.

(E) a new U.S. health care system.

GO ON TO THE NEXT PAGE

19. Which of the following statements about the U.S. elderly population is TRUE?

    (A) It is largely responsible for the nation's current housing shortage.
    (B) It is expected to double within the next 40 years.
    (C) It is the wealthiest segment of the U.S. population.
    (D) It represents almost 30 percent of the U.S. population.
    (E) It constitutes the population majority in the Sunbelt states.

20. According to the passage, the "baby boom" generation

    (A) has the highest life expectancy of any generation in U.S. history.
    (B) has a median age of 33.
    (C) includes approximately 75 million people born between 1946 and 1964.
    (D) perceives its aging parents as a financial burden.
    (E) is starting to enter the ranks of America's elderly.

21. According to demographic experts, the southward migration of retirees in the past three decades is

    (A) one cause of their relatively low incomes.
    (B) responsible for the shrinking of the U.S. workforce.
    (C) due to the availability of low-cost housing in the Sunbelt states.
    (D) attributed to overcrowded conditions in the north.
    (E) expected to diminish in the future.

22. According to the passage, the current divorce rate is

    (A) approximately 50 percent.
    (B) rising rapidly.
    (C) less than 40 percent.
    (D) slowly declining.
    (E) not affecting family structure.

23. The author states that over the next few decades, increasing numbers of "baby boomers" will

    (A) migrate west in search of employment.
    (B) benefit from early retirement opportunities.
    (C) join the elderly segment of the U.S. population.
    (D) fail to qualify for health insurance.
    (E) experience an increased birthrate.

24. What percentage of the total yearly federal expenditure in 1990 was spent on the U.S. elderly population?

    (A) 3 percent
    (B) 30 percent
    (C) 50 percent
    (D) 70 percent
    (E) 77 percent

25. All of the following are mentioned as having contributed to increased life expectancy EXCEPT

    (A) the availability of better medical care.
    (B) increased subsidies for the elderly.
    (C) improved sanitation techniques.
    (D) a decline in the birth rate.
    (E) the growing popularity of physical fitness.

26. According to the passage, the majority of elderly people in the United States

    (A) currently earn less than $20,000 per year.
    (B) will suffer some sort of disability between the ages of 65 and 75.
    (C) have been unable to purchase their own homes.
    (D) continue to work at least 20 hours per week.
    (E) do not depend on subsidies.

GO ON TO THE NEXT PAGE

27. Medicare was instituted in
    (A) 1946.
    (B) 1950.
    (C) 1964.
    (D) 1965.
    (E) 1935.

28. The fact that health care costs for disabled elderly Americans are expected to double in the next ten years suggests that
    (A) the federal government will be unable to finance a national health care system.
    (B) the Medicaid/Medicare system will probably become even more expensive in the future.
    (C) money will have to be borrowed from the Social Security fund in order to finance the Medicaid/Medicare system.
    (D) "baby boomers" will be unable to receive federal health benefits as they grow older.
    (E) the elderly received poor preventive care in the past.

29. Which of the following correctly describes the policy of early retirement?
    (A) It will transform the U.S. workforce over the next several decades.
    (B) It is a relatively recent phenomenon in U.S. history.
    (C) It is thought to have been a major cause in the decline of the U.S. economy.
    (D) It will become more popular in the 21st century.
    (E) It restructured the U.S. workforce prior to World War II.

30. According to the U.S. Census Bureau, today's elderly population is
    (A) larger than the current population of teenagers.
    (B) larger than the current population of "boomers."
    (C) smaller than the number of elderly people in 1950.
    (D) smaller than the number of elderly people in 1970.
    (E) larger than the projected elderly population in 2030.

31. The author speculates that in future decades, the typical U.S. family will probably be
    (A) divorce-free.
    (B) subsidized by Social Security.
    (C) multigenerational.
    (D) wealthier than today's family.
    (E) youth-oriented.

32. The author suggests that over the past three decades, many of today's elderly people
    (A) supplemented their incomes by working past the age of retirement.
    (B) lost their Social Security benefits.
    (C) suffered a serious physical disability.
    (D) relocated to a warmer climate.
    (E) lost their homes.

33. According to the author, the federal government has not yet instituted a program mandating health care for all U.S. citizens because
    (A) the federal deficit must first be eliminated.
    (B) such a program would be too expensive.
    (C) legislative lobbies have prevented it.
    (D) Medicaid and Medicare have made it unnecessary.
    (E) most U.S. citizens have private insurance.

GO ON TO THE NEXT PAGE

Radioisotopes have been in use in scientific research for the last 50 years. Understanding radioisotopes first requires a grasp of basic atomic structure.

The atom is composed of two parts: a nucleus, consisting of protons and neutrons, and a series of electron shells surrounding the nucleus. The mass of an atom is concentrated in the nucleus. *Mass number* refers to the mass of an atom and is defined as the number of protons plus the number of neutrons in the nucleus of that atom. Protons and neutrons have approximately the same mass. The *atomic number* of an atom is defined as the number of protons in the nucleus of that atom. In a neutral atom, the number of electrons in the shells surrounding the nucleus must be equal to the number of protons in the nucleus. Two atoms that have the same atomic number belong to the same *element*. Though they must have the same number of protons, atoms of the same element may contain different numbers of neutrons. Such atoms are called *isotopes*. In other words, isotopes of the same element have identical atomic numbers but different mass numbers. For example, oxygen-15 and oxygen-16 have mass numbers of 15 and 16, respectively; however, both have the same atomic number, 8.

Isotopes whose nuclear structures are unstable undergo radioactive decay. All elements with atomic numbers higher than 83 have only unstable isotopes. Nuclear decay manifests itself in the emission of one of three possible types of particle or ray: alpha, beta, or gamma. Alpha particles are helium nuclei containing 2 protons and 2 neutrons. Emission of such particles results in a decrease of mass number by 4 and a decrease of atomic number by 2. Beta particles are high-speed electrons, produced when neutrons are converted into protons. The result of this type of emission is an increase in the atomic number by 1 while the mass number remains the same. The third type of emission, the gamma ray, is a high-energy X-ray emitted by the nucleus.

The rate at which nuclei in a given radioactive substance decay is directly proportional to the number of nuclei in that substance. The half-life of an isotope is the amount of time required for one-half of the nuclei in any given radioactive sample to disintegrate.

Radioisotopes can be produced in cyclotrons and fission nuclear reactors. Cyclotrons accelerate rather than produce electrons and protons, which are then used as "bullets" to bombard non-radioactive targets. Electron and proton bullets must have a very high speed in order to overcome the repulsive forces of the electrons and protons of the targets. Fission reactors produce neutron bullets. Since neutrons are uncharged particles, they are not repelled by any part of the target atom and are therefore able to penetrate an atom much more easily than either protons or electrons. The use of neutrons thus allows a much wider variety of radioactive particles to be produced than when protons or electrons are used.

Radioactive emissions can be detected through the use of photographic film. Photographic film will darken upon exposure to radiation, indicating both the distribution and the total number of radioactive particles emitted by the sample being studied while it was in contact with the film. In a study of the uptake of radioactive material by a thin leaf, a photographic plate is pressed firmly against the leaf and kept in a totally darkened place. The more intense the radiation and the longer the exposure to it, the more the film will darken. Another means of detecting radiation, one more sensitive than film, is to use a Geiger counter. A Geiger counter operates by means of two electrodes sealed within a tube containing argon gas. The electrodes are held at a potential difference slightly less than the potential difference necessary for a charged particle to cross the gap between them. High-energy radioactive particles ionize the argon gas, allowing charge to bridge the gap between the electrodes, thereby producing a clicking noise in the instrument.

Geiger counters are not capable of detecting neutrons. Since neutrons are not charged, they are incapable of ionizing the argon gas and therefore cannot cause a current between the electrodes.

GO ON TO THE NEXT PAGE

Geiger counters will only indicate the presence of a radioactive material when they are receiving significantly more radiation than that normally present in the atmosphere. This atmospheric baseline is about 20 counts per second. The minimum number of atoms (N) that must be present in a radioactive sample for a Geiger counter to detect radiation is given by the formula $N = RT/0.693$, where T is the half-life of the radioactive material in seconds and R is a constant. R depends on both the atmospheric baseline and on the geometries of the Geiger counter and the sample. For a standard Geiger counter and an ordinary lab sample, about 10 percent of the radiation registers in the Geiger counter's tube. Based on this percentage, R can be calculated to be approximately 30.

The use of radioisotopes in research is based upon the fact that radioisotopes have the same chemical properties as their nonradioactive counterparts. In biological systems, radioactive substances will localize themselves in the same area as nonradioactive isotopes of the same element. Radioisotopes are introduced into an organism by mixing them with large quantities of nonradioactive substances in the diet.

In choosing a radioactive tracer, the half-life of the substance must be considered. Isotopes with very short half-lives will disintegrate too quickly to be detected. In addition, the shorter the half-life, the higher the intensity of the radiation. Too much radiation can damage the tissue it comes in contact with. It is for these reasons that carbon-14, which has a half-life of 5,730 years, is used rather than carbon-11, which has a half-life of only 20 minutes. Isotopes with very long half-lives emit radiation at a rate too small to be detected.

In the past, radioactive tracers have been used in experiments which disprove the notion that all ingested food is used as a supply of energy and then excreted from the body. Studies of the mouth utilizing radioactive phosphorus have shown that ions are constantly exchanged between the saliva and the teeth. Exchange is not limited to the outer surface of the teeth but includes the inner pulp. When the salivary glands are removed from an organism, the teeth are found to decay rapidly. In a similar experiment utilizing radioactive calcium, replacement of atoms in bone was shown to take place in the same manner. The only exception to this constant replacement of ions occurs in the case of the iron found in hemoglobin. In healthy organisms, ingested iron is not incorporated into the hemoglobin but rather stored in the form of a protein complex or excreted. These experiments, then, show that the body is in a state of dynamic equilibrium: atoms are constantly being replaced in the body.

Radioactive substances are also used in experiments involving blood. Blood with radioactivity of known intensity is injected into an organism, and after a suitable period of time, a sample of blood is taken and the radiation intensity is determined. This makes it possible to determine the amount of blood present in an organism.

34. The mass number of an atom containing 16 protons and 16 neutrons within its nucleus is

(A) twice the mass number of oxygen-16.

(B) equal to the mass number of oxygen-16.

(C) one-half the mass number of oxygen-16.

(D) one-quarter the mass number of oxygen-16.

(E) one-third the mass number of oxygen-16.

35. What is the advantage of using carbon-14 rather than carbon-11 in a biological experiment?

(A) It is easier to convert carbon-14 to carbon-12 than carbon-11 to carbon-12 by alpha emission.

(B) It is easier to convert carbon-14 to carbon-12 than carbon-11 to carbon-12 by beta emission.

(C) The half-life of carbon-14 is too short.

(D) The half-life of carbon-11 is too long.

(E) The radiation emitted by carbon-11 is too intense.

GO ON TO THE NEXT PAGE

36. The advantage of photographic film over the Geiger counter in determining radioactivity is that
    (A) film can discriminate between types of radiation.
    (B) film indicates the area where the radiation is absorbed.
    (C) atmospheric radiation does not interfere in film absorption.
    (D) the Geiger counter cannot determine the intensity of radiation.
    (E) film requires the use of an isotope.

37. The half-life of radon-222 is 3.8 days. Starting with 2 grams of radon, how much would be left after 7.6 days?
    (A) 0.5 gm
    (B) 1.0 gm
    (C) 1.5 gms
    (D) 0.25 gm
    (E) 0.40 gm

38. Phosphorus-32 emits a beta particle. It will become
    (A) aluminum-28.
    (B) phosphorus-32.
    (C) sulfur-32.
    (D) nickel-53.
    (E) antimony-51.

39. Photographic film badges are worn by workers in plants where radiation is present. The degree to which the film darkens indicates the
    (A) lowest level of radiation for the day.
    (B) type of radioactive emission.
    (C) normal atmospheric radiation.
    (D) total radiation absorbed over the period of time for which the badge is worn.
    (E) total level of gamete damage suffered by the worker.

40. Alpha particles have
    (A) 1 proton and 2 neutrons.
    (B) 2 protons and 1 electron.
    (C) 1 proton and 2 electrons.
    (D) 2 protons and 2 electrons.
    (E) 2 protons and 2 neutrons.

41. If a healthy organism is treated with iron, what will happen to the iron once it has entered the body?
    (A) It may be exchanged with the iron in hemoglobin.
    (B) It may be stored as a protein complex.
    (C) It may be used to manufacture white blood cells.
    (D) It may be used as a neurotransmitter.
    (E) It will cross the blood-brain barrier.

42. What is the reason that neutrons CANNOT be detected by a Geiger counter?
    (A) Neutral particles cannot ionize argon gas and therefore cannot cause a current to flow.
    (B) Neutrons are too heavy to move and cause a current between the electrodes.
    (C) Neutrons disintegrate at a rate equal to atmospheric radiation, and this rate is too slow to be detected by a Geiger counter.
    (D) Neutron emission is impossible.
    (E) Neutrons have too weak a charge.

43. The difference among isotopes of one element is in
    (A) the charge of the nucleus.
    (B) the electron configuration.
    (C) the number of neutrons.
    (D) the number of electrons.
    (E) the number of protons.

GO ON TO THE NEXT PAGE

44. In what respect is a Geiger counter more useful than photographic film in detecting radiation?

(A) A Geiger counter can detect the presence of neutrons.

(B) A Geiger counter is more sensitive than photographic film.

(C) A Geiger counter can measure atmospheric radiation, whereas photographic film cannot.

(D) A Geiger counter is less portable.

(E) A Geiger counter is more efficient than photographic film.

45. What disadvantage is there in using isotopes with very long half-lives as tracers as opposed to isotopes with shorter half-lives?

(A) Such isotopes can only be used in the treatment of hyperthyroidism.

(B) Such isotopes are cancerous.

(C) Such isotopes would not be able to enter the organism's bloodstream.

(D) The rate of emission from such isotopes is too small to be measured.

(E) Such isotopes are difficult to isolate.

46. Which of the following is an advantage nuclear reactors have over cyclotrons in producing radioisotopes?

(A) Neutrons are capable of producing a larger variety of radioactive substances.

(B) A proton or an electron can penetrate an atom more easily than can a neutron.

(C) A cyclotron cannot accelerate protons and electrons to high enough speeds to bombard atoms.

(D) Neutron bullets are repelled by target atoms.

(E) Nuclear reactors are more energy-efficient than cyclotrons.

47. What would be the BEST title for the first two paragraphs?

(A) The Detection of Radioactive Emissions

(B) A History of the Study of Atoms

(C) The Production of Radioisotopes

(D) Dangers of Radioactive Experimentation

(E) The Structure of the Atom

48. An isotope is radioactive if it can undergo

(A) beta decay only.

(B) alpha or beta decay.

(C) neither alpha nor beta decay.

(D) alpha, beta, or gamma emission.

(E) gamma decay.

49. What characteristic of radioisotopes allows them to be used in biological experiments?

(A) They have no side effects.

(B) They have the same chemical properties as their nonradioactive counterparts.

(C) They are inert.

(D) They are not harmful to the organism.

(E) They have extremely long half-lives.

50. All of the following statements concerning radioactive experiments with blood are true EXCEPT

(A) the amount of blood in an organism can be detected.

(B) radioactive blood is injected into an organism.

(C) there needs to be a waiting period before measuring the results.

(D) blood does not need to be drawn to obtain results.

(E) to determine accurate data, radiation intensity must be measured.

IF YOU FINISH BEFORE TIME IS CALLED, YOU MAY CHECK YOUR WORK ON THIS SECTION ONLY. DO NOT TURN TO ANY OTHER SECTION IN THE TEST. **STOP**

PHYSICS

40 questions – 50 minutes

Directions: Choose the best answer for each question from the five choices provided.

The values for the physical constants below are to be used as needed:

Gravitational acceleration at the surface of the Earth: $g = 10 \text{ m/s}^2$

Speed of light in a vacuum: $c = 3 \times 10^8 \text{ m/s}$

Charge of an electron: $e = 2.0 \times 10^{-19}$ Coulomb

1. Which vector represents the force exerted on q^+ by Q^+ and Q^-, which are equidistant from q^+?

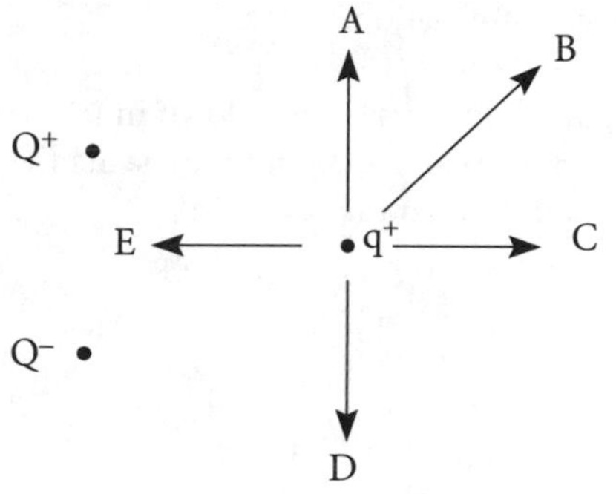

(A) A
(B) B
(C) C
(D) D
(E) E

2. If light is shone on a mirror as shown below, at which surfaces will the light be reflected?

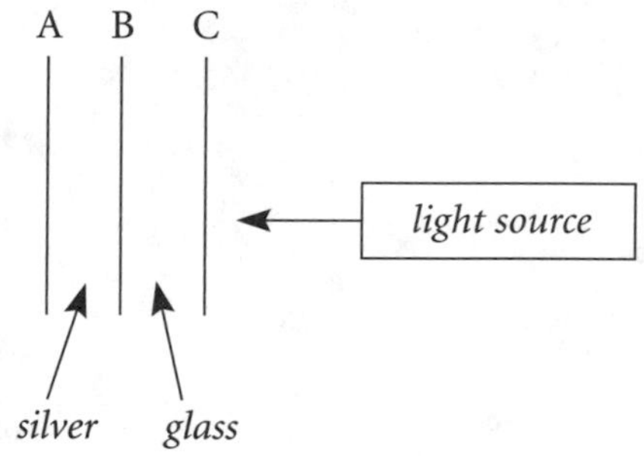

(A) A
(B) B
(C) C
(D) A and C
(E) A, B, and C

3. If 2 A pass through the 3-ohm resistor, what is the current passing through the 2-ohm resistor?

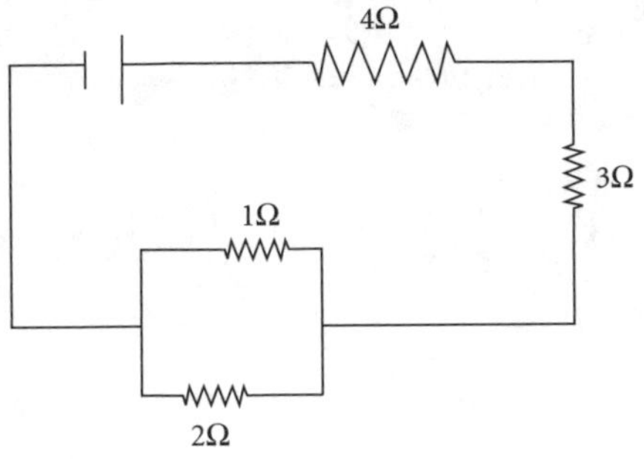

(A) $\frac{3}{2}$A

(B) 1A

(C) $\frac{4}{3}$A

(D) $\frac{2}{3}$A

(E) 2A

4. How do the frequency and wavelength of light change when it passes from air to water?

(A) The frequency decreases, and the wavelength remains the same.

(B) The wavelength decreases, and the frequency remains the same.

(C) Both the frequency and the wavelength decrease.

(D) Both the wavelength and the frequency remain the same.

(E) The wavelength increases, and the frequency decreases.

5. The operating temperature of a tungsten filament in an incandescent lamp is 2,450 K. If it were possible for this lamp to operate at a much higher temperature than 2,450 K, what would be the expected effect on the relative intensity values for the emitted electromagnetic wavelengths?

(A) Shorter wavelengths would increase in relative intensity.

(B) Longer wavelengths would increase in relative intensity.

(C) Shorter wavelengths would decrease in relative intensity.

(D) There would be no change in relative intensity.

(E) Cannot be determined from the given information.

6. A stick of wood bobs up and down in the water as shown below. Which diagram represents the stick at minimum acceleration?

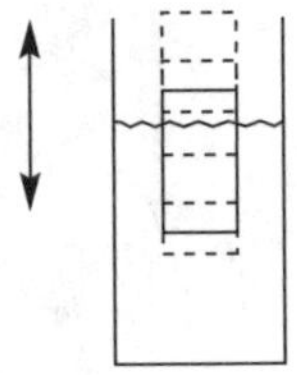

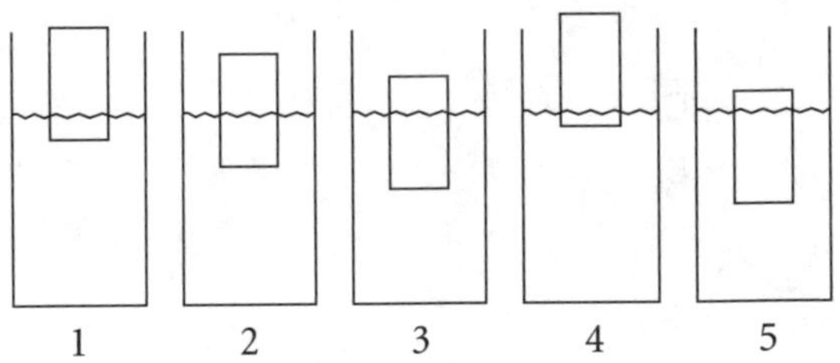

(A) 1

(B) 2

(C) 3

(D) 4

(E) 5

GO ON TO THE NEXT PAGE

7. Light is traveling through a medium whose index of refraction is n_1 and is incident on a medium whose index of refraction is n_2. What must be the minimal angle of incidence such that total internal reflection is achieved?

(A) $\sin^{-1}\left(\frac{n_2}{n_1}\right)$

(B) $\tan^{-1}\left(\frac{n_1}{n_2}\right)$

(C) $\sin^{-1}\left(\frac{n_1}{n_2}\right)$

(D) $\sin\theta_2\left(\frac{n_2}{n_1}\right)$

(E) None of the above

8. An element undergoes the following reaction: $X + \alpha \rightarrow {}^1_0n + Y \rightarrow {}^{30}_{14}Si + \beta^+$ (α is an alpha particle and β^+ is a positron, i.e., e.) What is the atomic number of X ?

(A) 11

(B) 12

(C) 10

(D) 14

(E) 13

9. A bat locates insects through reflection of sound-waves (echo) off objects, a process known as echolocation. A sound is emitted ahead of the bat in the same direction as the bat travels. Assuming that the bat's velocity and the frequency of the emitted sonar are constant, what is the character of the frequency received by the bat? (Consider locating a stationary object.)

(A) It is higher than that emitted by the bat.

(B) It is lower than that emitted by the bat.

(C) It is the same as that emitted by the bat.

(D) It is out of the range of the bat's detection.

(E) Its character cannot be determined from the above information.

10. A cubic block, with sides of length 5 cm, is floating partially submerged in water. The block is composed of an unknown substance. A second liquid of specific gravity 0.5, which is immiscible in water, is added to an additional depth of 6 cm. The block will

(A) completely sink into the water.

(B) remain partially submerged in water.

(C) float upward but remain below the surface of the upper liquid.

(D) float to the surface of the upper liquid.

(E) Cannot be determined from the information given.

11. Which of the following statements about steady fluid flow is TRUE in the pipe of constant cross section shown below?

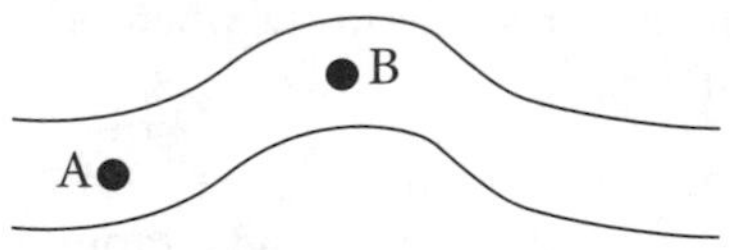

(A) The pressure at A is greater than the pressure at B.

(B) The pressure at B is greater than the pressure at A.

(C) The volume flow per unit time at A is greater than the volume flow per unit time at B.

(D) The volume flow per unit time at B is greater than the volume flow per unit time at A.

(E) Two of the above

12. When a solid cube is submerged upright in a liquid, the liquid exerts a pressure on

(A) the top of the cube.

(B) the top and bottom of the cube.

(C) the bottom of the cube.

(D) the bottom and sides of the cube.

(E) the top, bottom, and sides of the cube.

GO ON TO THE NEXT PAGE

13. An electric heater is adding 1,000 BTU/hour of heat to the water in a perfectly insulated swimming pool. If there are 186,000 L of water in the pool, if the water is initially at 20°C, and if all of the added heat is used to warm the water, what will the water temperature be after 2 hours? (1 BTU = 934 kcal)

(A) 21°C

(B) 25°C

(C) 29°C

(D) 30°C

(E) 35°C

Questions 14 and 15 refer to the following:

There are two massless, open-topped circular tubes, each of which rests on a scale. (The scales are identical.) The tubes are filled to a height H with a liquid of density ρ. One tube has a radius D, whereas the other has a radius 4D.

14. The ratio of the pressure at the bottom of the narrow tube to the pressure at the bottom of the wide tube is

(A) 1:1.

(B) 1:4.

(C) 4:1.

(D) 1:16.

(E) 16:1.

15. The ratio of the reading on the scale under the narrow tube to the reading on the scale under the wide tube is

(A) 1:1.

(B) 1:4.

(C) 4:1.

(D) 1:16.

(E) 16:1.

16. An electric dipole consists of two opposite charges of equal magnitude separated by a distance d. What is the direction of the electric field midway between the charges on a straight line joining the charges?

(A) The electric field is zero so it really has no direction.

(B) Toward the positive charge

(C) Toward the negative charge

(D) Perpendicular to the line joining the charges

(E) The direction of the field can't be determined without knowing the charge magnitudes.

17. A particle moves across the page from left to right in the presence of a uniform electric field directed toward the top of the page. Determine the type of charge and the direction of a uniform magnetic field that could result in zero net force on the particle.

I. A positive charge and magnetic field directed out of the page
II. A positive charge and magnetic field directed into the page
III. An uncharged particle and magnetic field directed into the page

(A) I only

(B) II only

(C) III only

(D) I and III

(E) I and II

GO ON TO THE NEXT PAGE

18. A 5-kg mass of water is cooled until it freezes at 0°C. What additional information is sufficient to determine the heat lost by this system?

    (A) The specific heat of water
    (B) The specific heat of water and the latent heat of fusion of water
    (C) The initial temperature of the water and the specific heat of water
    (D) The specific heat of water, the initial temperature of the water, and the latent heat of fusion of water
    (E) The specific heat of ice, the initial temperature of the water, and the latent heat of fusion of water

19. A converging lens is used as the lens of a movie projector, forming a greatly magnified image on a large screen. Which of the following must be TRUE, assuming that the film acts as a real object?

    (A) The image distance equals the object distance.
    (B) The image is real and upright.
    (C) The image is virtual and inverted.
    (D) The image distance is greater than the object distance.
    (E) The image is located at the focal point.

20. A real object is placed in front of a diverging mirror. Which of the following is always TRUE?

    (A) The image distance is positive.
    (B) The image distance is the same as the object distance.
    (C) The image is upright.
    (D) The image is inverted.
    (E) The image is real.

21. A microwave photon has a wavelength of 20 cm. A photon with a wavelength of 40 cm has

    (A) the same energy.
    (B) twice the energy.
    (C) half the energy.
    (D) one-quarter the energy.
    (E) four times the energy.

22. A nucleus emits a gamma ray. Which of the following is TRUE?

    (A) The nucleus gains energy.
    (B) The nucleus loses energy.
    (C) The atomic number decreases by one.
    (D) The atomic number decreases by two.
    (E) The number of electrons decreases by one.

23. A wave traveling along a string is described by the function y = Asin(kx–wt), where y is the displacement of the string from equilibrium and is measured in meters. What is the maximum displacement?

    (A) 1 meter
    (B) $\frac{\pi}{2}$ meters
    (C) 2π meters
    (D) A meters
    (E) A^2 meters

24. A long, straight wire carries a current that is directed into the page. The magnetic field due to this current is

    (A) directed into the page.
    (B) directed out of the page.
    (C) directed in a counterclockwise manner.
    (D) directed in a clockwise manner.
    (E) directed radially outward from the wire.

GO ON TO THE NEXT PAGE

25. Two sound waves of amplitudes A_1 and A_2 meet at a point where they are 180° out of phase. Assume the wave with amplitude A_1 exhibits a crest and the wave with amplitude A_2 exhibits a valley at this point. The displacement of the resulting wave is

 (A) 0.
 (B) $A_1 - A_2$.
 (C) $A_1 + A_2$.
 (D) $A_2 - A_1$.
 (E) $\frac{(A_1 + A_2)}{2}$.

26. A vessel used for deep-sea diving maintains an inside pressure equal to atmospheric pressure P_o. What maximum pressure must the hull be capable of withstanding at a depth of 1,000 m? Assume the density of seawater is ρ_s.

 (A) P_o
 (B) $P_o + 1{,}000\rho_s g$
 (C) $2P_o + 1{,}000\rho_s g$
 (D) $1{,}000\rho_s g$
 (E) $\rho_s g$

27. For a pond to freeze over on a hot day, which law would have to be violated?

 (A) The first law of thermodynamics
 (B) The second law of thermodynamics
 (C) Newton's first law
 (D) Newton's second law
 (E) Newton's third law

28. Two blocks of mass m and 2m and of equal volume are submerged in water. The ratio of their respective apparent weights while underwater is

 (A) 2:1.
 (B) 1:2.
 (C) 1:1.
 (D) 3:2.
 (E) Cannot be determined from the information given.

29. A cube of aluminum has been heated to its melting point but is still completely solid. If a little more heat is added

 (A) some of the aluminum will melt, and the temperature will increase.
 (B) some of the aluminum will melt, and the temperature will remain the same.
 (C) some of the aluminum will melt, and the temperature will decrease.
 (D) none of the aluminum will melt, but the temperature will increase.
 (E) none of the aluminum will melt, and the temperature will remain the same.

30. A car rolls off a horizontal cliff 125 m high, and lands 100 m from the base of the cliff. How fast was the car moving when it rolled off the cliff?

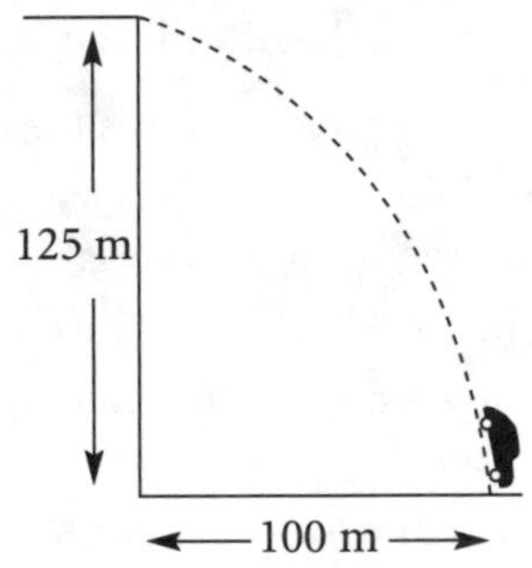

 (A) 8 m/s
 (B) 10 m/s
 (C) 16 m/s
 (D) 20 m/s
 (E) 33 m/s

GO ON TO THE NEXT PAGE

31. A 5-kg block moving with velocity v approaches a plane that is inclined at 30° to the horizontal and proceeds to slide up the plane. If the plane is 20 m long, the coefficient of kinetic friction, μ_k, is $\frac{1}{\sqrt{3}}$, and the block just reaches the top of the plane before coming to a stop, what must be the value of v ?

(A) $\frac{\sqrt{50}}{3}$ m/s

(B) 10 m/s

(C) 20 m/s

(D) $10\sqrt{3}$ m/s

(E) $\frac{20}{\sqrt{3}}$ m/s

32. A mass m_1 slides down a frictionless plane that is inclined at an angle θ_1 to the horizontal. A mass m_2 slides down a second frictionless plane that is inclined at an angle θ_2 to the horizontal. The ratio of the acceleration of m_1 to that of m_2 is

(A) $\frac{m_1\sin\theta_1}{m_2\sin\theta_2}$

(B) $\frac{\sin\theta_1}{\sin\theta_2}$

(C) $\frac{\cos\theta_1}{\cos\theta_2}$

(D) $\frac{\theta_1}{\theta_2}$

(E) None of the above

33. A ball is thrown on the Earth with an initial speed y and angle θ and travels a horizontal distance x meters. How far would it have traveled if the experiment were repeated on the moon where gravitational acceleration is $\frac{1}{6}$ that of the Earth?

(A) x meters

(B) 2x meters

(C) 6x meters

(D) 12x meters

(E) 36x meters

34. A bomber flying at 900 mph and an altitude of 6,400 ft drops a 2-ton bomb above point A on the ground. How far from point A will the bomb land?

(A) 3,200 ft

(B) 6,400 ft

(C) 2.5 miles

(D) 5.0 miles

(E) 7.5 miles

35. When blue light of wavelength 470 nm travels from a medium with index of refraction 1.5 to a medium with index of refraction 1.0

(A) its wavelength increases.

(B) its frequency increases.

(C) its speed decreases.

(D) its energy decreases.

(E) its energy increases.

GO ON TO THE NEXT PAGE

36. What is the effective resistance of the circuit below?

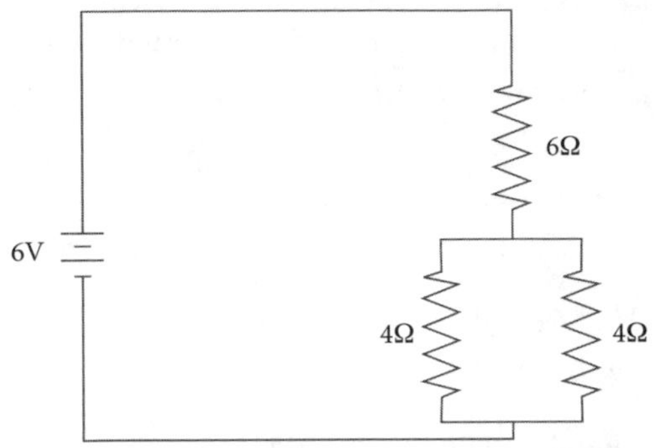

(A) 6 Ω
(B) 6.5 Ω
(C) 8 Ω
(D) 10 Ω
(E) 14 Ω

37. The circuit shown below consists of two capacitors C_1 and C_2 and a voltage supply V. The electric potential at point a is equal to the electric potential at point

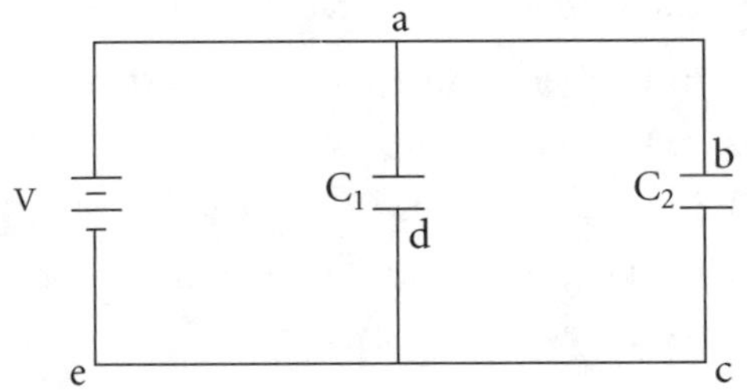

(A) b.
(B) c.
(C) d.
(D) e.
(E) None of the above

38. An object travels at 30 m/s for 5 s, then accelerates uniformly at 15 m/s^2 for 4 s. How far does the object travel?

(A) 120 m
(B) 240 m
(C) 390 m
(D) 480 m
(E) 510 m

39. Object A of mass M is released from height H, whereas object B of mass 0.5M is released from height 2H. What is the ratio of the velocity of object A to that of object B immediately before they hit the ground?

(A) 1:1
(B) $1:\sqrt{2}$
(C) 1:2
(D) 1:4
(E) $\sqrt{2}:1$

40. A projectile is launched at an angle of 60° to the horizontal with an initial speed of 5 m/s. What is the speed of the projectile at its highest point?

(A) 0 m/s
(B) 5 m/s
(C) 2.5 m/s
(D) $\frac{5}{2}\sqrt{3}$ m/s
(E) 9.8 m/s

IF YOU FINISH BEFORE TIME IS CALLED, YOU MAY CHECK YOUR WORK ON THIS SECTION ONLY. DO NOT TURN TO ANY OTHER SECTION IN THE TEST. **STOP**

QUANTITATIVE REASONING

50 questions—45 minutes

Directions: Choose the best answer for each question from the five choices provided.

1. An aquarium is filled with water. The aquarium has a base of $1\frac{1}{2}$ feet by 2 feet and a depth of $1\frac{1}{2}$ feet. If 1 gallon of water equals 231 cubic inches, how many gallons will it take to fill the aquarium?

   (A) 1,039.5
   (B) 51.3
   (C) 33.7
   (D) 29.9
   (E) 28.0

2. $1\frac{7}{8} \times 2\frac{1}{10} \times \frac{6}{7} = ?$

   (A) $3\frac{513}{280}$
   (B) $2\frac{3}{40}$
   (C) $3\frac{3}{8}$
   (D) 12
   (E) $1\frac{17}{24}$

3. Kate and Jim take a trip together. Jim drives half the distance at 40 miles per hour, and Kate drives the other half at 60 miles per hour. What is their average speed for the trip in miles per hour?

   (A) 45
   (B) 48
   (C) 50
   (D) 52
   (E) 54

4. A machine has two meshed gears, one with 24 teeth and the other with 40 teeth. If the smaller gear revolves 15 times, how many times does the larger gear revolve?

   (A) 3
   (B) 6
   (C) 9
   (D) 20
   (E) 25

5. If 23% of $\frac{2}{5}\left(\frac{190}{3x}\right) = 8$, what is x ?

   (A) $\frac{11}{6}$
   (B) $\frac{57}{6}$
   (C) $\frac{437}{200}$
   (D) $\frac{437}{600}$
   (E) $\frac{19}{6}$

6. If a heart beats 72 times every minute, how many times does it beat every second?

   (A) 0.83
   (B) 0.6
   (C) 1.5
   (D) 1.67
   (E) 1.2

GO ON TO THE NEXT PAGE

7. $\dfrac{6534}{\frac{3}{4}} = ?$

(A) $544\frac{1}{2}$

(B) $4{,}900\frac{1}{2}$

(C) 7,218

(D) 8,712

(E) 9,112

8. $a = \pi r^2 h$, $\pi = \frac{22}{7}$, $h = 14$, $a = 396$, $r > 0$, $2r = ?$

(A) 3

(B) 6

(C) 9

(D) $2\sqrt{3}$

(E) $2\sqrt{2}$

9. A number is larger than 5 by the same amount that it is smaller than 3 more than 14. What is the number?

(A) 14

(B) 12

(C) 10

(D) 11

(E) 13

10. A circle passes through the point (0, 0) and the point (10, 0). Which of the following could NOT be a third point on the circle?

(A) (2, 4)

(B) (8, 4)

(C) (2, −4)

(D) (5, 0)

(E) (1, −3)

11. If a is 25% of b and b is 60% of c, then $\frac{c}{a} = ?$

(A) $\frac{5}{12}$

(B) $\frac{20}{3}$

(C) $\frac{48}{5}$

(D) $\frac{12}{5}$

(E) $\frac{5}{3}$

12. A chemist needs to make a solution that is 60% alcohol. If she has 4 liters of a solution that is 35% alcohol, how many liters of 80% solution will she need to add?

(A) 2.5

(B) 3.75

(C) 4

(D) 5

(E) 5.5

13. $\frac{9}{8} - \frac{5}{12} + \frac{1}{2} - (?) = 1$

(A) 5

(B) $\frac{5}{24}$

(C) $\frac{29}{24}$

(D) $\frac{5}{12}$

(E) $\frac{7}{12}$

14. What is the approximate area of the largest circle that can be drawn inside of a square with an area of 1,000 square inches? $\left(\pi = \frac{22}{7}\right)$

(A) 785.7 square inches

(B) 873.0 square inches

(C) 99.4 square inches

(D) 990.1 square inches

(E) 314.1 square inches

GO ON TO THE NEXT PAGE

15. $\frac{a}{b} - \frac{b}{a} = ?$

(A) $\frac{ab}{a-b}$

(B) $\frac{ab}{b^2} - \frac{a^2}{ab}$

(C) $\frac{a^2 - b^2}{ab}$

(D) 0

(E) None of these

16. If 55% of $\frac{9z}{5} = 33$, $z = ?$

(A) $\frac{11}{5}$

(B) $\frac{165}{9}$

(C) $\frac{52}{99}$

(D) $\frac{363}{20}$

(E) $\frac{100}{3}$

17. What is the average of $\frac{1}{2}$, $\frac{2}{3}$, and $\frac{3}{4}$?

(A) $\frac{6}{36}$

(B) $\frac{23}{12}$

(C) $\frac{7}{12}$

(D) $\frac{23}{36}$

(E) $\frac{1}{4}$

18. 14 is to 35 as $2x$ is to 40. What is x?

(A) 4

(B) 7

(C) 8

(D) 2

(E) $\frac{40}{7}$

19. Diane and Sandy want to paint their room. Diane could paint the room by herself in 6 hours. Sandy could paint it by herself in 4 hours. If they work together, how many hours will it take them to paint the room?

(A) $2\frac{2}{5}$

(B) $2\frac{1}{2}$

(C) 3

(D) 5

(E) 10

20. If 8 mL of water are added to 32 mL of a 5% sugar solution, what % of the resulting solution is sugar?

(A) 2.5

(B) 4

(C) 4.5

(D) 5

(E) 6

21. The average of 5 scores is 9.6. If the highest and lowest scores are dropped, the average rises to 9.7. Compute the average of the highest and lowest scores.

(A) 9.35

(B) 9.45

(C) 9.55

(D) 9.65

(E) 9.75

22. $\frac{10 \text{ feet } (x) \text{ inches}}{9 \text{ feet } (3) \text{ inches}}$ approximates 1.2. $x = ?$

(A) 3

(B) 13.2

(C) 10

(D) 1.2

(E) 8

GO ON TO THE NEXT PAGE

23. Arrange the following numbers from the greatest to least.

a. $\frac{2}{3}$ b. $\frac{5}{11}$ c. $\frac{7}{9}$ d. $\frac{3}{4}$ e. $\frac{5}{8}$

(A) a, d, c, b, e
(B) b, d, e, a, c
(C) e, c, a, d, b
(D) c, b, e, d, a
(E) c, d, a, e, b

24. In a class, 70% of the students are girls. If the girls have an average height of 5 feet 4 inches and the boys have an average height of 5 feet 8 inches, approximately what is the average height of the entire class?

(A) 5 feet $4\frac{1}{2}$ inches
(B) 5 feet 5 inches
(C) 5 feet $5\frac{1}{2}$ inches
(D) 5 feet 6 inches
(E) 5 feet $6\frac{1}{2}$ inches

25. The cost if a ride at an amusement park rises from 75¢ to 90¢. After the rise, the number of riders decreases by 20%. What is the percent decrease in total revenues from the ride?

(A) 4%
(B) 5%
(C) 8.5%
(D) 16.67%
(E) 20%

26. $\frac{4a - 7a + 6a}{6ab} = ?$

(A) $\frac{-3}{b}$
(B) $\frac{3a}{b}$
(C) $\frac{5}{2a}$
(D) $\frac{1}{2b}$
(E) $\frac{a}{2b}$

27. Which is the largest?

(A) 0.636
(B) 0.163
(C) 0.36
(D) 0.136
(E) 0.3

28. On 150 flips of a coin, 48% of the time it landed heads. If the coin is flipped another 100 times, on what percent of those flips must it land heads to raise the percent of heads to 50%?

(A) 51%
(B) 53%
(C) 57%
(D) 52%
(E) 55%

29. Which is the smallest?

(A) 0.3
(B) $(0.3)^2$
(C) $\sqrt{0.03}$
(D) 0.03
(E) $\sqrt{0.3}$

GO ON TO THE NEXT PAGE

30. What is the number of degrees in the angle formed by the minute and hour hands of a clock at 4:50?

(A) 155
(B) 180
(C) 150
(D) 165
(E) 175

31. $10.5 \div 0.35 =$

(A) 0.3
(B) 0.03
(C) 300
(D) 30
(E) 3

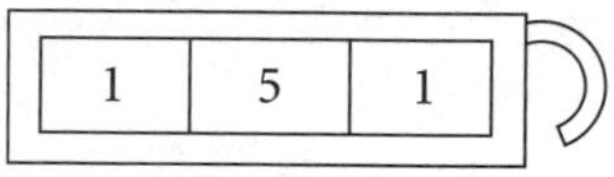

32. The lock above is at the correct setting when each of the three sections contains the correct digit from 1 to 5. How many of the possible settings will NOT open the lock?

(A) 63
(B) 24
(C) 124
(D) 215
(E) 14

33. A woman receives $286 gross pay for 48 hours work. This pay includes 8 hours of overtime at $1\frac{1}{2}$ times her normal hourly rate. Determine her normal hourly rate.

(A) $4.50
(B) $5.40
(C) $5.50
(D) $5.80
(E) $5.95

34. A fence 33 feet 4 inches long costs $99. What was the cost per foot of the fence?

(A) $3.33
(B) $3.03
(C) $2.97
(D) $3.00
(E) $2.47

35. If 1 ounce = 28 grams, $3\frac{1}{5}$ grams = (?) ounces.

(A) $\frac{1}{7}$
(B) $\frac{20}{7}$
(C) 8
(D) $\frac{4}{35}$
(E) $\frac{448}{5}$

36. $\frac{63}{3x} = 4\frac{2}{7}$. $x = ?$

(A) 0.1
(B) 4.29
(C) 5.3
(D) 2.1
(E) 4.9

37. An empty bottle weighs one-tenth of its filled weight. If the bottled is partially filled so that it weighs one-half of its filled weight, what fraction of the bottle is filled?

(A) $\frac{4}{9}$
(B) $\frac{4}{10}$
(C) $\frac{6}{10}$
(D) $\frac{45}{100}$
(E) $\frac{3}{4}$

GO ON TO THE NEXT PAGE

38. $x - y = 0.2z$

$x + z = 1.6y$

What % of $y = 0.4x$?

(A) 32%

(B) 33%

(C) 36%

(D) 40%

(E) 44%

39. $\frac{3y + 14 - y}{2y + 1} = 2.\ y = ?$

(A) 0

(B) $5\frac{1}{2}$

(C) 6

(D) 11

(E) 12

40. A 39-ounce box of cereal costs 91¢, and an 18-ounce box of the same cereal costs 48¢. What is the ratio of the cost per pound of the larger box to the cost per pound of the smaller box?

(A) 0.875:1

(B) 0.9:1

(C) 0.93:1

(D) 1.14:1

(E) 2:3

41. ( ) is to 8 as $\frac{x}{6}$ is to ( ).

(A) 16 … $\frac{x}{3}$

(B) 4 … $\frac{x}{12}$

(C) 12 … $\frac{x}{9}$

(D) 2 … $2x$

(E) $6x$ … 8

42. If a car dealer buys a car at 75% of the list price and sells it for 93% of the list price, what will the percent profit be?

(A) 18%

(B) 57%

(C) 13%

(D) 24%

(E) 21.2%

43. The volume of liquid in a container doubles every half hour. What is the percent increase in volume from 11:30 AM to 2:00 PM of the same day?

(A) 1,600%

(B) 160%

(C) 320%

(D) 3,100%

(E) 3,200%

44. Last year the ratio of teachers to students in a school was 1:8. This year the number of teachers increased by 10%, and the number of students also increased by 10%. What is the ratio of teachers to students this year?

(A) 1.1:8

(B) 2:9

(C) 1:8

(D) 1:8.8

(E) 11:18

45. $\sqrt{0.4761} = ?$

(A) 0.065

(B) 0.7

(C) 0.07

(D) 0.69

(E) 0.08

GO ON TO THE NEXT PAGE

46. If $\frac{8a}{9} = \frac{2b}{3}$ and $0.5b = \frac{4c}{5}$, how many $a = 24c$?

(A) 20

(B) 23

(C) 15

(D) $\frac{144}{5}$

(E) 18

47. In September a dentist saw $\frac{1}{3}$ more patients than he saw in August. In October, he saw $\frac{1}{5}$ more patients than he saw in September. If he saw 240 patients in October, how many did he see in August?

(A) 180

(B) 150

(C) 142

(D) 160

(E) 172

48. 90% of 40 = $\frac{5}{6}$ of (?)

(A) 36

(B) 33.33

(C) 43.2

(D) 45.6

(E) 75

49. Rebecca has twice as many toys as Jennifer. If Jennifer gives Rebecca four of her toys, then she will have one-fourth as many as Rebecca. How many toys does Rebecca have now?

(A) 6

(B) 10

(C) 16

(D) 20

(E) 24

50. If $c = \frac{2}{5}$, $\frac{1}{b} = 4$, and $a = 10$, what is $(b \cdot a) + \frac{1}{c}$?

(A) $2\frac{9}{10}$

(B) $40\frac{2}{5}$

(C) $42\frac{1}{5}$

(D) $42\frac{1}{2}$

(E) 5

IF YOU FINISH BEFORE TIME IS CALLED, YOU MAY CHECK YOUR WORK ON THIS SECTION ONLY. DO NOT TURN TO ANY OTHER SECTION IN THE TEST.

STOP

Full-Length Practice Test II: **Answer Key**

Survey of the Natural Sciences

1. C
2. B
3. B
4. D
5. A
6. D
7. B
8. B
9. B
10. E
11. D
12. B
13. C
14. B
15. B
16. C
17. A
18. E
19. D
20. B
21. B
22. D
23. B
24. B
25. A
26. C
27. E
28. A
29. C
30. B
31. C
32. A
33. D
34. C
35. D
36. E
37. B
38. D
39. C
40. D
41. D
42. E
43. B
44. D
45. A
46. C
47. C
48. D
49. C
50. D
51. D
52. C
53. C
54. D
55. A
56. B
57. D
58. D
59. C
60. E
61. C
62. E
63. E
64. C
65. A
66. D
67. B
68. A
69. D
70. C
71. E
72. C
73. C
74. D
75. E
76. E
77. D
78. C
79. A
80. A
81. D
82. E
83. C
84. B
85. C
86. E
87. A
88. D
89. C
90. E
91. D
92. A
93. B
94. C
95. B
96. B
97. A
98. A
99. B
100. A

Reading Comprehension

1. A
2. B
3. E
4. D
5. B
6. D
7. A
8. B
9. D
10. E
11. C
12. D
13. C
14. C
15. B
16. E
17. C
18. D
19. B
20. C
21. E
22. A
23. C
24. B
25. D
26. A
27. D
28. B
29. B
30. A
31. C
32. D
33. C
34. A
35. E
36. B
37. A
38. C
39. D
40. E
41. B
42. A
43. C
44. B
45. D
46. A
47. E
48. D
49. B
50. D

Physics

1. D
2. E
3. D
4. B
5. A
6. B
7. A
8. E
9. A
10. E
11. A
12. E
13. D
14. A
15. D
16. C
17. D
18. D
19. D
20. C
21. C
22. B
23. D
24. D
25. B
26. D
27. B
28. E
29. B
30. D
31. C
32. B
33. C
34. D
35. A
36. C
37. A
38. C
39. B
40. C

Quantitative Reasoning

1. C
2. C
3. B
4. C
5. D
6. E
7. D
8. B
9. D
10. D
11. B
12. D
13. B
14. A
15. C
16. E
17. D
18. C
19. A
20. B
21. B
22. B
23. E
24. B
25. A
26. D
27. A
28. B
29. D
30. A
31. D
32. C
33. C
34. C
35. D
36. E
37. A
38. E
39. C
40. A
41. C
42. D
43. D
44. C
45. D
46. A
47. B
48. C
49. D
50. E

Answers and Explanations

1. C	21. B	41. D	61. C	81. D
2. B	22. D	42. E	62. E	82. E
3. B	23. B	43. B	63. E	83. C
4. D	24. B	44. D	64. C	84. B
5. A	25. A	45. A	65. A	85. C
6. D	26. C	46. C	66. D	86. E
7. B	27. E	47. C	67. B	87. A
8. B	28. A	48. D	68. A	88. D
9. B	29. C	49. C	69. D	89. C
10. E	30. B	50. D	70. C	90. E
11. D	31. C	51. D	71. E	91. D
12. B	32. A	52. C	72. C	92. A
13. C	33. D	53. C	73. C	93. B
14. B	34. C	54. D	74. D	94. C
15. B	35. D	55. A	75. E	95. B
16. C	36. E	56. B	76. E	96. B
17. A	37. B	57. D	77. D	97. A
18. E	38. D	58. D	78. C	98. A
19. D	39. C	59. C	79. A	99. B
20. B	40. D	60. E	80. A	100. A

1. C

In a BB × bb cross, the F_1 generation genotype will be entirely heterozygous (Bb) and express the dominant phenotype. Therefore, (A) and (B) would appear in the F_1 generation. In the F_2 generation formed by crossing Bb × Bb, BB, Bb, and bb would be formed in a 1:2:1 ratio. Because the recessive could not appear in the F_1 generation but could appear in the F_2 generation (Bb × Bb cross), (C) is the only correct answer.

2. B

Distinctions between plants and animals include the following: (1) animals generally go through a larval stage—a developmental stage between the fertilized egg and the adult (i.e., the metamorphosis of tadpoles and caterpillars), whereas plants do not pass through intermediate larval stages; (2) plants are typically photosynthetic and sessile, and animals are generally heterotrophic and motile; (3) plant structure is adapted for maximum exposure to light, air, and soil by extensive branching, whereas animals are adapted for minimum surface exposure in that they are extremely compact; and (4) plant cells contain cell walls composed of cellulose.

3. B

The ectoderm primarily forms the skin, nervous system, and eyes, whereas the endoderm forms the digestive tract, the liver and the pancreas, the bladder, and the respiratory system. The mesoderm forms the musculoskeletal system and all other internal organs, such as the kidneys and the reproductive organs. (B) is the only answer that correctly associates those two with the retina and the lungs. (A) is incorrect because the heart is developed from mesoderm, and (C) is incorrect because the skeletal muscles are developed from the mesoderm. (D) and (E) are incorrect because the stomach muscles and uterus are also developed from the mesoderm.

4. D

The number of gametes can be calculated 2^n, where $n =$ the number of heterozygous genes. In this case, $n = 3$, so the number of gametes $= 2^3 \Rightarrow 8$.

5. A

Inbreeding occurs when one breeds animals that are closely related. (B) is incorrect; hybridization occurs when one breeds animals that are phylogenetically distinct to develop an animal that has characteristics of both parents. (C) is incorrect because cross-breeding is the crossing of two animals and can be used to determine phenotype when the genotype is known; or to determine genotype when the phenotype is known; or to investigate codominance, expressivity, or penetrance. (D) is incorrect; selective breeding is the creation of certain strains of specific traits by controlled breeding. (E) is incorrect; test breeding is breeding of an organism with a homozygous recessive to determine whether an organism is homozygous dominant or heterozygous dominant for a given trait.

6. D

Chlorophyll is a green pigment essential as an electron donor, and for light capture in photosynthesis. When photons of light strike chlorophyll molecules, those molecules transfer the energy of the light to their electrons. This energy (1) is then transferred to ADP to form ATP, (2) is transferred to NADP to form NADPH, and (3) splits H_2O into $2H^+$ and $\frac{1}{2}O_2$.

7. B

The allantois is found in the eggs of birds and reptiles and is used as a receptacle for nitrogenous wastes. The vessels of this structure also lie close enough to the surface of the shell to enable the exchange of gases. (A) is incorrect because the amnion is the innermost fluid-filled embryonic membrane; it forms a protective sac surrounding the embryos of birds, reptiles, and mammals. (C) is incorrect because the chorion is the outermost extra-embryonic membrane of reptiles and birds that separates the embryo from the albumin. (D) is incorrect because the umbilical cord connects the embryo to the placenta. Gas exchange occurs in the placenta. (E) is incorrect because the yolk sac contains food for the developing embryo.

8. B

A cell that is n (haploid) cannot undergo meiosis to become $\frac{1}{2}$n. (A), (C), and (D) are incorrect because there are a number of organisms that are haploid and these organisms undergo mitosis and divide and grow. An example of such an organism is a braconid wasp. These animals in the haploid form are males (n), and females (2n) are formed only when a female mates. (E) is incorrect because an organism, diploid or haploid, must be able to digest to maintain life.

9. B

(A) is incorrect because $NADH_2$ is formed from NAD during the Krebs cycle, and (C) and (D) have nothing to do with the Krebs cycle. Answer (E) is false because glycogen formation occurs only in hepatic cells and does not occur in every cell.

10. E

RNA is made up of a ribose sugar bound to a phosphate group, which is then bound to one of the four bases. (A) is incorrect because RNA is characterized by having uracil as one of its bases rather than thymine, and (B) is incorrect because DNA utilizes thymine rather than uracil. (C) is incorrect because RNA doesn't replicate in eukaryotic cells. Although in some retroviruses RNA will synthesize DNA, this is not known as the replication of DNA. (D) is incorrect because tRNA actually picks up the amino acids and brings them to the ribosome and the mRNA carries to the ribosome the message of the protein that is to be produced.

11. D

Enzymes are necessary to catalyze the reactions that allow the breakdown of glucose into ATP. (A) is incorrect because enzymes are typically proteins. (B) is incorrect because enzymes typically act most effectively at a physiological pH of 7–7.4, except for the enzymes that break down protein in the stomach, which act most effectively in an acidic environment. (C) is incorrect because enzymes do not always require a coenzyme to function. (E) is incorrect because enzymes are never irreversibly changed during a reaction. They just increase the rate of the reaction.

12. B

Homologous recombination occurs during metaphase I after tetrad formation. The farther apart two genes are, the more likely a homologous recombination will occur between them. Therefore, the genes that are farthest apart are most likely to cross over. Also, genes are more likely to recombine the farther away from the centromere they are.

13. C

A point or frameshift mutation in a gene may be evidenced by a corresponding mutation in the protein. (A) has nothing to do with how DNA might control the synthesis of a protein, and (B) is false because DNA actually directs amino acid synthesis by serving as the template that determines the sequence of the mRNA. (D) and (E) are both true but are not the best answers. Each of these answers could be merely coincidental and do not fully support the statement.

14. B

Ribosomes, the site of protein production, give the rough endoplasmic reticulum (ER) its characteristic appearance. The function of the ER is to transport proteins around the cells or for export out of the cell. Sections of the ER are lined with ribosomes where proteins are produced and then transported to the appropriate areas. (A) is incorrect because lysosomes are membrane-bound organelles in the cytoplasm that have very low pH, are filled with proteolytic enzymes, and are the site of degradation in the cell. (C) is incorrect because mitochondria are also membrane-bound organelles and are the site of cellular respiration. (D) is incorrect because the Golgi apparatus is also a membrane-bound organelle and follows the ER in the production of proteins. It is here that proteins are glycosylated and further post-translationally modified and packaged. (E) is incorrect because histones are proteins in the nucleus that bind to DNA like "beads on a string."

15. B

The eggs are released from the ovaries and are picked up by the fallopian tubes. In the case of fertilization, a haploid sperm will swim to the egg and fertilize it. The fertilized egg will then continue down the fallopian tube until it reaches the uterus, where it will implant. (C) is incorrect because fertilization in the uterus can occur but is rare and sometimes associated with complications such as cervical implantation. (D) and (E) would both disallow implantation of the fertilized egg into the uterus.

16. C

A characteristic difference between eukaryotes and prokaryotes is the presence of membrane-bound organelles in eukaryotes. (A), (B), and (D) are incorrect because both of these cell types have ribosomal RNA, plasma membranes, and ribosomes.

17. A

A totipotent cell is one that has the ability to differentiate and mature into any cell type. (B) and (C) are the opposite of totipotent. (D) is incorrect because the DNA of any cell is species-specific, so a totipotent cell will only be able to develop into a cell of that organism, and (E) is incorrect because these cells are usually unspecialized cells of multicellular organisms and are not found in unicellular organisms.

18. E

The endosymbiotic hypothesis states that blue-green algae entered into a symbiotic arrangement with early eukaryotic plants to develop into chloroplasts and bacteria entered into a similar arrangement with eukaryotic animal cells to become mitochondria. Chloroplasts and mitochondria have a plasma membrane (their inner membrane) and the ability to produce their own proteins without utilizing the cell's machinery. In addition, they have circular DNA, and their rRNA subunits are characteristic of prokaryotes.

19. D

Spermatogenesis occurs in the seminiferous tubule, and the sperm mature over a period of 2–4 days, in the epididymis. The epididymis leads to the vas deferens, which connects to the urethra to allow for ejaculation. The seminal vesicle, prostate gland, and Cowper's gland all contribute seminal fluid to lubricate, nourish, and buffer the sperm.

20. B

The electron transport chain is a complex carrier mechanism located on the inside of the inner mitochondrial membrane. During oxidative phosphorylation, ATP is produced when high-energy potential electrons are transferred from NADH and $FADH_2$ to oxygen by a series of carriers located in the inner mitochondrial membrane. As the electrons are transferred from carrier to carrier, free energy is released, which is then used to form ATP. The last carrier of the electron transport chain, cytochrome a3, passes its electron to the final electron acceptor, O_2. In addition to the electrons, O_2 picks up a pair of hydrogen ions from the surrounding medium, forming water.

21. B

Mesoderm produces the musculoskeletal system as well as the internal organs and the reproductive system. Ectoderm develops into the epidermis, the neural tissue, and the eyes. Endoderm develops into the digestive and respiratory tracts and the bladder.

22. D

Gastrulation begins with the blastula forming an inpocket into the pre-existing blastocoel. This invagination forms the archenteron, which will develop into the digestive tract. The hole that forms from the blastocoel is known as the blastopore and becomes the anus. Therefore, gastrulation forms the archenteron and the blastopore, but the blastocoel was already present.

23. B

Neurulation is the process of neural tube formation. The neural plate invaginates and forms a tube. A chemokine from an underlying mesodermal structure called the notochord (B) induces neurulation. The neural ectoderm (D) is formed during neurulation, and the neural crest (E) is formed after the neural tube. The endodermal layer (C) plays no role in neurulation, and neither does the archenteron (A), an endodermal structure that becomes the digestive tract.

24. B

Photosynthesis occurs in two steps. Step one is the light reaction in which visible light, especially that in the red/blue wavelengths, produces ATP and $NADPH_2$ through the splitting of CO_2 and H_2O. O_2 is produced during the splitting of water. During the dark cycle, carbohydrates such as glucose are synthesized when you have $NADPH_2$, ATP, and CO_2, and this will occur anytime these three compounds are present, regardless of the presence of light.

25. A

The blastula is the hollow-ball stage of embryonic development. It develops from the morula, a solid cluster of cells. The center of the blastula is termed the blastocoel. This invaginates during gastrulation to form the gastrula. At this stage, mesoderm is formed, and the archenteron and blastopore are formed. The next stage is called the neurula, and in this stage the ectoderm forms the nerve cord. Therefore (B), (C), (D), and (E) all correctly represent the stages of the embryonic development, and (A) is incorrect as the blastula is a hollow ball of cells.

26. C

Fat contains approximately 9 calories/gram while carbohydrates and proteins contain only 4 calories/gram. Sugar and starch are two forms of carbohydrates. Vitamins are coenzymes, which are typically not metabolized.

27. E

mRNA includes a coded base sequence called a codon. tRNA, which carries the amino acids to the mRNA and the ribosome, has a complementary strand called the anti-codon. Therefore, a tRNA with an anti-codon of AAC should match the mRNA codon UUG. Remember that in RNA, adenine bonds with uracil and guanine bonds with cytosine.

28. A

In the light reaction, light splits H_2O into excited electrons, H^+ and O_2. The excited electrons go on to form ATP, and H^+ is incorporated in the carbohydrates produced during the dark reaction. The O_2 is released into the environment as a waste product of this reaction. (B) is incorrect because CO_2 donates the carbon and the oxygen required for carbohydrate formation in the dark reaction. (C) and (D) are end products of photosynthesis, and answer (E) is incorrect because chlorophyll is involved in the initial capture of sunlight.

29. C

The number of genetically distinct offspring is found by multiplying the number of distinct gametes each parent can produce. The number of gametes can be calculated from the formula 2^n, where n = the number of heterozygous genes. The AaBbCc parent can produce 8 unique gametes ($2^3 = 8$), and the AaBBCc parent can produce 4 ($2^2 = 4$). Therefore, the possible number of different offspring is $8 \times 4 = 32$.

30. B

Identical twins are produced when a zygote produced by one egg and one sperm splits during the four- or eight-cell stage to develop into two genetically identical organisms. (A) is incorrect because identical twins will be the same gender but fraternal twins can also be the same gender. (D) is incorrect because these are termed fraternal twins and are no more genetically alike than siblings. (C) and (E) are impossible events.

31. C

In the light reaction, chlorophyll absorbs energy to split water into excited electrons, H^+ and O_2. The excited electrons make ATP through photophosphorylation. In the dark reaction, carbohydrates are produced, without the need for sunlight, by CO_2, the H^+ ions in the form of $NADPH_2$, and ATP. (B) is incorrect because that describes cellular respiration. (D) is incorrect because that does not occur; and (E) is incorrect because H_2O is split, not CO_2.

32. A

Multiple alleles describe more than two allele possibilities. In the ABO blood group, there are three alleles: A and B, which are codominant over the recessive allele O. There are four possible phenotypes, A, B, AB, and O, and six possible genotypes, AA, AO, BB, BO, AB, and OO. (B) refers to crossing organisms heterozygous for two traits such as AaBb × AaBb. This cross will have the characteristic 9:3:3:1 ratio of offspring. (C) refers to recessive alleles, which are not expressed unless they are homozygous. (D) refers to the fact that two genes will be inherited independently of each other if they are not linked physically on the chromosome. (E) refers to changes in genes through spontaneous changes in base sequence.

33. D

In the nucleus, DNA is produced during cell division, and RNA is transcribed. mRNA travels from the nucleus into the endoplasmic reticulum where it is translated on the ribosomes into polypeptides.

34. C

If a male is affected with red-green color blindness, his genotype would be $X^{cb}Y$. If he mated with a normal female, XX, their female offspring would be all $X^{cb}X$, receiving one good copy of the X chromosome from their mother and the color blindness gene from their father. Because this is a recessive trait, all the offspring (100%) would be carriers. The male offspring of this mating would all be XY (100% normal), receiving one good copy of the X chromosome from their mother and receiving their Y chromosome from their father.

35. D

Mutations in somatic cells affect only the individuals involved and no progeny, because they cannot be passed on to the next generation and will not affect gamete formation. These mutations are typically recessive although there are some instances of dominant negative mutations. The major concern about mutations in somatic cells is the development of tumors as a result of a protein that has lost its function due to a somatic mutation. This is the basis for tumors such as malignant melanomas caused by mutations to the DNA as a result of UV irradiation.

36. E

Nondisjunction is a failure of homologous pairs to separate after synapsis. The result is an extra chromosome or a missing chromosome for a given pair. For example, Down syndrome is due to an extra chromosome 21. The number of chromosomes in a case of single nondisjunction is $2n + 1$ or $2n - 1$. In Down syndrome, it is 47. Most of these embryos are aborted early in their development, and only a few, like Down syndrome trisomy 21, trisomy 13, and trisomy 18, are viable, albeit with developmental disorders. Breakage near the centromere might be induced by environmental factors such as mutagens, but would not be caused by nondisjunction.

37. B

DNA replication occurs during the S phase so that each daughter cell will receive a complete copy of the genome. DNA replication is semiconservative: half of the original DNA (one strand) is present in each of the new, or daughter, double-stranded DNA molecules. As always, purines bind to pyrimidines; more specifically, adenine binds to thymine whereas cytosine binds to guanine. Okazaki fragments are formed on the lagging strand so that although DNA is synthesized in the 5′ to 3′ direction in short segments, overall it is synthesized in the 3′ to 5′ direction.

38. D

Let R = dominant red color and r = recessive white color. There are two possible red genotypes for the unknown offspring: RR (pure homozygous red) and Rr (heterozygous red). The unknown offspring will be referred to as R_. If the cross in (A) were performed, crossing R_ with Rr (red plant with a white parent), then you would be able to determine the unknown genotype. If there were any white offspring, the unknown genotype must be Rr. If only red offspring resulted, then the genotype must be RR. If the cross in (B) were performed, crossing R_ with RR, you would not be able to determine the genotype. If the unknown allele was recessive, it would be masked by the homozygous dominant red genotype. The only phenotype that can result from a parent that is RR is red, so any white allele would never be exposed. If the cross in (C) were performed, crossing R_ with rr, you would be able to determine the unknown genotype of the offspring. If there were any white offspring, the unknown genotype must be Rr. If only red offspring resulted, then the genotype must be RR. Therefore (D), two of the above, is the correct answer.

39. C

AO × AB potentially will result in offspring with the genotypes AA, AB, AO, or BO. As you can see, OO homozygous blood type O is impossible in this mating.

40. D

Given that males have a frequency of color blindness of 1 in 12, you know that the gene frequency of the color-blindness allele is 1 in 12. Because females would require both copies of the color-blindness allele to be color blind, the frequency of color-blind females is $\frac{1}{12} \times \frac{1}{12}$, or $\frac{1}{144}$.

41. D

The density of a gas is the mass of the gas divided by the volume it occupies. For simplicity, we can assume a 1-mole sample of the gas, which occupies 22.4 L at STP. If XY_2 were in fact the molecular formula, then the mass of one mole would be 14 grams and the density would be

$$\frac{14\text{ g}}{22.4\text{ L}} = \frac{0.63\text{ g}}{\text{L}}$$

Because the density is given to be approximately twice as much, it follows that the molecular weight must be twice as much and, therefore, that the molecular formula must be twice the empirical formula, or X_2Y_4.

As for the wrong choices, (A) and (C) can be dismissed for not being integral multiples of the empirical formula, XY_2. The calculation done above could have been repeated on each of the remaining choices, or avoided by a rough approximation on the remaining choices:

$$\frac{14\text{ g}}{22.4\text{ L}} < \frac{1\text{ g}}{\text{L}}, \frac{28\text{ g}}{22.4\text{ L}} > \frac{1\text{ g}}{\text{L}}, \frac{56\text{ g}}{22.4\text{ L}} > \frac{2\text{ g}}{\text{L}}$$

42. E

To answer this question correctly, first write and balance the equation for the combustion described:

$$C_3H_8 + 5\ O_2 \rightarrow 3\ CO_2 + 4\ H_2O$$

For every mole of propane, 5 mol of oxygen will be required. The formula weight of propane is 44 g/mol ($3 \times 12 + 8 \times 1$), so 88 g will be 2 mol and, therefore, 10 mol of oxygen will be required. At 32 g/mol, 10 mol of O_2 is 320 g.

43. B

According to the periodic table provided with the test, the atomic weight of bromine is 79.9 g/mol. Because 1.204×10^{24} is twice Avogadro's number, 1.204×10^{24} atoms correspond to 2 mol, and the total mass of this number of bromine atoms will be 2 x 79.9 g/mol, or 159.8 g. Note that a rough approximation allows you to dismiss (A), (D), and (E). The question then becomes "more or less than 160?"

44. D

The element has an atomic number of 16, corresponding to 16 protons in its nucleus. A neutral atom of X would thus have 16 electrons surrounding its nucleus. To acquire a –2 charge, an atom of X must acquire two extra electrons, bringing the total number of electrons on the X^{2-} ion to 18. Note that wrong answer (A) corresponds to the number of electrons that must be added to produce the –2 charge, rather than the total number of electrons as requested. (B) and (C) would be correct if we had been asked for the number of electrons in a 4+ or 2+ cation, respectively, rather than the 2– anion. (E) might have been correct if the question had asked for the total number of nucleons rather than for the number of electrons. Note that the atomic weight of the element is an extraneous piece of information that is not necessary for the problem.

45. A

Given that Mg is 2.4312% of the chlorophyll, a 100-g sample of chlorophyll will contain 2.4312 g of magnesium. Because the atomic weight of magnesium is close to 24.312 g/mol, this 2.4312 g will correspond to about one-tenth of a mole, or 6.022×10^{22} atoms. The wrong answers here result from errors in the placement of the decimal point.

46. C

This is a limiting reactant problem, recognizable as such because the quantities of both reactants are given. As occasionally happens, we can recycle some scratchwork from an earlier question. The reaction is the same as that used in question 42, and the same balanced equation applies:

$$C_3H_8 + 5\ O_2 \rightarrow 3\ CO_2 + 4\ H_2O$$

Having found that 320 g of oxygen were required for complete combustion of 88 g of propane in the earlier question, it follows that oxygen will be the limiting reactant here, with only 160 g available. This corresponds to 5 mol of oxygen (molecular weight = 32 g), which in turn implies that 3 mol of carbon dioxide are produced. After determining the formula weight of CO_2 to be 44 g/mol, an answer of 132 g, or (C), is reached.

47. C

The valence, or outermost, electrons are those involved in bonding; it is these same electrons that will determine the chemical properties of an element, simply defined as its ability to combine with other elements or compounds. The number of valence electrons, as offered in (C), is then what most affects the general behavior of an element in the presence of another substance. Elements with a large number of valence electrons (i.e., those found toward the right side of the periodic table), are nonmetallic, with large ionization energies and electronegativities, for instance, and are thus likely to combine with metals (with a relatively small number of valence electrons) to form ionic compounds.

(A) is incorrect because the electrons in an *s* orbital will affect chemical behavior only if the *s* orbital in question is part of the valence shell; inner *s* orbitals, however, house core electrons which are not involved in bonding. (B) is wrong in that it refers to the protons contained in the nucleus of the atom; the nucleus itself is not involved directly in bond formation, i.e., it does not directly influence chemical interactions, or behavior. (D), although correctly identifying electrons as the influential factor, distorts the truth in saying that it is the total number of electrons, rather than the number in the valence shell. Finally, (E) refers to atomic mass, which, like the number of protons in (B), is wrong in that nuclear rather than chemical properties will be affected by this factor.

48. D

Atomic radii are greatest toward the lower left-hand corner of the periodic table, with cesium, Cs, the largest naturally occurring atom. Atomic radius decreases as one moves from left to right across the table, disqualifying (A), (C), and (E). (B) can be eliminated because atomic size increases, along with principal quantum number, as one moves downward in the periodic table, leaving us with (D), the credited choice.

49. C

This question on VSEPR theory and molecular geometries can be answered by drawing the proper Lewis structure and applying the theory or, more conveniently, by comparing the given compound to a more familiar reference compound. The former approach requires that the Lewis structure be correctly composed of a central nitrogen atom bonded to three surrounding fluorine atoms, with one lone pair of electrons remaining on the nitrogen atom.

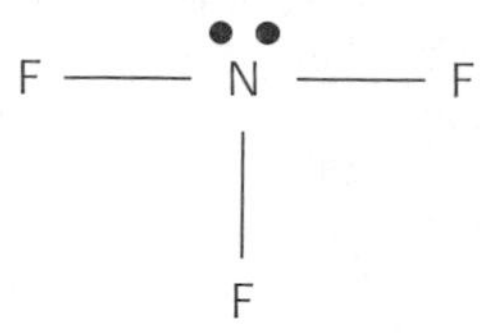

Because four regions of electron density surround the central atom, the electronic geometry is tetrahedral, but because only three of these regions are composed of bonded electrons, the molecular geometry is trigonal pyramidal. In short, the nitrogen trifluoride molecule is of the general formula AB_3U and, thus, has the electronic and molecular geometries associated with this general formula. To approach this problem by comparison to a reference compound, NF_3 is just like NH_3, except that the H atoms have been replaced by F atoms. Because ammonia is a trigonal pyramid, it follows that NF_3 will be as well.

50. D

In general, a cation is smaller than a neutral atom of the same element because the removal of an electron or electrons to form the cation leaves fewer electrons to shield each other from the attractive force of the nucleus. The remaining electrons on the cation are thus drawn in closer to the nucleus, resulting in a reduction in size. Conversely, anions are generally larger than the corresponding neutral atoms due to an increased number of electrons shielding the attractive nuclear force and repelling each other. When attempting to compare the sizes of ions of different elements, it is generally most convenient to compare them to an intermediate species. In this example, each answer choice offers an isoelectronic series of atoms and ions—i.e., each entry in (A), (B), (C), and (D) has 54 electrons, the xenon configuration. With the same number of electrons being attracted to a different nuclear charge, it follows that size will decrease in the same order as atomic number and, therefore, the positive charge of the nucleus increases. Only (D) provides the elements in increasing atomic number order from Te, number 52, through La, number 57.

51. D

This question is testing some basic concepts of quantum mechanics, the relationship between the principal and azimuthal quantum numbers n and l. The secondary, or azimuthal, quantum number l can take on any value from zero to $(n - 1)$; when $n = 4$, l can thus have the values 0, 1, 2, 3, as stated in (D).

52. C

This question on reaction stoichiometry requires us to recognize which of the two reactants is the limiting reactant. The equation is provided in its fully balanced form, and we can see that magnesium nitride reacts with water in a 1:6 ratio. Thus 2 mol of magnesium nitride would require 12 mol of water to react fully, which is more than is available in this case. Water is therefore the limiting reactant. Because 2 mol of ammonia are produced for every 6 mol of water, 9 mol of water should yield 3 mol of ammonia. (D), which is incorrect, most likely results from ignoring the limiting reactant aspect of the problem.

53. C

This question may appear to be testing bonding, but it can be answered based on periodic trends. Metallic character increases toward the left side of the periodic table. Sodium and magnesium are both active metals and thus combine with hydrogen to form ionic hydrides. (This is true for any Group IA or IIA metal.) Nitrogen, on the other hand, is a nonmetal and thus combines with hydrogen to form a molecular compound held together by covalent bonding.

54. D

Because 8.0 grams of hydrogen correspond to 4 moles, and they undergo combustion completely, the heat released will be twice that of the reaction as written, which describes the combustion of 2 moles of hydrogen gas: $\Delta H = 2 \times 115.60 \text{ kcal} = 231.2 \text{ kcal}$.

55. A

This question requires you to interpret the given electron configuration. Adding the superscripts first, we can see that there are 20 electrons all together. This finding is sufficient to dispose of (C), (D), and (E) because they have 21, 19, and 18 electrons, respectively. Calcium does have 20 electrons when neutral; to distinguish between (A) and (B), we will thus need to inspect the order of orbital occupancy. According to the Aufbau principle, 20 electrons should result in the electron configuration $1s^2 2s^2 2p^6 3s^2 3p^6 4s^2$. By occupying the $3d$ subshell instead of the $4s$ subshell, the given configuration indicates an excited state, and (A) is correct.

56. B

This question can be answered by applying the relationship $\Delta H_{rxn} = \Delta H^o_f(\text{products}) - \Delta H^o_f(\text{reactants})$. Recalling that ΔH^o_f for any element is zero, we can substitute values as follows:

$$\begin{aligned} \Delta H_{rxn} &= H^o_f(CO_2) - \tfrac{1}{2} H_f(O_2) - H^o_f(CO) \\ &= (-94.05) - (0) - (-26.41) \\ &= -94.05 + 26.41 = -67.64 \end{aligned}$$

Note the potential for approximation: $-100 + 25 = -75$ is close enough for the choices offered. (A) and (D) result if you add the values instead of subtracting them, whereas (C) and (D) come from losing track of the minus sign.

57. D

Increasing pressure would be the result of a decrease in volume (V), an increase in temperature (T), or an increase in the number of moles of gas (n) in the container. Because we are asked about the number of molecules of gas B in an identical container at the same temperature, we can focus on this last variable. To raise the pressure from 25 to 125 torr, or five times as much, we need five times as many moles, or equivalently, five times as many molecules. Because we began with one mole of gas A, we need five moles of gas B; converting moles to molecules, we get $(5 \text{ mol}) \times (6.02 \times 10^{23} \text{ molecules/mol}) = 3 \times 10^{24}$ molecules, as stated in (D). (A) results if we misread the question stem and solved for the number of moles instead of the number of molecules, (B) if we forgot to multiply by five, (C) if we messed up the exponent in our calculation, and (E) if we gave up too soon. Note that (B) and (C) could have been eliminated upon the realization that if the pressure is higher, the number of molecules must be greater than that contained in the original sample of gas A.

58. D

Gas volume is proportional to the number of moles of gas present in the sample, all other things being equal. As such, we can predict the required volume by finding the number of moles, or vice versa. Given that 1.0 mL of blood produces 0.15 mL of oxygen, we can extrapolate that 100 mL of the same blood will produce 15 mL of the gas under the same conditions of temperature and pressure. Because one mole of an ideal gas occupies 22.4 L at STP, it follows that 1 mmol of the gas will occupy 22.4 mL, also at STP. The following calculation is therefore valid:

$$15 \text{ mL} \times \frac{1 \text{ mmol}}{22.4 \text{ mL}} = \frac{15}{22.4} \text{ mmol}$$

59. C

This question asks us to apply Le Châtelier's principle to determine which of the choices offered will increase the yield of iodine or, in other words, shift the equilibrium to the right. Because the reaction shown has oxygen as a reactant, addition of oxygen should produce the desired result. (A) is incorrect because the reaction has heat shown as a product; raising the temperature would thus shift the equilibrium to the left. (B) is wrong because addition of a catalyst has no effect on the ultimate position of the equilibrium but only on its rate of attainment. (D) is incorrect because water is a product; adding H_2O would thus shift the equilibrium toward the reactant side, decreasing the yield of iodine. Finally, (E) is wrong because there are more moles of gas shown on the reactant side of the given reaction; an increase in pressure would thus shift toward production of product, while a decrease in pressure would shift the equilibrium to the left.

60. E

This question on periodic trends can be translated to "Which of the following is closest to the upper right-hand corner of the periodic table?", excluding the last column of the table. Chlorine, (E), is above bromine, (D), and far to the right of lithium and sodium, (B) and (C), respectively. Although helium, (A), is furthest in the upper right direction, it is an inert gas and thus does not have a propensity to accept electrons. Remember that the periodic trend of electron affinity, as well as that of electronegativity, does not apply to the rare gases.

61. C

An exothermic reaction is one for which heat is emitted (i.e., one for which ΔH is negative). The sign of ΔH is not directly transferred to ΔG, which also depends partially on the sign and magnitude of ΔS (the entropy change) and on the value of T (the absolute temperature), because $\Delta G = \Delta H - T\Delta S$.

62. E

The balanced equation is:

$$8\,KMnO_4 + 3\,NH_3 \rightarrow 3\,KNO_3 + 8\,MnO_2 + 5\,KOH + 2\,H_2O$$

Adding up the coefficients on the reactant and product sides, then subtracting as the question dictates, yields $(3 + 8 + 5 + 2) - (8 + 3) = 18 - 11 = 7$.

63. E

This question requires us to determine an empirical formula from a given mass ratio. Because the ratio is given as 6 g of carbon for 1 g of hydrogen, and because the atomic weight of carbon is 12 g/mol, it would probably be most convenient just to double the whole ratio. The ratio then becomes 12 g of C for every 2 g of H, or 1 mol C for every 2 mol H. (A) and (B) can be eliminated because they do not contain the correct ratio of carbon to hydrogen content. One may also question whether (A) is a valid empirical formula because it conveys structural information—the presence of a hydroxyl group making it a methanol molecule—that should not be present in an empirical formula, which merely gives the simplest whole number ratio of the atoms present in the compound. (C) and (D) can also be eliminated because the subscripts can be reduced further, making them invalid as empirical formulas. Note that one may easily jump erroneously to (C) as the answer if one does not keep in mind the definition of an empirical formula. (E) lists the atoms in the simplest whole number ratio possible and has the correct proportion of carbon to hydrogen, making it the correct choice. Notice that it was never claimed that the compound contains only carbon and hydrogen!

64. C

This thermodynamics question can be answered by applying the fundamental relationship $\Delta H_{rxn} = \Delta H_f(\text{products}) - \Delta H_f(\text{reactants})$. Recalling that ΔH_f for any element is zero, we can substitute values as follows:

$$\Delta H_{rxn} = 3\,\Delta H^o_f(H_2O, g) + \Delta H^o_f(W, s) - \Delta H^o_f(WO_3, s) - 3\,\Delta H^o_f(H_2, g) = 3(-57.798) + (0) - (-200.84) - 3(0) = -173.39 + 200.84 = 27.45$$

Note that the approximation $-180 + 200 = 20$ is quite sufficient to distinguish among the choices offered.

65. A

The magnetic number, m_l, can take on any of the integral values from negative l to positive l inclusive. When $l = 3$, m_l can thus have the values −3, −2, −1, 0, 1, 2, 3, as are listed in (A).

66. D

As one descends the column in the periodic table, the principal quantum numbers of the valence shells, and hence the atomic and ionic radii, increase. (D), beryllium, located at the top of Group IIA, is thus the smallest of the ions listed. The increasing order of ionic radius is $Be^{2+} < Mg^{2+} < Ca^{2+} < Sr^{2+}$; the remaining choices are thus incorrect, because each of the other ions is larger than Be^{2+}.

67. B

The value of the equilibrium constant is dependent on temperature. (A), (C), and (E) may change the relative concentrations of the species at equilibrium but would not change the numerical value of K; thus these three choices are incorrect. (D) doesn't affect the position of equilibrium at all, making it incorrect as well.

68. A

It is a general and very nonquantitative rule that many reactions will double their rates for each 10° increase in temperature. This somewhat oddball question can probably best be answered by dismissing the incorrect choices because the stem gives little hint as to what to predict for an answer. (B) is incorrect because, although velocity of particles does increase with increasing temperature, it is unlikely to double for a small temperature rise. (C) can be dismissed because increasing temperature will usually expand a substance; with an increase in volume, the concentration actually decreases. (D) is wrong because the pressure of a gas is proportional to its absolute temperature; a 10°C rise in temperature will thus only double the pressure if the initial temperature was 10 K, a very unlikely temperature for a gas. (The ideal gas law is unlikely to apply at such a low temperature anyway.) Finally, (E) is wrong because in an endothermic reaction, as the question stem indicated, heat is absorbed and not evolved.

69. D

This question requires that you calculate the formula weight of quinine from the given formula and then convert the given mass, in grams, to the number of molecules via Avogadro's number. The formula weight is the sum of the atomic weights of the atoms in the formula, thus, the formula weight of quinine is

$$20\ (12) + 24\ (1) + 2\ (14) + 2\ (16)$$
$$= 240 + 24 + 28 + 32 = 324 \text{ g/mol.}$$

There are thus $\frac{16.2}{324}$ moles of quinine in the sample.

We can observe that $\frac{16.2}{324}$ is $\frac{1}{20}$; the answer should therefore be about $\frac{1}{20}$ of Avogadro's number, 6×10^{23}.

70. C

Metallic character is the result of the combination of low ionization energy, electron affinity, and electronegativity that increase toward the lower left-hand corner of the periodic table. (Remember that cesium, Cs, is the most metallic naturally occurring element!) The question can thus be translated as, "which of the following lists elements, in order, from upper-right to lower-left on the periodic table?" The four elements listed in the choices are all in the same column of the table, Group IVA, and so we need only to check the vertical arrangement of these elements, which should then be from top to bottom. Descending the column now, the order is Si, Ge, Sn, Pb, the same as that in (C).

71. E

The key here is that bond length decreases as bond order increases (single > double > triple). Thus, reduction of the bond to a lower bond order will result in a longer bond, which is given only in (E). However, even if you did not remember this fact about bonding, there still is a hint here that could help you guess the correct answer. No one would expect you to memorize the exact bond lengths in question, because this is really mindless trivia. However, you could guess that you need to see the trend. There are three choices that are reductions in bond length (none of which you are expected to know!), so you could discount (A), (B), and (C). The only unique answers are (D), no change, and (E), elongation. Because the student might imagine that there should be some difference between the two bond lengths, (E) is the logical choice. The form of the question itself often suggests an answer.

72. C

The slowest and, hence, rate-determining step in an S_N1 reaction is the formation of the carbocation. Molecules that form stable carbocations are therefore more likely to undergo S_N1 reactions. Remember, carbocation stability decreases in this order: tertiary > secondary > primary > methyl. (A) is a primary bromide and would not be expected to react via the S_N1 mechanism at all. (B), (D), and (E) are secondary and will also not be expected to react as readily as (C), the most substituted (tertiary) bromide.

73. C

Obviously, rotation must occur for configuration A to transform into configuration B. However, double bonds, composed of a σ and a π bond, are not free to rotate (hence eliminating (E)), whereas single bonds composed of one π bond have rotational freedom. Therefore, the π bond must be broken, and rotated around the central carbon-carbon σ bond to yield configuration B after reforming the π bond. (A) and (D) are incorrect because breaking the σ bond alone does not alter the stable geometry of the molecule: unlike σ orbitals, π bonds do not have cylindrical symmetry, and rotation about one would disrupt the favorable overlap. (B) is incorrect because the σ bond does not need to be broken.

74. D

The *sp* hybridization is found only on atoms that are bonded to two other species (each bonded group can be replaced by a lone pair of electrons). With more substituents, more atomic orbitals must be deployed for hybridization to accommodate the expanded valency. (A), (B), and (C) are all sp^2 hybridized (three different bonding partners), whereas (E) is sp^3 hybridized (four bonding partners).

75. E

The first step in identifying the compound with the most stereoisomers is to determine the number of chiral centers in each molecule. (A) and (D) have three chiral centers each, while choices (B), (C), and (E) have four, as asterisked below:

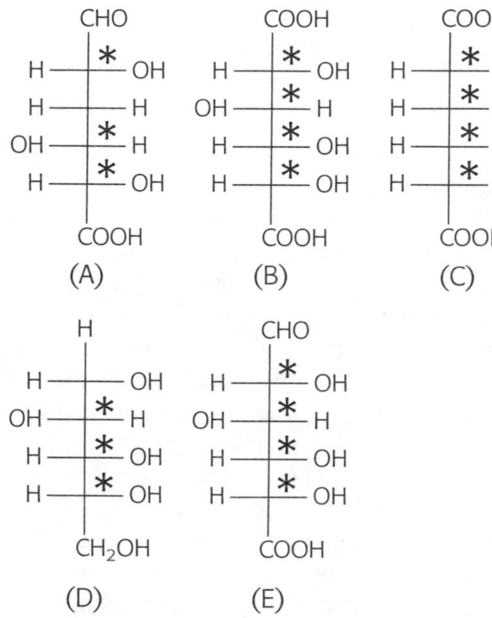

(A) and (D) are thus eliminated. The presence of four chiral centers generally implies the existence of $2^4 = 16$ stereoisomers, except in the cases of *meso* structures, which despite possessing chiral centers are nonetheless superimposable upon their mirror images. The presence of *meso* compounds means that certain enantiomeric pairs are actually identical structures and, thus, the number of stereoisomers would be lowered. (C) in fact is a *meso* compound, as it is seen easily that it possesses a plane of symmetry and is therefore superimposable upon its mirror image. (B), being itself a stereoisomer of (C), will likewise possess fewer than 16 stereoisomers. (E), in contrast, has different groups attached on each end (an aldehyde on one and a carboxylic acid on the other), and there is no possibility that any of its stereoisomers will be a *meso* compound. It will therefore possess the full 16 stereoisomers allowed by its four chiral centers and is the correct choice.

76. E

Methyl acetate is an ester composed of acetate (the acid half) and methanol (the alcohol part). (A) is incorrect; it is acetic acid. (B) is simply sodium acetate, a common buffering salt. (C) is dimethyl ether. (D) and (E) are both esters. However, the name should give the clue that one methyl group is present. (D) is incorrect because ethyl acetate (or ethyl ethanoate), a common solvent, does not have a methyl group. Only (E) corresponds to methyl acetate.

77. D

Properties that stabilize the S_N1 carbocation intermediate or destabilize the S_N2 transition state will favor S_N1 reactions. (A) is incorrect because polar rather than nonpolar solvents will help stabilize the ionic (charged) intermediate, favoring S_N1 mechanisms. (B) is incorrect because temperature does not specifically affect either reaction type one way or the other (although high temperature tends to favor elimination reactions over substitutions in general). (D) is correct because a higher concentration of nucleophile will affect only S_N2 reaction kinetics, whereas S_N1 kinetics is independent of nucleophile concentration. (C) is incorrect because weak nucleophiles will have a hard time displacing the leaving group. This will favor the formation of the carbocation intermediate *before* nucleophilic attack, which is an S_N1 reaction. Obviously, (E) must be incorrect due to the discussion above.

78. C

Atoms in the ground state have their electrons in the lowest energy configuration. Upon absorbing energy, one or more of the electrons will get promoted into an orbital of higher energy, increasing the energy of the electronic configuration. This does not involve the necessary loss of the electron in question (although it could), which eliminates (A), (B), and (E). In principle, the number of core electrons could also decrease if a core electron is excited to the valence level, but again, this is not a requirement for excitation. The energy is increased and not decreased, so (D) is also incorrect.

79. A

As an uncharged organic molecule, dimethylpropylamine could dissolve at least partially in most organic solvents, eliminating (C) and (D). In aqueous solutions, the amine moiety could act as a base by accepting a proton and acquiring a positive charge, making an ammonium ion, which would be soluble to some extent in water. For this to happen, there must be a supply of protons, whether from the water itself or from an acid. Either dilute or concentrated acid would suffice, thus eliminating (B) and (E). A KOH solution would be very proton-poor, which would leave the amine unprotonated and uncharged. When uncharged, organic molecules are not very soluble in water, so (A) is correct.

80. A

Both cyclohexane and benzene have six carbons. Cyclohexane and other saturated six-member ring structures are found predominantly in the chair formation, but benzene is an unsaturated ring that has a planar geometry. This eliminates (B) and therefore (E) as well. (C) and (D) are also incorrect because benzene is not as stable as cyclohexane thermodynamically. Note that one often says that benzene is stabilized by the resonance delocalization of the π electrons. This does not mean, however, that it is more stable than its fully hydrogenated analog cyclohexane; the extra stability is in reference to nonconjugated trienes.

81. D

The first step in arriving at the correct IUPAC name for an alkane is the identification of the longest unbranched carbon chain in the molecule. In this case, there are many possible choices for the carbon skeleton (because of the equivalence of the four methyl groups), but they all contain three carbon atoms, so the root name for this molecule would be propane. The only possible candidates then become (C) and (D). Prefixes like *iso*, *neo*, and *sec*- are used in the IUPAC system to label substituents but are not used in naming the backbone; therefore, (D) is correct. One can verify that after singling out a carbon skeleton, the two remaining methyl groups will be attached to the middle carbon atom of the three (i.e., the one numbered two), so 2,2-dimethyl propane is indeed the IUPAC name for the molecule. It should be pointed out that none of the other choices is a valid IUPAC name for *any* compound. Incidentally, the compound is more commonly known as neopentane, and this common name is also recognized by the IUPAC.

82. E

Enantiomers are nonsuperimposable mirror-image isomers of chiral compounds. As mirror images, they occur in pairs, so (D) cannot be correct. The Fischer projections can be rotated in the page, or both pairs of substituents can be exchanged, without changing the chirality of the compound.

If compound I is rotated 180° in the page, it gives compound II. These two compounds are therefore identical and are not enantiomers. Compound I is the mirror image of compound III (imagine holding a mirror between compounds I and III), so they are enantiomers. Because I and II are identical, II and III must also be enantiomers.

83. C

The Lewis structure of benzene shows a ring structure with three double bonds and three single bonds. However, this is one case where the inadequacy of the Lewis dot structure approach is revealed. The alternating double bonds drawn are actually π bonds occupied by electrons delocalized about the ring. All six bonds in benzene are equivalent and possess characteristics intermediate between those of single and double bonds. (A) and (B) are therefore incorrect. (D) is incorrect because although benzene is often drawn as two resonant structures where the positions of the single and double bonds have been exchanged, this is merely an attempt to fix the inadequacy of the Lewis structures. No one resonant structure is an accurate depiction of benzene at any one instant of time, and in particular resonant structures should never be thought of as mixtures of different species.

84. B

The oxygen atom has six valence electrons and needs to form two bonds to share two extra electrons to form a stable octet. Therefore, oxygen usually has two unshared electron pairs and two bonds (two single bonds, as in the water molecule, or a double bond, as in the carbonyl group). Oxygen has three bonds here but has done so at the expense of its other unshared electron pair. According to the rule of assigning formal charges to atoms in a molecule, formal charge = valency – half the number of bonding electrons – number of unshared electrons. Thus, in the case of oxygen here, the formal charge $= 6 - \left(\frac{1}{2} \times 6\right) - 2 = 1$. (A) is incorrect because carbon, with a valency of four, here participates in four bonds and does not possess any lone pairs. Its formal charge is therefore zero. (C) is incorrect because this type of structure is common for six-ringed structures with oxygen, notably the anomeric carbon of monosaccharides undergoing glycosidic reactions. (D) and (E) are incorrect for the reasons given above.

85. C

The first step toward naming alkanes is to identify the longest carbon chain, which in this case contains nine carbon atoms. This eliminates (B) and (D). The substituents should then be named alphabetically, keeping the numbers of the substituents as small as possible. Here, the substituents are 1,2 dimethylpropyl (using the same rules again to identify the longest chain) and a methyl group. The compound is named 5-(1,2-dimethylpropyl)-2-methyl nonane, which is (C).

86. E

Aromatic compounds are cyclic, planar compounds with $(4n + 2)$ π electrons (where n is any non-negative integer). This is known as Hückel's rule. Compound I is benzene with 6 π electrons ($n = 1$) and is therefore aromatic. Compound II, naphthalene, has 10 or $(4 \times 2 + 2)$ π electrons and is also aromatic. Compounds III (furan) and IV (pyrrole) are both examples of heterocyclic compounds (cyclic compounds having elements other than carbon in the ring backbone). The oxygen in furan has two lone pairs of electrons. One of the two pairs would participate in the delocalized π cloud, which together with the two double bonds drawn would yield a total of 6 π electrons, thus making furan aromatic. (The other lone pair will occupy an sp^2 orbital orthogonal to the π system.) The nitrogen in pyrrole has a lone pair of electrons that is part of the π system, and thus pyrrole is also aromatic with 6 π electrons. The correct answer must then be all of the above, or (E).

87. A

Boiling points for similar compounds are determined by the amount of hydrogen bonding, dipole moment, and molecular weight, in that order. Hydrogen-bonding and dipole moments increase the attraction molecules have among themselves, which raises the boiling point. Compounds I and III, as carboxylic acids, contain both polar carbonyl groups and hydroxyl groups that are capable of hydrogen bonding. They will thus have the strongest intermolecular interactions and, consequently, the highest boiling points. Because compound III is one methylene unit larger than compound I, it should have the higher boiling point of the two. After these two comes compound IV, which, as an alcohol with a hydroxyl group, is also capable of hydrogen bonding. Compound V is next. It is slightly heavier than compound II but, more importantly, will have a dipole moment because of the high electronegativity of the bromine atom, which will give bromine a slight negative charge. Compound II, a straight chain alkane, has the lowest boiling point. Arranging this information from lowest to highest, we have II, V, IV, I, and III, which is (A). Note that a rudimentary knowledge of what governs boiling points is sufficient to rule out other choices without the need to arrange the five compounds precisely. Straight-chain unbranched alkanes do not possess strong polarity and will be expected to have the lowest boiling points among the compounds, thus eliminating (D) and (E). Compound III is expected to have a higher boiling point than compound I because of its additional methylene group (but otherwise similar chemical functionality). With these two pieces of information alone, one can arrive at the correct answer of (A).

88. D

Amides are amine groups directly bonded to a carbonyl carbon. (A) is a primary amine, with the alkyl group attached to it being an ether. (B) is a secondary amine. Neither of these choices contains a carbonyl group, which is necessary. (C) is a ketone with a tertiary amine substituent: it would be an amide if the intervening methylene group between the carbonyl carbon and the nitrogen were removed.

89. C

Stereoisomers are isomers that arise from the different spatial arrangements of groups attached to double bonds or chiral centers. In this case, the compound has two carbon atoms that are stereocenters (second and third). Each will have either *R* or *S* designations. The possible isomers are then *S,S*, *S,R*, *R,S*, or *R,R*, which is (C). Note that if the two halogens are the same, then the number of stereoisomers will be 3, because then *R,S* would be identical to *S,R*, known as a *meso* compound.

90. E

Overlapping orbitals that are perpendicular to the axis of the bond are features of π bonds. Because the overlap is not cylindrically symmetric, rotation about the interatomic axis would break such bonds. Double bonds consist of one σ and one π bond, whereas triple bonds consist of one σ and two π bonds. (The two π bonds in a triple bond are perpendicular to each other.) (A) and (B) are incorrect because σ bonds, found in single bonds, are formed when the overlap is along the axis joining the atoms. (C) and (D) are incorrect because double and triple bonds differ only in the number of π bonds, not in their nature.

91. D

The compound in question has the common name neopentyl chloride (A) but also has a name assigned under the IUPAC guidelines. (You are expected to know certain common names.) To identify the IUPAC name, one first observes that the longest unbranched chain contains three carbon atoms, and thus the compound is a propane. In numbering the carbon atoms, one tries to minimize the numbers of those with substituents. In this case, we have a chlorine attached to one end and two methyl groups attached to the middle carbon atom, and given a choice between 1,2 and 2,3, we opt for the former. Alphabetizing the substituents, one arrives at the IUPAC name 1-chloro-2,2-dimethylpropane, which is (B). Both (A) and (B) can be names for the compound shown, and so (D) is correct.

92. A

A secondary amine consists of a nitrogen attached to one hydrogen atom and two alkyl groups. (B) is a tertiary, (C) a primary, and (D) a quaternary amine. (E) is ammonia, which is technically not an amine at all.

93. B

The greater the number of alkyl groups attached to the sp^2 hybridized carbons (i.e., the more substituted they are), the more stable the alkene. Molecule IV has two methyl groups on each side of the double bond and will thus be the most stable among the five, followed by molecule II, which has two methyl groups on one side and one on the other. Next comes molecule I, which has one methyl group on each side. (It is worthwhile to point out that the *trans* configuration would be more stable then the *cis* one, but this aspect is irrelevant here.) Molecule V has only one methyl group on one side, whereas molecule III has none and will therefore be the least stable. Thus, stability in increasing order would go III, V, I, II, IV, which is indicated in (B). Note once again that one can pick out the correct answer without having to determine the entire sequence: knowing that III is the least stable and IV is the most stable would be sufficient.

94. C

The complete oxidation of any hydrocarbon (or carbohydrate) composed solely of carbon, hydrogen, and oxygen is a combustion reaction leading to the products CO_2 and H_2O. (A) is incorrect because combustion reactions such as this are always exothermic. This is the basis of energy sources such as natural gas, propane, octane, etc. (B) is incorrect because the compound listed is an alkane, not an alkene. (D) and (E) do not have the right products.

95. B

Because each carbon of acetylene has two bonding partners (one carbon and one hydrogen), it is *sp* hybridized. The rest of the choices are all true and therefore incorrect. Acetylene, or ethyne, has the molecular formula C_2H_2 (alkynes in general have the molecular formula C_nH_n), and is a linear molecule with a triple bond (one σ and two π bonds). Because it is also symmetric, the (already weak) polarity of the C–H bonds cancel each other vectorially, so the molecule does not have a net dipole moment, making it relatively nonpolar: it is only slightly soluble in water. (A), (C), (D), and (E) are therefore all true.

96. B

Resonance is a mechanism by which molecules are stabilized by delocalization of charges. (A) and (D) are incorrect because all aromatic compounds owe their stability (compared with nonconjugated alkenes and alkynes) to resonance of their conjugated, or alternating, double bonds. (C) is incorrect because organic acid anions, such as the acetate ion depicted here, stabilize their negative charge between the two oxygen atoms of the acid moiety. Finally, (E) is incorrect because one can draw an equivalent resonance structure in which the positive charge of the molecule switches to the other end and the double bond jumps to the other carbons. The π electrons of the double bond are thus delocalized over all three carbon atoms. Only (B), having no double bonds or charges to delocalize, is without stabilizing resonance forms.

97. A

The ion in (A), an allyl cation, is the only one of the choices that has a resonance form that can delocalize the positive charge and thereby stabilize the cation:

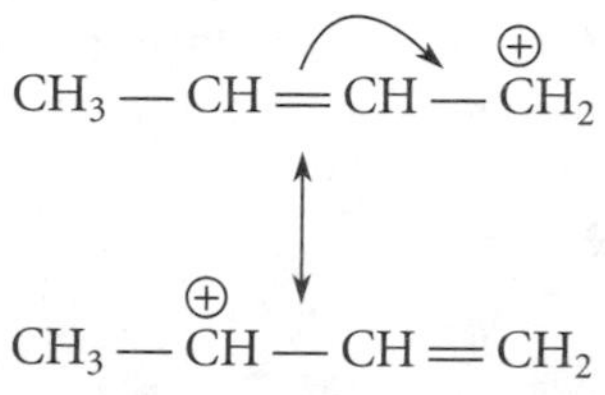

In (B) and (C), the double bond is unable to participate in charge delocalization because of the intervening sp^3 hybridized carbon, which disrupts the π system. In (C), the phenyl group and the double bond are conjugated but do not affect the positive charge. The same is true for the phenyl group in (D). (If the intervening methylene group were removed we would have the very stable benzyl cation.) (E), a vinyl cation, is also incorrect because the π bond is perpendicular to the empty *p* orbital of the carbon atom bearing the positive charge; stabilization through delocalization thus cannot take place.

98. A

Of the compounds listed, only alcohols are capable of hydrogen bonding, which is the most important factor when discussing the melting/boiling points of organic compounds. (B), (C), and (D) all may possess dipole moments that will cause them to boil at higher temperatures than that of an alkane (E) of similar molecular weight. However, the dipole interactions are much weaker than are hydrogen-bonding interactions.

99. B

This is a simple matter of evaluating the effects of steric hindrance upon molecule stability. The two phenyl groups are very bulky substituents (much larger than the bromine atoms) and will strive to be as far away from each other as possible. (A) and (C) both will have more steric repulsion than (B), because the phenyl groups will be fighting to occupy the same space. The phenyl rings can, of course, relieve part of the steric repulsion by rotating out of the plane of the double-bonded carbons, but then this means we will have to give up the favorable delocalization of the π electron system that we have in (B).

100. A

This is a textbook S_N2 reaction in which the oxygen atom on the ethoxide ion acts as a nucleophile and displaces the iodine. The iodide ion is a good leaving group, and ethoxide is a good nucleophile. The methyl species is sterically unhindered, and the ethoxide is not a very bulky base (which would have favored E2 over S_N2). The resultant products are $C_2H_5OCH_3$ (ethyl methyl ether) and iodide ion that may complex with the positive sodium ion, depending on the solvent. This reaction is, in fact, a Williamson ether synthesis.

Answers and Explanations

1. A	11. C	21. E	31. C	41. B
2. B	12. D	22. A	32. D	42. A
3. E	13. C	23. C	33. C	43. C
4. D	14. C	24. B	34. A	44. B
5. B	15. B	25. D	35. E	45. D
6. D	16. E	26. A	36. B	46. A
7. A	17. C	27. D	37. A	47. E
8. B	18. D	28. B	38. C	48. D
9. D	19. B	29. B	39. D	49. B
10. E	20. C	30. A	40. E	50. D

1. A

The passage states clearly that the speech pathologist and the orthodontist deal with problems of improper speech in different contexts, one functional and the other structural. While it may be argued that orthodontists need more training than speech pathologists, the passage does not address this issue. In addition, the passage does not indicate that orthodontics and speech therapists are contraindicated in cases of lisping or that one works better on adolescents. Orthodontics corrects structural anomalies, not functional disorders. Therefore, choice (A) is the correct answer.

2. B

The author of the passage states that the purpose of passive methods of speech therapy is to direct the child's articulatory organs into the proper position for making a correct sound. Speech therapy itself supposes the development of new sounds, and passive therapy methods involve close personal contact between therapist and child. However, passive methods of speech therapy are not effective in cases of severe malocclusion.

3. E

One of the main benefits of speech therapy is that it takes what is already there—the child's vocal anatomy—and teaches the child to utilize it effectively. As a result, surgery is often unnecessary, as described in choice (E). Choice (A) is incorrect because many patients do achieve desired results, especially with problems of sibilant articulation. Choice (B) is wrong because in many cases speech defects can be treated without the use of orthodontic equipment. Choice (C) is also incorrect because the passage does not mention lack of emotional support as a cause of speech defects. The correlation of speech problems and learning disabilities is not addressed in the passage and has little foundation.

4. D

The author states that the cardinal rule of speech therapy is that the patient must learn an entirely new sound to compensate for the one he or she is incapable of articulating. It is quite possible that the child with a speech disorder may be better served if orthodontic treatment is completed before speech therapy is initiated, thereby preserving the anatomy during the therapeutic process. While active methods of speech therapy are important, the passive methods of speech therapy are equally critical. Therefore, choice (D) is correct.

5. B

The author states that the active methods of speech therapy are deductive in nature, as they begin with sounds that the child can already make, and work toward the sound that is to be learned. Passive methods retrain the articulatory organs. While the use of mirrors for speech therapy is often associated with passive methods, it is not this characteristic that is essential to active speech therapy. The use of active therapy does not obviate the use of passive therapy. Thus, choice (B) is correct.

6. D

It can be inferred from the passage that problems with the articulation of sibilants generally appear late in the child's language development because the *s* sounds are the last to appear in the course of development. The correction of sibilants can be performed using active speech therapy, but not always easily, and can be completed without the use of surgery. Usually, the sibilant mispronunciations lie in the manner in which the child verbalizes the *s* sound, not in the anatomy. Therefore, choice (D) is correct.

7. A

The passage states that class I malocclusions are treated with fixed or removable appliances that help turn or straighten irregular teeth. These methods, as the passage further describes, are uniformly effective. Therefore, choice (A) is correct.

8. B

During the description of active speech therapy, the author provides the caveat that the speech therapists must avoid the demonstration of perfect pronunciation because it is of no use to the patient and predisposes the patient to tension and nervousness. While it may be argued that choice (A) is a viable option, the speech therapist should be more aware of the proper pronunciation shortcoming rather than the treatment of a class III malocclusion with the subsequent referral of the patient to a surgeon. Speech therapists often associate articulative mechanisms with particular sounds and more often than not can correct lisps without the help of orthodontists. Therefore, choice (B) is correct.

9. D

The author states that the recommended attitude of therapy is the combined use of orthodontists and speech therapists, rendering results faster and more positive. The author believes that the benefit from speech therapy can often come when orthodontic work is not performed; however, in many cases orthodontics aid in the process of speech therapy. While orthodontic treatment is sometimes detrimental to the progress speech therapy alone has made, it is never contraindicated to the treatment of structural vocal defects. The passage does not mention the use of modern advances in dental surgery for the treatment of speech disorders. Therefore, choice (D) is correct.

10. E

The passage states that an appliance for class II malocclusion must be worn for at least 13 hours a day. To save the child more emotional embarrassment, this appliance is worn at night. The night brace is also worn in class III malocclusion, but this was not presented as an answer choice. Treatment of problems with sibilant articulation involving night braces is not discussed in the passage. Therefore, choice (E) is correct.

11. C

The passage states that as a form of preventive dentistry, orthodontics is concerned with the correction of dental anomalies for the purpose of heading off future difficulties. It is not speech pathology, or functional therapy, or sibilant modification; these therapies are initiated by speech therapists. Therefore, choice (C) is correct.

12. D

Class II and class III malocclusive defects are described at length in the passage and are compared almost as opposites of one another. Class II defects involve an underdevelopment of the lower jaw, while class III children demonstrate an overdeveloped lower jaw. Therefore, choice (D) is correct.

13. C

Active methods of speech therapy, which begin with sounds that the child can already make, are often desired in lisping because the child is usually able to pronounce some of the *s* sounds. Usually, these children do not need orthodontic treatment; active speech therapy is sufficient. Therefore, choice (C) is correct.

14. C

An example the author gives of initiating passive speech therapy is for a therapist to show a child how to approximate the position of the front teeth. This is in accordance with learning the proper alignment of the front teeth. Listening to recordings and performing exercises to increase tongue flexibility are not passive processes, nor is recognizing that changing one's speech habits is an emotional process as well as a physical one. Wearing a night brace would be a treatment prescribed by a orthodontist, not a speech therapist.

15. B

The class II malocclusion, according to the passage, involves an underdevelopment of the lower jaw, with upper molars falling in front of the lower ones. Therefore, choice (B) is correct.

16. E

In the description of class I malocclusions, the author argues against the use of removable appliances. Removable appliances, he claims, may be neglected, which can bring progress to a halt. Class II malocclusive patients often suffer from "buck teeth." In addition, the passage does not mention the irritation of removal devices to gums or the age of patients with fixed appliances. Therefore, choice (E) is correct.

17. C

The passage states the number of U.S. citizens 85 years old and older is growing six times as fast as the rest of the population. It makes no mention of these citizens being predominantly male; instead, it argues that the majority of these individuals are female. The author does note that hundreds of thousands of senior citizens have migrated to the Sunbelt states over the last 30 years. Yet he never delineates what percentage of these seniors is over 85. Further, there is no indication in the passage that those 85 and older primarily live in the Sunbelt states. In addition, the 85-year-old and older population is not solely responsible for the high cost of medical care. The passage indicates that it is the disabled elderly (hence, not just those 85 and older) and people without insurance of all ages who are contributing to high costs. Finally, there is no indication in the passage that those 85 and older on average garner an annual income between $20,000 and $50,000. The facts that "77 percent of elderly Americans have annual incomes of less than $20,000" and that "most elderly Americans come to depend heavily on federal and state subsidies...as their earning power declines and their need for health care increases" seem to imply that, if anything, those 85 and older most likely do not earn average annual incomes between $20,000 and $50,000.

18. D

The author indicates in lines 84–86 that "by the year 2030, there'll only be two workers for every person 65 and older." While the passage mentions the threat to Social Security by constant borrowing to pay interest on the national debt, the author never indicates that there will be no money left in Social Security by 2030. The passage never indicates that there will be a ratio of 81 men for every 100 women in the U.S. by 2030; rather, it reveals that by the age of 65, there are only 81 men left for every 100 women. Choice (C) is simply incorrect. The passage reveals that by the year 2030, there will be 65 million senior citizens (not 51 million). Finally, while the last paragraph of the passage indicates that in the next few decades the U.S. population may demand a less expensive health care system, it never specifically says that there will be a new system in place in 2030.

19. B

The author states in lines 131–133 that "the elderly population will double within the next 40 years." There is no indication in the passage that there is a current housing shortage (much less that the elderly are responsible for such a shortage) or that the elderly are the wealthiest segment of the U.S. population (in fact, the passage reveals that most elderly come to rely heavily on federal and state subsidies). In addition, the passage never mentions that the elderly account for 30 percent of the U.S. population; rather, it reflects that by 1990 "spending on the elderly accounted for 30 percent of the annual federal budget." Finally, although there has been a large flux of senior citizens into Sunbelt states over the last 30 years, there is no evidence in the passage that seniors constitute the majority of the population in these states.

20. C

The passage defines the "baby boom" generation as the generation born after World War II. It goes on to state that between 1946 and 1964 (the baby boom period), more than 75 million Americans were born. The baby boom generation does not have the highest life expectancy of any generation; rather, the newest generation does, owing to medical advances, etc. The median age of the U.S. population (in general) at the start of the 1990s was 33; there is no indication in the passage of the median age of the baby boom generation. In addition, there is no evidence that the baby boom generation regards its parents as a financial burden. In fact, the passage seems to imply that many of the baby boom generation's parents are taking care of them. As the author indicates, "today's elders often find themselves acting as family bankers," and most own their homes while their children encounter difficulty in financing a home. Finally, baby boomers have not yet reached the ranks of the elderly; as the passage indicates, "in less than two decades, they will join the ranks of America's elderly."

21. E

According to the author, demographic experts predict that the southward migration of the elderly will diminish in the future, since surveys have found that the great majority of people 55 and older would prefer not to relocate. The passage does not correlate southward migration with relatively low incomes or with the shrinking of the U.S. workforce. This shrinking, rather, has been attributed to the fact that the number of available young workers is decreasing. In addition, there is no indication that seniors migrated south because of the availability of low-cost housing. Finally, there is no evidence in the passage that seniors migrated to the south because of overcrowded conditions in the north.

22. A

The author states that presently one out of every two marriages ends in divorce; thus, the current divorce rate is approximately 50 percent (not less than 40 percent). In addition, there is no indication in the passage that the divorce rate is rising rapidly or slowly declining. Finally, the current divorce rate is affecting family structures, as the author states that with the present occurrence of divorce, "a significant number of today's grandparents are suddenly faced with the task of raising or helping to raise their grandchildren."

23. C

The passage specifically indicates that "in less than two decades, they [the baby boom generation] will join the ranks of America's elderly." There is no evidence that baby boomers will migrate west in search of employment or that baby boomers (specifically) will fail to qualify for health insurance. The passage clearly states that early retirement will probably "become a thing of the past" and that "[a]s the number of available younger workers shrinks, elderly people will become more attractive as prospective employees." Finally, an increased birthrate for this generation in the future is wrong, as the passage reveals that millions of baby boomers have already entered middle age and that in the next two decades they will join the ranks of the elderly.

24. B

According to the passage, "by 1990, spending on the elderly accounted for 30 percent of the annual federal budget."

25. D

The author lists a myriad of factors that contribute to increased life expectancy, including improved public sanitation, the ever-increasing popularity of physical fitness, federal and state aid for the poor and senior citizens, and advances in medicine. No mention is made of a decline in birth rate.

26. A

According to the passage, 77 percent of the elderly earn less than $20,000 per year. While the passage notes that the cost of providing care for disabled elderly will double in the next decade, there is no indication that a majority of the elderly suffer a disability between the ages of 65 and 75. In addition, the author states that approximately 75 percent of today's elderly own their own homes. It can also be construed that a majority of the elderly no longer work. The passage states that at present, only 15 percent of 65-year-old men work, that the median retirement age is now 61, and that early retirement flourished over the last four decades. Finally, the elderly do depend on subsidies, and in large numbers. According to the passage, "[a]s their earning power declines and their need for health care increases, most elderly Americans come to depend heavily on federal and state subsidies."

27. D

Medicare was instituted in 1965. Note: Do not become confused by the date 1935, which is the year in which Social Security was instituted.

28. B

The author states that the cost of caring for disabled elderly Americans is expected to double in the next decade alone. This cost will add to the continuous upward spiral of medical costs that threaten the Medicaid/Medicare system. In all likelihood, then, these systems will become increasingly expensive. There is no indication in the passage that the government will be unable to finance a national health care system; in fact, the only obstacles that the author notes to such a system are the medical establishment and various special interest groups. In addition, there is no evidence that the government will have to (or be able to) borrow from Social Security to finance Medicaid/Medicare. It may be argued that baby boomers will be unable to receive federal health benefits as they grow older if costs continue to escalate. Yet, according to the passage, this group will not be without federal health benefits, as it will probably demand a national health care system over the next few decades. Finally, while the passage does note the improvement of medicine in the recent past, there is no indication that the ensuing increase in health care costs of the elderly can be correlated with poor care in the past.

29. B

It can be inferred from the passage that the process of early retirement is a relatively recent phenomenon. The author supports this inference by stating that in 1950, about 50 percent of all 65-year-old men still worked; today, only 15 percent of them do. Early retirement will not transform the workforce of the future; rather, it is said to have transformed the workforce of the past 40 years. In addition, it will most likely not become more popular in the next century, as the passage states that it will soon become a thing of the past. There is no indication that early retirement is correlated with a decline in the U.S. economy. Finally, there is no proof in the passage that early retirement restructured the U.S. workforce prior to World War II; instead, the passage reflects that early retirement transformed the workforce after WW II.

30. A

The passage states that elders—those people 65 and older—now outnumber teenagers for the first time in American history. It can be inferred that today's elderly population is not larger than the current population of baby boomers, as the passage notes that the reason the elderly population will be even larger in the future is that the baby boom generation will be entering the ranks of senior citizens. The elderly population of today is larger than that of 1950 or 1970; the passage states that "the population of elders has doubled in just 40 years." Finally, the elderly population of today will not be larger than the projected elderly population of the year 2030. As the passage indicates, "the elderly population will double within the next 40 years."

31. C

The author of the passage states that one offshoot of the aging of America will be a gradual restructuring of the family unit away from the traditional nuclear family and toward a multigenerational family dominated by elders, not by their adult children. Thus, the typical U.S. family will not be youth-oriented. In addition, there is no specific indication that this family type will be wealthier than today's family structure or that this family unit will be subsidized by Social Security. Finally, the passage never mentions that the typical future family structure will be free from divorce (in fact, the opposite could be argued, as the author states that one of every two marriages today ends in divorce).

32. D

The author states that over the past 30 years, hundreds of thousands of senior citizens migrated south to Sunbelt states. There is no indication in the passage that many seniors worked past the age of retirement, lost their Social Security benefits, or suffered a serious physical disability. Finally, there is no evidence that many of the elderly lost their homes over the past 30 years; on the contrary, the passage notes that 75 percent of today's elderly own their own homes.

33. C

The author argues that a nationalized health care system has not been implemented in the United States because the medical establishment and various special interest groups have so far blocked legislation aimed at creating one. There is no indication in the passage that the federal deficit, the efficacy of Medicare/Medicaid, or expense is the impediment to a national health care system. Finally, according to the passage, millions of U.S. citizens cannot afford private health insurance (which is an argument for nationalizing health care).

34. A

As described in the passage, mass number refers to the mass of an atom and is defined as the number of protons plus the number of neutrons in the nucleus of that atom. Therefore, an atom that contains 16 protons and 16 neutrons should have a mass number of 32, or twice the mass number of oxygen-16.

35. E

The paragraph states that carbon-14 rather than carbon-11 is used in biological experiments because carbon-14 has a half-life of 5,730 years while carbon-11 has a half-life of only 20 minutes. The short half-life causes it to disintegrate too quickly to be detected and emit too intense a radiation, which may be detrimental to tissue with which it comes into contact.

36. B

As the passage describes, the Geiger counter merely indicates the presence of a radioactive material when it receives significantly more radiation than that normally present in the atmosphere. In contrast, radioactive emissions detected via photographic film are indicated both with respect to the total number of radioactive particles emitted by the sample as well as by the distribution.

Therefore, choice (B) is correct because the film can indicate the area where the radiation is absorbed.

37. A

The half-life of a material is the time in which half of that initial substance will decay. Radon-222, with a half-life of 3.8 days, will decay by one half every 3.8 days. Therefore, with an initial 2 grams, only 1 gram will remain after 3.8 days. After another 3.8 days, or 7.6 days total, only 0.5 grams will remain.

38. C

The passage describes a beta particle as a high-speed electron that is produced when neutrons are converted to protons. While this type of emission will raise the atomic number by 1, the mass number will remain the same. Therefore, phosphorus-32 emitting a beta particle will result in the formation of an atom with 1 higher proton number but the same mass number. This would be sulfur-32 (proton number of 33, mass number of 32).

39. D

The passage states that photographic films will darken when exposed to radiation of higher intensity or for longer duration. Therefore, the degree to which photographic film badges worn by workers in plants where radiation is present darken represents the total radiation absorbed over the period of time for which the badge is worn.

40. E

The passage states that alpha particles are helium nuclei that contain 2 protons and 2 neutrons.

41. B

Ingested iron, as the passage argues, is not incorporated into the hemoglobin but is stored in the form of a protein complex or excreted. This makes choice (B) the appropriate answer.

42. A

Geiger counters are composed of two electrodes sealed in a tube containing argon gas. High-energy radioactive particles ionize the argon gas and allow charges to bridge the gap between the electrodes. The result of this process is the clicking noise of a Geiger counter. The passage states that Geiger counters are incapable of detecting neutrons because neutrons are not charged. This is because uncharged atomic components cannot ionize argon gas and, therefore, cannot cause a current between the electrodes of a Geiger counter. Therefore, choice (A) is correct.

43. C

Isotopes, as defined in the passage, are elements with the same number of protons and different numbers of neutrons. The distinction of an isotope has nothing to do with the charge of the nucleus, the electron configuration, or the number of electrons.

44. B

Although the photographic film can detect location of radiation (something the Geiger counter cannot), it is less sensitive than the Geiger counter. Choice (A) is incorrect, as a Geiger counter cannot detect the presence of neutrons, and Geiger counters are not able to detect atmospheric radiation (choice C). The Geiger counter is more portable than photographic film. The efficiency of the Geiger counter and the film is not discussed.

45. D

The passage states the disadvantages of using isotopes with short half-lives: 1) short half-lives result in disintegration of isotopes that cannot be detected, and 2) the intensity of radiation emitted by isotopes with short half-lives is more damaging to tissue. However, in contrast, the disadvantage of the isotopes with long half-lives is that they often emit radiation at a rate too small to be detected.

46. A

Cyclotrons accelerate electrons and protons, while fission reactors produce neutron bullets. Because neutrons are uncharged particles, they are not repelled by any part of a target atom and can therefore penetrate an atom much more easily than either protons or electrons. It follows that the use of neutrons allows for a much wider variety of radioactive particles to be produced than when protons or electrons are used.

47. E

The first two paragraphs of the passage describe the general structure and nomenclature used when describing an atom. Therefore, choice (E) is the most logical answer. The history of the study of atoms is not delineated within the passage, and the detection of radioactive emissions and the production of radioisotopes, while addressed in the passage, are not discussed within the first two paragraphs. Dangers of radioactive experiments are also not touched upon in the first two paragraphs of this passage.

48. D

The passage states that isotopes whose nuclear structures are unstable undergo radioactive decay. It further states that this nuclear decay can manifest itself in the emission of one of three possible types of particles or rays: alpha, beta, or gamma.

49. B

The passage states that the use of radioisotopes in research is based upon the fact that radioisotopes have the same chemical properties as their nonradioactive counterparts. For example, in biological systems, radioactive substances will localize themselves in the same area as nonradioactive isotopes of the same element. Therefore, choice (B) is correct. Choice (A) is a poor possibility because isotopes with short half-lives have significant side effects stemming from tissue damage. Additionally, these isotopes are not inert; they emit radiation. Often, they can be harmful to the organism being studied. Isotopes with very long half-lives emit radiation at a rate too small to be detected.

50. D

Look for the false statement in these choices. In the final paragraph, the author discusses the use of radioisotopes in experiments that involve blood. Choice (D) is incorrect because blood does need to be taken in this type of experimentation to determine the radiation intensity. Since radiation intensity must be measured, choice (E) is a true statement. Choice (A) is correct—this is the purpose of the experiment. The second sentence states that radioactive blood is injected into the organism, making choice (B) a correct statement. Choice (C) is a true statement because blood must be drawn after "a suitable period of time."

Answers and Explanations

1. D	11. A	21. C	31. C
2. E	12. E	22. B	32. B
3. D	13. D	23. D	33. C
4. B	14. A	24. D	34. D
5. A	15. D	25. B	35. A
6. B	16. C	26. D	36. C
7. A	17. D	27. B	37. A
8. E	18. D	28. E	38. C
9. A	19. D	29. B	39. B
10. E	20. C	30. D	40. C

1. D

The force on q^+ due to Q^+ is directed along the line joining the two and also directed away from Q^+ because the two charges repel. The force on q^+ due to Q^- is directed along the line joining the two and toward Q^- because the two charges attract. The net force due to the two charges is the vector sum of the force due to each. So we have to sum two vectors, one of which is directed toward the bottom right part of the page and the other toward the bottom left part of the page. Clearly the net vector will be directed generally downward.

2. E

The system is a simple schematic of a mirror, which consists of a piece of glass and a silver backing. In general, whenever light reaches an interface, some of it is reflected and the rest of it is transmitted (and refracted). The proportion of light that is reflected depends on such factors as the relative indices of refraction of the two media, the angle of incidence, and the wavelength of the light. Reflection, then, occurs at all three interfaces, although with different intensities.

3. D

From Kirchhoff's first law, we know that if 2 A pass through the 3Ω resistor, then 2 A must also pass through the combination of the 2Ω and 1Ω resistors. We then have $2 = I_1 + I_2$, where I_1 is the current through the 1Ω resistor and I_2 is the current through the 2Ω resistor. Because the resistors are in parallel, we also know that the voltage drop across each is the same, so $I_1(1) = I_2(2)$ (i.e., the voltage drop is IR). Substituting for I_1 in the first equation we have $2 = 2I_2 + I_2 = 3I_2 \Rightarrow I_2 = \frac{2}{3}$ A.

4. B

When light passes from one medium to another, its frequency remains the same and its wavelength changes. The only answer choice consistent with this is (B). For completeness, let's see just how the wavelength changes. We should remember that the index of refraction of water is greater than that of air. Also recall that $v = \frac{c}{n}$, where n is the index of refraction and v is the speed of light in the medium. But it's also true that $v = \lambda f$, so we have $\lambda f = \frac{c}{n} \Rightarrow \lambda = \frac{c}{nf}$. Thus, given constant frequency, we see that wavelength decreases when index of refraction increases. Another way to think about this is to remember that speed always decreases when going through a medium with greater index of refraction. Given fixed frequency, speed can only decrease when wavelength decreases.

5. A

All objects radiate electromagnetic radiation because of their nonzero absolute temperature. Also, the intensity of radiation is proportional to the temperature. Given that the energy of radiation, E, is related to frequency by $E = hf$, higher temperature means higher frequency of radiation. Because the speed of the radiation is simply the speed of light, c, we also have that $c = \lambda f$. So higher frequency means shorter wavelength. Thus, higher temperature means a greater intensity of shorter wavelength radiation.

6. B

From the top figure, we see that the equilibrium configuration of the stick is such that approximately half the stick is submerged. In this case, equilibrium means that the downward force of gravity is exactly balanced by the upward buoyant force, resulting in zero acceleration. Consider figure 1. Because less of the stick is submerged than at equilibrium, we know that the upward buoyant force is smaller than the downward gravitational force, so there will be a net downward force and thus a nonzero acceleration. In figure 2, the stick has the same configuration as at equilibrium, which means no net force and, thus, zero acceleration. (B) is then the correct answer choice. For completeness, consider the other choices. Figure 3 shows a scenario where a greater portion of the stick is submerged than at equilibrium. This means the buoyant force will be greater than the force of gravity and there will be a net upward force and, thus, nonzero acceleration. Figure 4 is essentially the same general case as figure 1, and figure 5 is the same general case as figure 3.

7. A

Total internal reflection occurs when the angle of refraction equals 90°. From Snell's law, we have $n_1\sin\theta_1 = n_2\sin\theta_2$. Total internal reflection means $\sin\theta_2 = \sin 90° = 1$. Thus, the minimal angle of incidence for total internal reflection is found from $n_1\sin\theta_1 = n_2$, which implies $\theta_1 = \sin^{-1}\left(\frac{n_2}{n_1}\right)$.

8. E

Notice that the end products of the given reaction are a nucleus with atomic number 14 and a positron, which is a particle with atomic number 1. Because atomic number must balance on both sides of a reaction, we know that the atomic number of nucleus Y is 15. Now notice that Y is produced from nucleus X and an alpha particle. Recall that an alpha particle is just a helium nucleus. So the atomic number of X plus 2 must equal 15 (the atomic number of the neutron, n, is 0), which means the atomic number of X is 13.

9. A

Consider what must occur for the bat to receive an echo. The sound emitted by the bat must reflect off an object and then be received by the bat. Reflection occurs because the incident soundwave causes the molecules at the surface of the object to oscillate, giving rise to a reflected sound wave. Consider the frequency of the sound received at the position of the stationary object. According to the Doppler effect, this frequency will be greater than the frequency produced by the bat because the bat is moving toward the stationary object. The reflected frequency (echo) is then higher than the frequency emitted by the bat. Because the bat is moving toward this reflected sound wave, the frequency perceived by the bat is even higher than the frequency of the echo. The net effect is that the bat receives a frequency higher than the original frequency emitted.

10. E

We're given that a certain block floats in water but not given any information that would allow us to determine the density of the block, other than to know that the density of the block is less than the density of water (because the block floats). The second liquid mentioned has a specific gravity of 0.5, which means that its density is $\frac{1}{2}$ the density of water. Without any information to determine the density of the block, we don't know if the block's density is greater or less than that of the second liquid. In other words, if the block's density is less than that of the liquid, it will float to the top. If the block's density is greater than that of the liquid, the block will sink to the bottom of the liquid and be partially submerged in the water. We conclude that we have insufficient information to determine what happens to the block.

11. A

Recall that pressures in flowing fluids are described by Bernoulli's equation and volume flow rates by the continuity equation. Specifically, the continuity equation states that the volume flow rate is a constant; thus, we can eliminate (C) and (D). Now recall that Bernoulli's equation states $P_1 + \frac{1}{2}\rho v_1^2 + \rho g y_1 = P_2 + \frac{1}{2}\rho v_2^2 + \rho g y_2$, where 1 and 2 refer to any two points in the fluid flow. Let's consider 1 and 2 to be A and B, respectively. Because the cross section is constant, we know the velocity at A is the same as the velocity at B (this follows from the continuity equation). Thus, we have $P_A + \rho g y_A = P_B + \rho g y_B$. Now notice that $y_B > y_A$, which implies (from the equation) $P_A > P_B$.

12. E

The pressure in a liquid exists in all directions, so there will be pressure on the top, the bottom, and the sides of the cube.

13. D

Heat added to a substance is related to the change in temperature of the substance via the equation $\Delta Q = mc\Delta T$, where m is the mass of the substance, c is the specific heat, ΔQ is the heat added, and ΔT is the change in temperature (final minus initial). The specific heat of water is 1 cal/(gm·°C), 1 L = 1,000 cm^3, and the density of water is 1 g/cm^3. The volume of the pool is then 1.86×10^8 cm^3, which corresponds to a mass of $m = \rho V = (1)(1.86 \times 10^8) = 1.86 \times 10^8$ g. The total amount of heat added is 1,000 BTU/hour × 2 hour = 2,000 BTU = (2,000)(934 kcal) = 1.868×10^6 kcal = 1.868×10^9 cal. So our equation becomes $1.868 \times 10^9 = (1.86 \times 10^8)(1)\Delta T$; $\Delta T = 10$. Given an initial temperature of 20°C, we have a final temperature of 30°C.

14. A

The pressure at a depth H below the surface of a liquid is given by $P = P_0 + \rho g H$, where P_0 is the pressure at the surface, and ρ is the density of the liquid. Notice that this expression has no reference to the dimensions of the container holding the liquid. Because both tubes are filled to the same height, the pressure at the bottom of each will be the same.

15. D

To determine the scale reading, we'll have to compute the weight of the liquid in each tube. The weight of the liquid is simply m*g*, where m is the mass of the liquid. Expressing mass in terms of density by $m = \rho V$, we have weight equals $\rho g V$. So given equal liquid densities, weight is simply proportional to volume of liquid. Now recall that the volume of a cylinder is base × height = $\pi r^2 H$, where r is the radius of the cylinder (tube). The narrower tube has volume $V_1 = \pi D^2 H$, and the wider tube has volume $V_2 = \pi(4D)^2 H = 16\pi D^2 H$. The ratio of V_1 to V_2 is then 1:16, which is also the ratio of the weights.

16. C

The electric field of a collection of charges is the vector sum of the electric fields due to each of the separate charges. Recall that electric fields point away from positive charges and toward negative charges. Consider any point along the line joining the positive and negative charge. The electric field due to the positive charge is directed away from the positive charge, which means it's directed toward the negative charge. Likewise, the electric field due to the negative charge is directed toward the negative charge. Thus, the total electric field is the sum of two vectors, both directed toward the negative charge. The result is clearly a vector directed at the negative charge.

- - - - - -► electric field due to negative charge
———► electric field due to positive charge

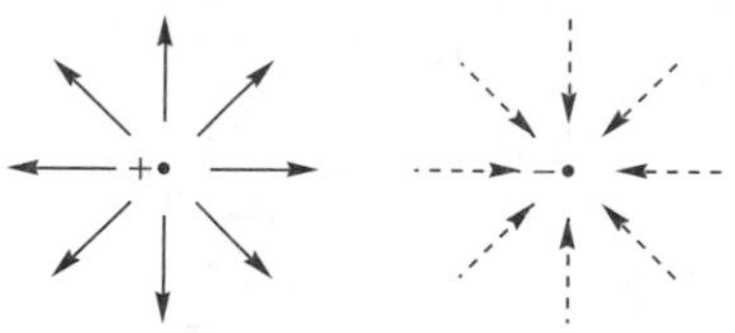

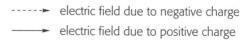

Midway between charges, the field is:

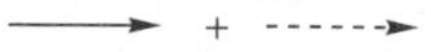

17. D

To solve this problem, we have to consider the combined effect of an electric and a magnetic field. The total force on a given particle will be the vector sum of the forces due to the electric and magnetic fields. Uncharged particles, of course, experience no force from either field; thus, we immediately determine that III is a true statement. We then eliminate (A), (B), and (E). Consider choice I. A positive charge will experience a force in the direction of an electric field (i.e., toward the top of the page). If this charge moves across the page from left to right and a magnetic field is directed out of the page, then the right-hand rule gives a magnetic force down the page. The sum of the electric and magnetic fields, in this case, can equal zero, resulting in no net force. Choice I is correct, which means (D) is correct. For completeness, choice II will give an electric force toward the top of the page and a magnetic force toward the top of the page. The net force will then be toward the top of the page, which means the net force isn't zero.

18. D

When an object loses heat, its temperature changes according to $Q = mc\Delta T$, where c is the specific heat and ΔT is the change in temperature. We're given the mass and final temperature but not the specific heat of water or the initial temperature. From this information we can rule out (A), (B), and (E). We're told, however, that the water turns to ice. Thus, in addition to the heat lost in cooling the water to 0°C, the water loses latent heat as it turns to ice. The latent heat is given by mL, where L is the latent heat of fusion of water. Thus we require the initial temperature, the specific heat of water, and the latent heat of fusion of water.

19. D

Consider (A), which states that the image distance equals the object distance. If this is true, then the magnification has magnitude 1, because $m = -\frac{i}{o}$, where i is the image distance and o is the object distance. Because we're told the image is greatly magnified we can safely rule out this choice. (B) says the image is real and upright. A real image means that $i > 0$. Given $o > 0$, we have $m < 0$, which gives an inverted image. So we rule out (B). (C) can be ruled out because a virtual image wouldn't be projected on a screen. (D) is correct because $i > o$ will give a magnification. For completeness, we rule out (E) because an image at the focal point implies o is infinity, which implies $m = 0$ (i.e., the image is a point).

20. C

Image formation by a diverging mirror is governed by the equation $\frac{1}{o} + \frac{1}{i} = \frac{1}{f}$ where *o* is the object distance, i is the image distance and f is the focal length and is negative. A real object means $o > 0$, which then implies (via the above equation) $i < 0$. Consider the answer choices. (A) is clearly false because we've found $i < 0$. In general the image distance is different than the object distance, so we can rule out (B). From the equation $m = -\frac{i}{o}$, and the fact that $i < 0$, we determine that $m > 0$, which means the image is upright. Thus (C) is true. (E) is ruled out because it's actually the same as (A).

21. C

Because all the answer choices deal with the energy of a photon, we need an expression that relates energy and wavelength. Recall $E = hf$ is the equation relating energy and frequency. For a photon, frequency and wavelength are related via $c = \lambda f$. Substituting for frequency in the energy equation, we have $E = hc/\lambda$. Thus, energy is inversely proportional to wavelength. Doubling the wavelength will result in halving the energy.

22. B

A gamma ray is simply a ray of energy. Thus, when a nucleus emits a gamma ray, the atomic number and the mass number remain the same, but the gamma ray carries away energy. The result is that the nucleus loses energy and becomes more stable.

23. D

The maximum displacement is given by the maximum of the function Asin(kx-wt). The maximum of any sine function is always 1. Thus, the maximum of the given function is simply A, which means that the maximum displacement is A meters.

24. D

This problem requires a direct application of the right-hand rule for determining the direction of magnetic fields produced by currents. The rule says to put the thumb of the right hand along the direction of the current and then the fingers of the right hand curl in the direction of the field. For a current directed into the page, this gives a magnetic field that curls in a clockwise sense.

25. B

When two waves are 180° out of phase and meet, they exhibit destructive interference. This means that one wave has a crest and the other a valley at this point. For an amplitude of A, a crest means a displacement of A, and a valley means a displacement of –A. The displacement of the superposition of the two waves is then the sum of the displacements of each wave. The wave with amplitude A_1 exhibits a crest so it contributes a displacement of A_1. The wave with amplitude A_2 exhibits a valley, so it contributes a displacement of $-A_2$. The resulting displacement is $A_1 - A_2$. Note that (A) is correct only if the two interfering waves have the same amplitude. If the amplitudes are different, as is the case here, the destructive interference is not total.

26. D

The absolute pressure at a depth of 1,000 m is $P_o + 1{,}000\rho_s g$. This pressure must be balanced by an equal and opposite pressure to avoid a breach of the hull of the vessel. Given that the inside cabin pressure is P_o, the hull must be capable of withstanding the remaining pressure of $1{,}000\rho_s g$.

27. B

According to the second law of thermodynamics, heat spontaneously flows from a hot body to a cold body but not the other way around. For the pond to freeze it must lose heat. Regardless of the initial water temperature, at some point in the freezing process heat will be flowing spontaneously (without outside intervention) from a colder body (the pond) to a warmer body (the air). This violates the second law of thermodynamics.

28. E

The apparent weight of an object is the difference between the downward gravitational force on the object (mg) and the upward buoyant force on the object. Recall that the upward buoyant force is given by ρgV, where ρ is the density of the liquid and V is the volume of the liquid displaced. Because both blocks are of equal volume and are completely submerged, they will both experience the same upward buoyant force F_B. The apparent weight of the mass m block is then $W_1 = mg - F_B$, and the apparent weight of the mass 2m block is then $W_2 = 2mg - F_B$. The ratio of the apparent weights is $\frac{mg - F_B}{2mg - F_B}$ and thus can't be determined without knowledge of F_B.

29. B

Recall that when a solid melts into a liquid, the phase transition occurs at a constant temperature; and that heat must be added at this constant temperature simply to cause this transition to occur. Physically, this latent heat is used to break the interatomic bonds that form the structure of the solid. So adding a bit more heat to the block will cause some of the aluminum to melt, but the temperature will remain at the melting point.

30. D

To determine the initial speed of the car, we can use the equation describing the horizontal motion of the car (i.e., $x = v_{ox}t$, where v_{ox} is the initial speed). We're given a horizontal range of $x = 100$ m, so to find speed, we simply need to know the amount of time required to hit the ground. To summarize, $v_{ox} = 100/t$, where t is the time to hit the ground. To find t, we'll use the equation describing the vertical motion of the car. The equation is $y = 125 - \frac{1}{2}gt^2$, where we take the ground as $y = 0$. We have $t = 5$ s. We then find $v_{ox} = \frac{100}{5} = 20$ m/s.

31. C

A fairly simple way to solve this problem is to use the equation $v^2 = v_o^2 + 2ad$. We know that when the block has gone a distance of 20 m, its speed is zero. So we have $0 = v_o^2 - 40a \rightarrow v_o = \sqrt{40a}$. Note that we have used a minus sign in front of acceleration because we know the acceleration up the plane is negative (deceleration). To find the acceleration we'll use Newton's second law, $F = ma$. The two forces on the object are the component of gravity down the plane and the frictional force, which is also down the plane. The gravitational force is given by $mg\sin30° = (5)(10)(0.5) = 25$ N. The frictional force is given by $\mu N = \mu mg\cos30° = \left(\frac{1}{\sqrt{3}}\right)(5)(10)\left(\frac{\sqrt{3}}{2}\right) = 25$ N. Thus, the total force down the plane is 50 N. So the acceleration is $a = 50/5 = 10$ m/s^2. We then have $v_o = \sqrt{400} = 20$ m/s.

32. B

To determine acceleration, we'll use Newton's second law, $a = F/m$. The acceleration experienced by a mass sliding down an inclined plane is directed down the plane and due to the component of the object's weight down the plane. This component is given by $mg\sin\theta$, where θ is the angle of the incline. We then have $a = mg\sin\theta/m = g\sin\theta$. The ratio of the accelerations is then given by $g\sin\theta_1/g\sin\theta_2 = \sin\theta_1/\sin\theta_2$.

33. C

First let's see what determines the range of a projectile. Recall the equation for horizontal motion of a projectile is $x = v_{ox}t$, where v_{ox} is the initial horizontal velocity. The range in the *x* direction is simply $x = v_{ox}T$, where T is the amount of time the projectile is in the air. The amount of time in the air is determined by the equations for the vertical motion. Specifically, the vertical velocity is given by $v_y = v_{oy} - gt$, where v_{oy} is the initial vertical velocity. We should recall that in the absence of air resistance, a projectile takes as much time to fall from its maximum height as it does to reach the maximum height. The time to reach the maximum height is found by setting $v_y = 0$ and solving for t, which gives a time of v_{oy}/g. Thus, the total time of flight is twice this, or $T = 2v_{oy}/g$, so we see that range in the x direction is proportional to T and, thus, inversely proportional to g. Thus, if g is reduced by a factor of $\frac{1}{6}$, the range is increased by a factor of 6.

34. D

We'll treat the bomb as a two-dimensional projectile whose initial velocity is only in the horizontal direction and of magnitude 900 mph. We're asked for the horizontal range of the projectile, which is obtained from $x = v_{ox}T$, where T is the time the projectile is in the air and $v_{ox} = 900$ mph. To find the time in the air, we use the equation for vertical motion. In the present case this becomes $y = 6{,}400 - \frac{1}{2}gt^2$, where we take the ground as $y = 0$ and where the initial vertical velocity is zero. Recalling that $g = 32$ ft/s^2, and setting $y = 0$, we have $0 = 6{,}400 - 16T^2 \Rightarrow T = 20$ s. The horizontal range is then $x = 20v_{ox}$ To convert from mph to ft/s use 1 mph = 5,280 ft/3,600 s, so 900 mph $= \frac{(900)(5280)}{3600}$ ft/s. The horizontal range is then $x = \frac{(20)(900)(5280)}{3600}$ ft $= \frac{(20)(900)}{3600}$ miles = 5 miles.

35. A

The light is traveling from a medium with a higher refractive index to one with a lower refractive index. The speed of light is therefore increased. (The lower the index of refraction, the higher the speed of light in that medium.) $v = f\lambda$, where v is the speed, f the frequency, and λ the wavelength. Because v increases, either f or λ (or both) must increase. Frequency does not change upon entering a new medium, as this is a property characteristic of the source of light and is independent of the medium. Therefore the wavelength must increase.

36. C

The two parallel 4-ohm resistors give an effective resistance of $\frac{1}{\left(\frac{1}{4}+\frac{1}{4}\right)} = \frac{1}{\left(\frac{2}{4}\right)} = 2$ ohms. This is in series with the 6-ohm resistor, giving an effective resistance of $6 + 2 = 8$ ohms for the circuit.

37. A

Point b is connected to point a without any circuit element in between. The electrical potential energy must therefore be the same at these two points, so they are at the same potential.

38. C

Calculate the distance traveled over the constant velocity and uniform acceleration stretches separately and then combine them to get the total distance traveled:

$$x = v\Delta t_1 + \left(v_i\Delta t_2 + \frac{1}{2}a\Delta t_2^2\right)$$

↓ constant v ↓ constant a

Thus v is the constant velocity of 30 m/s; Δt_1 is the time over which this constant speed applies (i.e., 5 s), and v_i is the initial speed when the object first starts to accelerate and is therefore the same as the constant speed of 30 m/s, Δt_2 is 4 s, and a is 15 m/s^2. Putting this all together

$$x = (30 \times 5) + (30 \times 4 + 0.5 \times 15 \times 16)$$
$$= 150 + (120 + 120) = 390 \text{ m}$$

Don't be fooled by (B), which is the distance traveled over the uniform acceleration stretch.

39. B

Immediately before it hits the ground, an object has zero potential energy. All of its initial energy has been converted into kinetic energy, and this application of energy conservation allows us to determine the correct answer choice. Object A has an initial gravitational potential energy of MgH. It is released (rather than thrown down or tossed up), so its initial kinetic energy is zero. Immediately before it hits the ground, its kinetic energy is

$$\frac{1}{2}Mv_A^2 = MgH$$
$$v_A = \sqrt{2gH}$$

As for object B, its initial potential energy is $(0.5M)g(2H) = MgH$ as well. Its velocity immediately before it hits the ground is

$$\frac{1}{2}\left(\frac{1}{2}M\right)v_B^2 = MgH$$
$$v_B = 2\sqrt{gH}$$

The ratio of v_A to v_B is therefore

$$\sqrt{2gH}: 2\sqrt{gH} = \sqrt{2}:2 = 1:\sqrt{2}$$

40. C

The key to this problem is to realize that at its highest point, the velocity of the projectile is completely in the horizontal direction. Recall that for projectile motion, the horizontal velocity is actually constant because there is no force acting along the horizontal direction. Thus, the velocity at the highest point equals the horizontal component of the initial velocity. From the information given, the initial horizontal velocity is $5\cos60°$ m/s. Thus, the speed at the highest point is $5\cos60°$ m/s $= (5 \times \frac{1}{2})$ m/s $= 2.5$ m/s.

Answers and Explanations

1. C	11. B	21. B	31. D	41. C
2. C	12. D	22. B	32. C	42. D
3. B	13. B	23. E	33. C	43. D
4. C	14. A	24. B	34. C	44. C
5. D	15. C	25. A	35. D	45. D
6. E	16. E	26. D	36. E	46. A
7. D	17. D	27. A	37. A	47. B
8. B	18. C	28. B	38. E	48. C
9. D	19. A	29. D	39. C	49. D
10. D	20. B	30. A	40. A	50. E

1. C

Because the dimensions of the aquarium are in feet whereas the unit gallon is defined in terms of cubic inches, we want either to convert the number of feet in each dimension of the aquarium to inches or convert the number of cubic inches in a gallon to the number of cubic feet in a gallon. Because converting the number of cubic inches in a gallon to the number of cubic feet in a gallon involves fractions, we'll convert the dimensions of the aquarium from feet to inches instead.

The base of the aquarium has dimensions of $1\frac{1}{2}$ feet by 2 feet, and the depth is $1\frac{1}{2}$ feet. There are 12 inches in a foot, so the dimensions of the base are $1\frac{1}{2} \times 12$, or 18 inches, and 2×12, or 24 inches. The depth is $1\frac{1}{2} \times 12$, or 18 inches. The volume of a rectangular box is length × width × height, so the volume of the aquarium in cubic inches is $18 \times 24 \times 18 = 432 \times 18 = 7{,}776$. Because the volume of the aquarium is 7,776 cubic inches and there are 231 cubic inches in a gallon, the number of gallons needed to fill the aquarium is $\frac{7776}{231} = \frac{2592}{77}$. You can tell by estimation that this is a little more than 30, and the only answer choice that is a little more than 30 is (C). Therefore (C), 33.7, must be correct. If you work accurately with $\frac{2592}{77}$, you'll find that $\frac{2592}{77} = 33\frac{51}{77}$, and $33\frac{51}{77}$ to the nearest tenth is 33.7.

2. C

Here you want to find the value of $1\frac{7}{8} \times 2\frac{1}{10} \times \frac{6}{7}$. Notice that $1\frac{7}{8}$ is about 2 and $2\frac{1}{10}$ is also about 2. So $1\frac{7}{8} \times 2\frac{1}{10} \times \frac{6}{7}$ is approximately $2 \times 2 \times \frac{6}{7} = 4 \times \frac{6}{7} = \frac{24}{7} = 3\frac{3}{7}$. Notice that choice (A), $3\frac{513}{280}$, is greater than 4 because the fractional part of this number, $\frac{513}{280}$, is greater than 1. The only answer choice that is close to $3\frac{3}{7}$ is (C), $3\frac{3}{8}$, so (C) must be correct.

You can also solve this question by converting the mixed numbers $1\frac{7}{8}$ and $2\frac{1}{10}$ to improper fractions and then doing the multiplication. To convert a mixed number to an improper fraction, multiply the whole number part by the denominator and then add the numerator. The result is the new numerator over the same denominator. So to convert $1\frac{7}{8}$ to an improper fraction, first multiply 1 by 8 and then add 7 to get the new numerator 15. The denominator is the denominator 8 of the original mixed number, so $1\frac{7}{8} = \frac{15}{8}$. Similarly, $2\frac{1}{10} = \frac{2 \times 10 + 1}{10} = \frac{20 + 1}{10} = \frac{21}{10}$.

Now we're ready to find the product.

$$1\frac{7}{8} \times 2\frac{1}{10} \times \frac{6}{7}$$

$$= \frac{15}{8} \times \frac{21}{10} \times \frac{6}{7}$$

Cancel the factors of 7 in 7 and in 21: $= \frac{15}{8} \times \frac{3}{10} \times \frac{6}{1}$

Cancel the factors of 5 in 15 and in 10: $= \frac{3}{8} \times \frac{3}{2} \times \frac{6}{1}$

Cancel the factors of 2 in 2 and in 6: $= \frac{3}{8} \times \frac{3}{1} \times \frac{3}{1}$

$$= \frac{27}{8}$$

$$= 3\frac{3}{8}$$

3. B

Because there are no actual distances specified in the question, you can pick a value for the distance and work with it. Be sure to pick a number that's easy to work with. Here, you want half of the distance to be a multiple of 40 and 60. Because the smallest common multiple of 40 and 60 is 120, let each half-distance be 120 miles, i.e., we're letting the distances that Jim and Kate each drive be 120 miles. Use the formula Distance = Rate × Time. Because Jim drove for 120 miles at 40 miles per hour, the time he spent driving was $\frac{\text{Distance}}{\text{Rate}} = \frac{120}{40} = 3$ hours. Because Kate drove for 120 miles at 60 miles per hour, the time she spent driving was $\frac{\text{Distance}}{\text{Rate}} = \frac{120}{60} = 2$ hours. The total distance driven was 120 + 120 = 240 miles, and the total time driving was 3 + 2 = 5 hours, so the average speed for the trip was $\frac{\text{Total distance}}{\text{Total time}} = \frac{240}{5} = 48$ miles per hour.

4. C

Because a tooth of one gear always touches a tooth of the other gear, the number of teeth of one gear multiplied by the number of times it revolves always equals the number of teeth of the other gear multiplied by the number of times it revolves. Let N be the number of times the larger gear revolves. Then 40 × N = 24 × 15, so $N = \frac{24 \times 15}{40} = \frac{6 \times 15}{10} = \frac{3 \times 15}{5} = 3 \times 3 = 9$.

5. D

First convert 23% to a fraction. Whenever you convert a percent to a fraction (and also whenever you convert a percent to a decimal), you divide the percent by 100%, having the percent symbols drop out. So $23\% = \frac{23\%}{100\%} = \frac{23}{100}$. The word *of* immediately after 23% means "times." We have the equation $\frac{23}{100} \times \frac{2}{5}\left(\frac{190}{3x}\right) = 8$. Now solve this equation for x.

$$\frac{23}{100} \times \frac{2}{5}\left(\frac{190}{3x}\right) = 8$$

$$\frac{23}{100} \times \frac{2}{5} \times \frac{190}{3x} = 8$$

$$x = \frac{23}{100} \times \frac{2}{5} \times \frac{190}{3 \times 8}$$

$$= \frac{23}{100} \times \frac{2}{5} \times \frac{190}{24}$$

Now find what this value of x equals.

$$x = \frac{23}{100} \times \frac{2}{5} \times \frac{190}{24}$$

Cancel a factor of 10 from the 100 and the 190: $= \frac{23}{10} \times \frac{2}{5} \times \frac{19}{24}$

Cancel a factor of 2 from the 10 and the 2: $= \frac{23}{5} \times \frac{1}{5} \times \frac{19}{24}$

$$= \frac{23 \times 19}{5 \times 5 \times 24}$$

$$= \frac{437}{600}$$

6. E

There are 60 seconds in a minute, so if a heart beats 72 times in 1 minute, it beats 72 times in 60 seconds. Thus in 1 second, the heart beats $\frac{72}{60} = \frac{12}{10} = 1.2$ times.

7. D

To divide by a fraction, you invert the fraction and multiply. To divide by $\frac{3}{4}$, you invert the $\frac{3}{4}$, getting $\frac{4}{3}$, and then multiply by $\frac{4}{3}$.

Thus, $\frac{6{,}534}{\frac{3}{4}} = 6{,}534 \times \frac{4}{3} = 2{,}178 \times 4 = 8{,}712$.

8. B

Plug the values of π, h, and a into the equation and solve for the value of r. (This formula is actually a geometric formula, however, if you don't recognize it, it doesn't matter. In geometry, π, with its usual meaning, is often approximated by $\frac{22}{7}$; however, in the solution, π can just be considered to be replaced by $\frac{22}{7}$.) Be careful to answer what the question requires; find the value of 2r and choose the answer choice that indicates the value of 2r.

$$a = r^2h$$
$$396 = \frac{22}{7}r^2(14)$$
$$22(2)r^2 = 396$$
$$44r^2 = 396$$
$$r^2 = \frac{396}{44}$$
$$r^2 = 9$$
$$r = 3 \text{ or } r = -3$$

Because $r > 0$, $r = 3$, So $2r = 2(3) = 6$. The value of 2r is 6 and (B) is correct.

9. D

Translate the English of the question stem into math. You will obtain an equation that can be solved for the value of the number. Call the number N. "A number is larger than 5 by" means "N – 5." Next, "the same" means "=", so now we have "N – 5 =." There are several steps in translating "amount that it is smaller than 3 more than 14." The word "it" refers to the number N, so "amount that it is smaller than 3 more than 14" means "amount that N is smaller than 3 more than 14." "3 more than 14" means "3 + 14." So "amount that it is smaller than 3 more than 14" means "(3 + 14) – N." So "A NUMBER is larger than 5 by the same amount that it is smaller than 3 more than 14" means that N – 5 = (3 + 14) – N. Now solve this equation for N.

$$N - 5 = (3 + 14) - N$$
$$N - 5 = 17 - N$$
$$2N - 5 = 17$$
$$2N = 22$$
$$N = \frac{22}{2}$$
$$N = 11$$

10. D

A circle can be drawn that goes through any three points that do not all lie on a straight line. If three points do lie on a straight line, no circle can be drawn that goes through all three of these points. The points (0, 0) and (10, 0) both have a y-coordinate of 0, so these two points are on the x-axis, which is the line with the equation $y = 0$. Look for a point among the answer choices, that is on the x-axis. Look for this point by looking for a point with a y-coordinate of 0. (D), (5, 0), has a y-coordinate of 0. Thus (5, 0) could not be a point on a circle passing through the two points (0, 0) and (10, 0).

11. B

Translate the information in the question stem into math and then try to find the value of $\frac{c}{a}$. "is" means "equals," so "a is" means "a =". The fractional equivalent of 25% is $\frac{1}{4}$. Now, "of" means "times," so "25% of b" means "$\frac{1}{4} \times b$" or "$\frac{1}{4}b$" and "a is 25% of b" means that $a = \frac{1}{4}b$. The translation of "b is 60% of c" is similar. The fractional equivalent of 60% is $\frac{3}{5}$, so "b is 60% of c" means that $b = \frac{3}{5}c$. Now we have the two equations $a = \frac{1}{4}b$ and $b = \frac{3}{5}c$. Because we want to find the value of $\frac{c}{a}$, use the equation $b = \frac{3}{5}c$ and substitute $\frac{3}{5}c$ for b into the equation $a = \frac{1}{4}b$. When we do this we'll be left with an equation that only contains the variables a and c. We can then try to solve this equation for the value of $\frac{c}{a}$. Substituting $\frac{3}{5}c$ for b into the equation $a = \frac{1}{4}b$ gives us $a = \frac{1}{4}(\frac{3}{5}c)$. Now solve this equation for the value of $\frac{c}{a}$.

$$a = \frac{1}{4}\left(\frac{3}{5}c\right)$$
$$a = \frac{1}{4} \times \frac{3}{5} \times c$$
$$a = \frac{3}{20} \times c$$
$$1 = \frac{3}{20} \times \frac{c}{a}$$
$$20 = 3 \times \frac{c}{a}$$
$$\frac{20}{3} = \frac{c}{a}$$

Therefore, $\frac{c}{a} = \frac{20}{3}$ and (B) is correct.

12. D

Call the number of liters of an 80% solution that are needed x. The new solution will then contain 4 + x liters. The 4 liters of solution that are 35% alcohol contain (35% of 4) liters of alcohol. Because the answer choices are all decimals, convert 35% to a decimal. Whenever you convert a percent to a decimal (also whenever you convert a percent to a fraction), you divide the percent by 100%, and the percent symbols cancel. Therefore, $35\% = \frac{35\%}{100\%} = \frac{35}{100} = \frac{7}{20} = 0.35$ and the 4 liters of solution that are 35% alcohol contain 0.35(4), or 1.4 liters of alcohol. The x liters of solution that are added are 80% alcohol. The decimal equivalent of 80% is 0.8, so the x liters of solution that are 80% alcohol contain 0.8x liters of alcohol. Therefore, the 4 + x liters of solution will contain 1.4 + 0.8x liters of alcohol. Now these 4 + x liters of solution are to be 60% alcohol, and the decimal equivalent of 60% is 0.6, so we can write down this equation:

$\frac{1.4 + 0.8x}{4 + x} = 0.6$. Now solve this equation for x.

$$\frac{1.4 + 0.8}{4 + x} = 0.6$$

$$1.4 + 0.8x = 0.6(4 + x)$$

$$1.4 + 0.8x = 2.4 + 0.6x$$

$$0.8x = 1.0 + 0.6x$$

$$0.2x = 1$$

$$x = \frac{1}{0.2} = \frac{10}{2} = 5$$

Therefore, 5 liters must be added, and (D) is correct.

13. B

The value represented by the question mark must be found. First, add and subtract the fractions on the left side. To add and subtract fractions, find a common denominator. Let's try to find the least common multiple of 12, 8, and 2. (Actually, because 8 is a multiple of 2, the least common multiple of 12 and 8 must be the least common multiple of 12, 8, and 2.) We could find the least common denominator here by taking multiples of the largest denominator, 12, until we get multiples of the other denominators, 8 and 2. Of course, 12 itself, which is 12 times 1, is not a multiple of 8. Try 12 times 2: 12 times 2 is 24, and 24 is a multiple of both 8 (24 = 8 × 3) and 2 (24 = 2 × 12). Now convert each of the fractions to an equivalent fraction with a denominator of 24:

$$\frac{9}{8} = \frac{9}{8} \times \frac{3}{3} = \frac{9 \times 3}{8 \times 3} = \frac{27}{24}$$

$$\frac{5}{12} = \frac{5}{12} \times \frac{2}{2} = \frac{5 \times 2}{12 \times 2} = \frac{10}{24}$$

$$\frac{1}{2} = \frac{1}{2} \times \frac{12}{12} = \frac{1 \times 12}{2 \times 12} = \frac{12}{24}$$

and then

$$\frac{9}{8} - \frac{5}{12} + \frac{1}{2} = \frac{27}{24} - \frac{10}{24} + \frac{12}{24} = \frac{27 - 10 + 12}{24} = \frac{29}{24}$$

Therefore, $\frac{29}{24} - (?) = 1$ and

$$? = \frac{29}{24} - 1 = \frac{29}{24} - \frac{24}{24} = \frac{29 - 24}{24} = \frac{5}{24}.$$

(B) is correct.

14. A

The area of a square is equal to the length of its side squared, and the area of this square is 1,000 square inches. If we call the length of a side of this square x, then $x^2 = 1{,}000$. Therefore, $x = \sqrt{1{,}000}$. We could simplify this radical by finding a perfect square that is a factor of the quantity 1,000 under the radical sign, but there is no need to because we will be squaring a quantity closely related to $\sqrt{1{,}000}$ when we find the area of the circle, so the radical symbols will drop out. The diameter of the largest circle that can be drawn inside this square is equal to the length of the side of the square. The diameter of this circle is $\sqrt{1{,}000}$. The diameter of a circle is always twice its radius, and equivalently, the radius of a circle is always $\frac{1}{2}$ of its diameter. The radius of the largest possible circle here is therefore $\frac{1}{2}\sqrt{1{,}000}$. The area of a circle with a radius r is πr^2, so the area of this circle is $\pi\left(\frac{1}{2}\sqrt{1{,}000}\right)^2$. Use the approximation $\frac{22}{7}$ for π. Then $\pi\left(\frac{1}{2}\sqrt{1{,}000}\right)^2$ is approximately

$$\frac{22}{7}\left(\frac{1}{2}\sqrt{1{,}000}\right)^2 = \frac{22}{7} \times \frac{1}{2} \times \sqrt{1{,}000} \times \frac{1}{2} \times \sqrt{1{,}000}$$

$$= \frac{22}{7} \times \frac{1}{2} \times \frac{1}{2} \times \sqrt{1{,}000} \times \sqrt{1{,}000}$$

$$= \frac{22}{7} \times \frac{1}{4} \times 1{,}000$$

$$= \frac{5{,}500}{7}$$

$$= 785\frac{5}{7}$$

Clearly, $785\frac{5}{7}$ is much closer to (A), 785.7, than to any other choice, so (A) must be correct. (When you're taking the test, you should not spend time converting $785\frac{5}{7}$ to a decimal and round the result to the nearest tenth. However, if you did convert $785\frac{5}{7}$ to a decimal and round the result to the nearest tenth, you would get 785.7. Never do such computations unless they are necessary.)

15. C

To subtract the algebraic expressions, find a common denominator for the two fractions. The fraction $\frac{a}{b}$ has the denominator b and the fraction $\frac{b}{a}$ has the denominator a. The common denominator to use here is the lowest common denominator, which is the product of the denominators, ab. Now convert each fraction to an equivalent fraction having a denominator ab and then do the subtraction.

$$\frac{a}{b} - \frac{b}{a} = \left(\frac{a}{b} \times \frac{a}{a}\right) - \left(\frac{b}{a} \times \frac{b}{b}\right)$$
$$= \frac{a^2}{ab} - \frac{b^2}{ab}$$
$$= \frac{a^2 - b^2}{ab}$$

(C) is correct.

16. E

First, convert 55% to a fraction. Whenever you convert a percent to a fraction (also whenever you convert a percent to a decimal), you divide the percent by 100%, thus the percent symbols cancel. $55\% = \frac{55\%}{100\%} = \frac{55}{100} = \frac{11}{20}$. The word "of" means "times," so "55% of" means "55% times," which is "$\frac{11}{20}$ times"; thus, you have the equation $\frac{11}{20}\left(\frac{9z}{5}\right) = 33$, which you can solve for z.

$$\frac{11}{20}\left(\frac{9z}{5}\right) = 33$$

Multiply the fractions on the left side: $\frac{11(9z)}{20(5)} = 33$

$$\frac{99z}{100} = 33$$

Divide both sides by 33: $\frac{3z}{100} = 1$

Multiply both sides by 100: $3z = 100$

Divide both sides by 3: $z = \frac{100}{3}$

17. D

The average formula is Average $= \frac{\text{Sum of the terms}}{\text{Number of terms}}$ (i.e., the average of a group of terms is the sum of the terms divided by the number of terms). The average of the numbers $\frac{1}{2}, \frac{2}{3}$, and $\frac{3}{4}$ is the sum of these three fractions divided by 3,

so the average of these numbers is $\frac{\frac{1}{2} + \frac{2}{3} + \frac{3}{4}}{3}$. To find the sum of the fractions in the numerator, $\frac{1}{2} + \frac{2}{3} + \frac{3}{4}$, find a common denominator for the fractions $\frac{1}{2}, \frac{2}{3}$, and $\frac{3}{4}$. You could find the lowest common denominator by taking multiples of the largest denominator, 4, until you get multiples of the other denominators, 3 and 2: 4 times 1 is 4, and 4 is not a multiple of 3. Try 4 times 2. 4 times 2 is 8, and 8 is not a multiple of 3. Now try 4 times 3: 4 times 3 is 12, and 12 is a multiple of both 2 ($12 = 2 \times 6$) and 3 ($12 = 3 \times 4$). Now convert each of the fractions to an equivalent fraction with a denominator of 12.

$$\frac{1}{2} = \frac{1}{2} \times \frac{6}{6} = \frac{1 \times 6}{2 \times 6} = \frac{6}{12}$$
$$\frac{2}{3} = \frac{2}{3} \times \frac{4}{4} = \frac{2 \times 4}{3 \times 4} = \frac{8}{12}$$
$$\frac{3}{4} = \frac{3}{4} \times \frac{3}{3} = \frac{3 \times 3}{4 \times 3} = \frac{9}{12}$$

So $\frac{1}{2} + \frac{2}{3} + \frac{3}{4} = \frac{6}{12} + \frac{8}{12} + \frac{9}{12} = \frac{6 + 8 + 9}{12} = \frac{23}{12}$.

Finally, the average is

$$\frac{\frac{1}{2} + \frac{2}{3} + \frac{3}{4}}{3} = \frac{\left(\frac{23}{12}\right)}{3} = \frac{23}{12} \times \frac{1}{3} = \frac{23 \times 1}{12 \times 3} = \frac{23}{36}$$

(D) is correct.

18. C

This is a proportion question. "14 is to 35" just means the ratio of 14 to 35, "2x is to 40" just means the ratio of 2x to 40, and "14 is to 35 as 2x is to 40" means that the ratio of 14 to 35 is equal to the ratio of 2x to 40. Now write the corresponding equation with the ratios replaced by fractions.

$$\frac{14}{35} = \frac{2x}{40}$$

Now solve this equation for x. $\frac{14}{35} = \frac{2x}{40}$

On the right side, divide the numerator and denominator by 2: $\frac{14}{35} = \frac{x}{20}$

On the left side, divide the numerator and denominator by 7: $\frac{2}{5} = \frac{x}{20}$

Cross multiply: $2(20) = 5x$

Simplify the left side: $40 = 5x$

Divide both sides by 5: $\frac{40}{5} = x$

$8 = x$

Therefore, $x = 8$ and (C) is correct.

19. A

Write the rate of each person in terms of rooms painted per hour, add these rates, and then find how long it would take working at this combined rate to paint 1 room. Diane can paint 1 room in 6 hours, so her rate of painting rooms is $\frac{1}{6}$ rooms per hour. Sandy can paint one room in 4 hours, so her rate of painting rooms is $\frac{1}{4}$ rooms per hour. The rate at which both of them paint when they work together is $\frac{1}{6} + \frac{1}{4}$ rooms per hour. Now $\frac{1}{6} + \frac{1}{4} = \frac{2}{12} + \frac{3}{12} = \frac{2+3}{12} = \frac{5}{12}$, so their rate when they work together is $\frac{5}{12}$ rooms per hour. The number of hours it takes them to paint one room is the reciprocal of $\frac{5}{12}$, which is $\frac{12}{5}$. None of the answer choices is $\frac{12}{5}$; however, $\frac{12}{5} = 2\frac{2}{5}$. (A) is correct.

If it was not immediately clear to you why if the combined rate is $\frac{5}{12}$ rooms per hour, then the time needed to paint 1 room, in hours, is the reciprocal of $\frac{5}{12}$, you can use the formula Work = Rate × Time, and here, work = 1 room, rate $= \frac{5}{12}$ rooms per hour, and the time in hours is unknown. Therefore, 1 room $= \left(\frac{5}{12} \text{ rooms per hour}\right) \times$ time, time $= \frac{1}{\left(\frac{5}{12}\right)}$ hours, and the number of hours is indeed the reciprocal of $\frac{5}{12}$.

20. B

To find the percent of the resulting solution that is sugar, we need the number of milliliters of sugar in the resulting solution and the total number of milliliters of the resulting solution. The number of milliliters of sugar in the resulting solution is the number of milliliters in the original solution, because the 8 milliliters of water that are added contain just water and no sugar. Therefore, the number of milliliters of sugar in the resulting solution is 5% of 32. To find 5% of 32, convert 5% to a decimal. Whenever you convert a percent to a decimal (and also whenever you convert a percent to a fraction), you divide the percent by 100%, having the percent symbols cancel. Therefore, $5\% = \frac{5\%}{100\%} = \frac{5}{100} = \frac{1}{20} = 0.05$, and 5% of 32 is 0.05(32), which is 1.6. The total number of milliliters in the resulting solution is the original 32 plus the added 8, so the total number of milliliters of resulting solution is 40. The fraction of the resulting solution that is sugar is $\frac{1.6}{40}$. The percent of the resulting solution that is sugar is the fraction of the resulting solution that is sugar, $\frac{1.6}{40}$, converted to a percent. To convert a fraction (or a decimal) to a percent, multiply that fraction (or decimal) by 100%. The percent of the resulting solution that is sugar is $\frac{1.6}{40} \times 100\% = \frac{1.6}{4} \times 10\% = \frac{1.6}{2} \times 5\% = 0.8 \times 5\% = 4\%$.

21. B

You need to know the average formula: Average $= \frac{\text{Sum of the terms}}{\text{Number of terms}}$. In this question, it is convenient to work with the sums of the scores, so you should therefore work with the average formula in the rearranged form Sum of the terms = Average × Number of terms. The average of the five scores is 9.6, and the sum of the five scores is 9.6 × 5, or 48. When the highest and lowest scores are dropped, the average rises to 9.7 and the sum of the remaining three scores is 9.7×3, or 29.1. The sum of the highest and lowest scores can be found by subtracting from the sum of all five scores the sum of the three scores that remain when the highest and lowest scores are removed. The sum of the highest and lowest scores is $48 - 29.1$, which equals 18.9. The average of the highest and lowest scores is $\frac{18.9}{2}$, which equals 9.45.

22. B

If $\frac{10 \text{ feet } (x) \text{ inches}}{9 \text{ feet } 3 \text{ inches}}$ approximates 1.2, then 10 feet (x) inches is approximately 1.2(9 feet 3 inches). The first thing we will do is rewrite 1.2(9 feet 3 inches) more simply in terms of feet and inches. Now 1.2(9 feet 3 inches) is 1.2(9 feet) plus 1.2(3 inches). 1.2(9 feet) = 10.8 feet. There are 12 inches in a foot, so in 0.8 feet there are 0.8(12), or 9.6 inches, and thus 1.2(9 feet) = 10 feet plus 9.6 inches. 1.2(3 inches) = 3.6 inches. So 1.2(9 feet 3 inches) equals 10 feet plus 9.6 inches plus 3.6 inches, which equals 10 feet plus 13.2 inches. Because 10 feet (x) inches is approximately 1.2(9 feet 3 inches), we can say that 10 feet (x) inches is approximately 10 feet plus 13.2 inches. There is no need to rewrite 10 feet plus 13.2 inches as an integer number of feet plus some number N of inches where N is less than 12. Notice that 10 feet (x) inches is approximately equal to 10 feet plus 13.2 inches, so among the answer choices, (B) is clearly closest to 13.2.

23. E

One way to solve this is by looking for pairs of fractions that are relatively easier to compare, then making these less difficult comparisons of fractions, and then eliminating answer choices as soon as you can. First, $\frac{2}{3}$ is $\frac{1}{3}$ less than 1 whereas $\frac{3}{4}$ is $\frac{1}{4}$ less than 1. Because $\frac{1}{4}$ is less than $\frac{1}{3}$, $\frac{3}{4}$ is closer to 1 than $\frac{2}{3}$, i.e., $\frac{3}{4}$ is greater than $\frac{2}{3}$. So d, representing $\frac{3}{4}$, must be on the list before a, representing $\frac{2}{3}$. (A) and (C) have a occurring before d, i.e., they incorrectly say that $\frac{2}{3}$ is greater than $\frac{3}{4}$. Eliminate (A) and (C). Next, $\frac{5}{8}$ and $\frac{5}{11}$ both have the same numerator. Whenever you have two fractions (that both have positive numerators and positive denominators) that have the same numerator, the fraction with the smaller denominator is the larger fraction. So $\frac{5}{8}$ is greater than $\frac{5}{11}$. So e, representing $\frac{5}{8}$, must be on the list before b, representing $\frac{5}{11}$. (B) and (D) have b on their lists before e; that is, they incorrectly say that $\frac{5}{11}$ is greater than $\frac{5}{8}$. Eliminate (B) and (D). Now that all four incorrect answer choices have been eliminated, you know that (E) must be correct.

This question could have been solved with other comparisons. For example, $\frac{5}{11}$ is the only fraction less than $\frac{1}{2}$ because it is the only fraction whose denominator is greater than twice its numerator. Therefore $\frac{5}{11}$ is the smallest fraction, and b, representing $\frac{5}{11}$, must be last on the list. You can eliminate (A), (B), and (D), which do not have b for the last entry on their lists. Next, $\frac{3}{4}$ is greater than $\frac{5}{8}$ because $\frac{3}{4} = \frac{6}{8}$, and $\frac{6}{8}$ is greater than $\frac{5}{8}$, so d, representing $\frac{3}{4}$, must be on the list before e, representing $\frac{5}{8}$. (C) has e on the list before d, i.e, this choice incorrectly says that $\frac{5}{8}$ is greater than $\frac{3}{4}$. Therefore eliminate (C). Now that all four incorrect choices have been eliminated, you know that (E) must be correct.

24. B

Because 70% of the students are girls, the other 30% of the students are boys. The average height of the girls has 70% of the total average, whereas the average height of the boys has the other 30% of the total average. Because the average height of the girls contributes so much more to the total, you know that the average of the entire class will have to be closer to the average height of the girls than to the average height of the boys. You therefore know that the average of the entire class will have to be less than 5 feet 6 inches, which is midway between 5 feet 4 inches and 5 feet 8 inches. You can eliminate choices (D) and (E). Now let's find the overall average. The decimal equivalent of 70% is 0.7, and the decimal equivalent of 30% is 0.3. The average height is

0.7(5 feet 4 inches) + 0.3(5 feet 8 inches)
= 0.7(5 feet) + 0.7(4 inches) + 0.3(5 feet) + 0.3(8 inches)
= [0.7(5 feet) + 0.3(5 feet)] + [0.7(4 inches) + 0.3(8 inches)]
= (0.7 + 0.3)(5 feet) + (2.8 inches + 2.4 inches)
= (5 feet) + (5.2 inches)

This is closest to (B), 5 feet 5 inches, so (B) must be correct.

25. A

This question can be solved by picking a number appropriately. The number to pick here is for the number of riders. Always pick a number that is easy to work with. Say that the original number of riders was 10. Then because the original cost of the ride was 75¢, the original total revenue was 75(10), or 750¢. There is no need to convert this to dollars. After the price rose to 90¢, the number of riders decreased by 20%. The fractional equivalent of 20% is $\frac{1}{5}$, so the number of riders decreased by $\frac{1}{5}$. The new number of riders was $10 - \frac{1}{5}(10) = 10 - 2 = 8$. The new total revenue was 90(8), or 720¢. The total revenue decreased from 750¢ to 720¢. The decrease in total revenues was 750 − 720 = 30¢. The fractional decrease is always found by dividing the amount of decrease by the *original whole*. The fractional decrease is $\frac{30}{750} = \frac{1}{25}$. The percent decrease is just the fractional decrease converted to a percent. To convert a fraction (or decimal) to a percent, multiply that fraction (or decimal) by 100%. The fractional decrease is $\frac{1}{25} \times 100\%$, which is 4%. Notice that you could find the percent decrease from 750 to 720 in one step according to the formula

$$\text{Percent decrease} = \frac{\text{Original value} - \text{New value}}{\text{Original value}} \times 100\%.$$

Used here,
percent decrease

$$= \frac{750 - 720}{750} \times 100\% = \frac{30}{750} \times 100\% = \frac{1}{25} \times 100\% = 4\%.$$

26. D

The expression $\frac{4a - 7a + 6a}{6ab}$ is to be simplified.

First combine the terms in the numerator: $\frac{4a - 7a + 6a}{6ab} = \frac{3a}{6ab}$

Now cancel a factor of 3 from the numerator and denominator: $\frac{3a}{6ab} = \frac{a}{2ab}$

Now cancel a factor of a from the numerator and denominator: $\frac{a}{2ab} = \frac{1}{2b}$

(D) is correct.

27. A

To compare two decimal numbers that are between 0 and 1, look at the tenths digit first. If the tenths digit in one number is larger, that number is larger. If the tenths digit is the same in both numbers, look at the hundredths digit next. If the hundredths digit in one number is larger, that number is larger. If the hundredths digit is the same in both numbers, look at the thousandths digits. If the thousandths digit in one number is larger that number is larger. If the thousandths digits are the same, look at the ten-thousandths digits. Continue this way until a comparison has been made. Looking at the numbers of the answer choices, the tenths digit of choice (A) is 6, whereas the tenths digits of the other choices are all less than 6. Therefore (A), 0.636, is largest.

28. B

Of the first 150 flips, 48% were heads: 48% of 150 is $\frac{48}{100} \times 150 = \frac{24}{50} \times 150 = 24 \times 3 = 72$. If the coin is flipped another 100 times, it will have been flipped a total of 150 + 100 = 250 times. If the overall percent of heads is to be 50%, then 50% of all the 250 tosses must be heads. The fractional equivalent of 50% is $\frac{1}{2}$, so $\frac{1}{2}$ of 250, or 125 heads, must have been tossed. Because 72 heads were tossed in the first 150 flips, 125 − 72 or 53 heads must be tossed in the next 100 flips. Of the next 100 tosses, 53 (i.e., 53%) must be heads. (B) is correct.

29. D

The easiest to compare are (A) and (D), so let's compare these first. Because 0.03 is less than 0.3, eliminate (A). (C) and (E) are relatively easy to compare: 0.03 is less than 0.3, and $\sqrt{0.03}$ is less than $\sqrt{0.3}$ because there is a smaller number under the radical sign of $\sqrt{0.03}$ than under the radical sign of $\sqrt{0.3}$. We can eliminate (E). Now (D) can be compared with (B) if the value of (B) is found: $(0.3)^2 = 0.3 \times 0.3 = 0.09$, so 0.03 is less than $(0.3)^2 = 0.09$. Eliminate (B). We're down to just (C) and (D). Now (D), 0.03, can be compared to (C), $\sqrt{0.03}$, if you know about the properties of numbers between 0 and 1. The number 0.03 is less than $\sqrt{0.03}$ because a positive number between 0 and 1 is less than the positive square root of that number. (For example, $\frac{1}{4}$ is less than $\sqrt{\frac{1}{4}} = \frac{1}{2}$.) Eliminate (C). Now that all four incorrect choices have been eliminated, we know that (D) must be correct.

30. A

In this solution, the positions of the minute hand and the hour hand at different times will be described in terms of the number of degrees they have moved clockwise away from a vertical line drawn from the center of the clock to the 12 on top. At 4:00, the minute hand points to the 12 on top whereas the hour hand points to the 4. The hour hand is $\frac{4}{12}$ of 360°, or $\frac{1}{3}(360) = 120°$ clockwise from the vertical line described. Now let's see where the minute and hour hands wind up after 50 minutes. In 1 hour (60 minutes), the minute hand will move 360°, and 50 minutes is $\frac{50}{60}$ of an hour, which is $\frac{5}{6}$ of an hour. Therefore, in 50 minutes, the minute hand will move $\frac{5}{6}$ of 360°, which is 300°. At 4:50, the minute hand has moved clockwise 300° from the vertical line described. In 1 hour, the hour hand moves clockwise from one number on the clock to the next number. There are 12 numbers on the clock, so in 1 hour, the hour hand moves $\frac{1}{12}$ of 360°, which is 30°. We have seen that 50 minutes is $\frac{5}{6}$ of an hour, so in 50 minutes, the hour hand will have moved clockwise $\frac{5}{6}$ of 30°, or 25°. At 4:00, the hour hand, which was pointing at the 4, was 120° clockwise away from the vertical line described; therefore at 4:50, the hour hand will be 120 + 25, or 145° clockwise away from the vertical line described. The minute hand is 300° away from this vertical line, so the minute hand and the hour hand form an angle of measure 300 − 145, or 155°. Because this 155° angle is less than 180°, we have found the smaller of the two angles formed by the hour and minute hand, and (A) is correct.

31. D

Because you're dividing 10.5 by a positive number less than 1, the result must be greater than 10.5, so you can eliminate (A), (B), and (E). Using a little estimation, 10.5 is about 10 and 0.35 is about $\frac{1}{3}$, so $10.5 \div 0.35$ is approximately $10 \div \frac{1}{3}$, which equals $10 \times \frac{3}{1}$, or 30. Choice (C), 300, is much too large, so eliminate (C). Now that all four incorrect choices have been eliminated, we know that (D) must be correct. Note that our approximation, $10 \div \frac{1}{3}$, of $10.5 \div 0.35$, happened to be the exact value of $10.5 \div 0.35$, but this was just a coincidence.

You could also actually do the division in $10.5 \div 0.35$. Multiply both numbers by a power with a base of 10 to get rid of all the decimal points. Because 10.5 has one digit to the right of the decimal point whereas 0.35 has two digits to the right of the decimal point, multiply both numbers by 10^2, or 100.

Then, $10.5 \div 0.35 = (10.5 \times 100) \div (0.35 \times 100) = 1{,}050 \div 35 = 30$.

32. C

There is only one correct setting. To find the number of possible settings that will not open the lock, find the total number of possible settings and subtract 1 from that number. In the section furthest to the left, any integer from 1 through 5 can be placed. Similarly, in the middle and right sections, any integer from 1 through 5 can be placed in each section. Therefore, the total number of settings is $5 \times 5 \times 5 = 25 \times 5 = 125$, and the number of settings that will not work is 125 − 1, or 124.

33. C

Let R be her normal hourly rate, in dollars per hour. The pay is in two types. The first 48 – 8 or 40 hours are at the normal rate of R dollars per hour. The final 8 hours are paid at a rate of $1\frac{1}{2}$R dollars per hour. In the first 40 hours, she earns R × 40, or 40R dollars. In the final 8 hours, she earns $1\frac{1}{2}R \times 8$, or 12R dollars. Altogether she earns 40R + 12R or 52R dollars. She earned 286 dollars, so 52R = 286 and $R = \frac{286}{52} = 5\frac{26}{52} = 5\frac{1}{2} = 5.50$. (C) is correct.

34. C

First, convert 33 feet and 4 inches to feet. There are 12 inches in a foot, so in 1 inch there is $\frac{1}{12}$ of a foot and in 4 inches there is $4 \times \frac{1}{12} = \frac{1}{3}$ of a foot. Therefore, 33 feet and 4 inches is 33 feet and $\frac{1}{3}$ of a foot, which is $33\frac{1}{3}$ feet. To find the cost in dollars per foot of a $99 fence that is $33\frac{1}{3}$ feet long, divide $99 by $33\frac{1}{3}$ feet. It is easier to divide 99 by the simplest improper fraction equal to $33\frac{1}{3}$, so first convert $33\frac{1}{3}$ to that improper fraction. $33\frac{1}{3} = \frac{3 \times 33 + 1}{3} = \frac{99 + 1}{3} = \frac{100}{3}$. Finally, the cost in dollars per foot is

$$\frac{99}{\left(\frac{100}{3}\right)} = 99 \times \frac{3}{100} = \frac{297}{100} = 2.97.$$ (C) is correct.

35. D

To find out how many ounces there are in $3\frac{1}{5}$ grams, first find the number of ounces that there are in 1 gram and then multiply this number by $3\frac{1}{5}$. Because 1 ounce = 28 grams, dividing both sides by 28 gives $\frac{1}{28}$ ounce = 1 gram (i.e., in 1 gram there is $\frac{1}{28}$ of an ounce, in $3\frac{1}{5}$ grams there is $3\frac{1}{5} \times \frac{1}{28}$ of an ounce). All that remains to be done is work out the value of $3\frac{1}{5} \times \frac{1}{28}$. First, convert $3\frac{1}{5}$ to an improper fraction. $3\frac{1}{5} = \frac{3 \times 5 + 1}{5} = \frac{15 + 1}{5} = \frac{16}{5}$. Then, $3\frac{1}{5} \times \frac{1}{28} = \frac{16}{5} \times \frac{1}{28} = \frac{4}{5} \times \frac{1}{7} = \frac{4}{35}$. Therefore, there is $\frac{4}{35}$ of an ounce in $3\frac{1}{5}$ grams, and (D) is correct.

It is often helpful to check and see if the answer you got looks reasonable, and our answer of $\frac{4}{35}$ here certainly does look reasonable. Notice that if 1 ounce = 28 grams, then $3\frac{1}{5}$ grams, which is much less than 28 grams, must be less than 1 ounce and our answer does look reasonable. Notice that (B), (C), and (E), which are all greater than 1, can be eliminated just from knowing that $3\frac{1}{5}$ grams must be less than 1 ounce.

36. E

Solve the equation $\frac{63}{3x} = 4\frac{2}{7}$ for x.

	$\frac{63}{3x} = 4\frac{2}{7}$
Cancel a factor of 3 from the 63 and the 3 on the left:	$\frac{21}{x} = 4\frac{2}{7}$
Convert $4\frac{2}{7}$ on the right to an improper fraction:	$\frac{21}{x} = \frac{4 \times 7 + 2}{7}$
	$\frac{21}{x} = \frac{30}{7}$
Cross multiply:	$21(7) = (x)(30)$
Multiply each side:	$147 = 30x$
Divide both sides by 30:	$\frac{147}{30} = x$
Cancel a factor of 3 from the 147 and the 30:	$\frac{49}{10} = x$
Convert $\frac{49}{10}$ to a decimal:	$4.9 = x$

37. A

This is a good question to solve by picking numbers. Always pick numbers that are easy to work with. Let the empty bottle weigh 10 units. This weight of 10 is $\frac{1}{10}$ of the weight of the bottle when it is full, so when the bottle is full the weight of the bottle is 100 units. This weight of 100 is the sum of the weight of 10 of the empty bottle and the weight of the contents that fill the bottle. So the weight of the contents that fill the bottle is 100 – 10, or 90 units.

If the bottle is filled so that it weighs $\frac{1}{2}$ of its full weight, the bottle is filled so that it weighs $\frac{1}{2}$ of 100, or 50. To find the actual weight of the amount put in the bottle, subtract the weight 10 of the empty bottle from the weight 50 of the partially filled bottle, and the weight of the amount in the partially filled bottle is 50 – 10, or 40. The weight of the contents in a completely filled bottle is 90, and the weight of the contents in this partially filled bottle is 40. Therefore, the fraction of the bottle that is filled is $\frac{40}{90}$, which is equal to $\frac{4}{9}$. (A) is correct.

38. E

It's important that we understand what the question requires. We have to determine what percent 0.4x is of y. Let's begin with an easier question. What fraction of y is 0.4x? Well, $\frac{0.4x}{y}$ is the fraction of y that 0.4x is. To find the percent that 0.4x is of y, convert $\frac{0.4x}{y}$ to a percent. Let's use the equations to find the value of the fraction $\frac{0.4x}{y}$, and then we'll convert this fraction to a percent.

There are two equations with the three variables x, y, and z. Because we are trying to find the value of the expression $\frac{0.4x}{y}$ (and then convert this to a percent), let's try to manipulate the equations to get a new equation which does not contain the variable z. Let's solve the first equation, $x - y = 0.2z$, for z. All we must do to solve the first equation, $x - y = 0.2z$, for z is divide both sides of this equation by 0.2, and then $\frac{x-y}{0.2} = z$. Now $0.2 = \frac{1}{5}$, so $\frac{x-y}{\left(\frac{1}{5}\right)} = z$, $(x - y) \times \frac{5}{1} = z$, and $z = 5(x - y)$. Now substitute $5(x - y)$ for z into the other equation, $x + z = 1.6y$, and then $x + 5(x - y) = 1.6y$. We would like to solve this equation for the value of $\frac{0.4x}{y}$ and then convert this to a percent. Let's first try to solve this equation for the value of $\frac{x}{y}$. If we can do this, then we can find the value of $\frac{0.4x}{y}$, and finally we can convert this to a percent.

$$x + 5(x - y) = 1.6y$$
$$x + 5x - 5y = 1.6y$$
$$6x - 5y = 1.6y$$
$$6x = 6.6y$$
$$\frac{6x}{y} = 6.6$$
$$\frac{x}{y} = \frac{6.6}{6}$$
$$\frac{x}{y} = 1.1$$

Because $\frac{x}{y} = 1.1$, $\frac{0.4x}{y} = 0.4\left(\frac{x}{y}\right) = 0.4(1.1) = 0.44$. All we must do is convert 0.44 to a percent. $0.44 = \frac{44}{100} = 44\%$. (E) is correct.

39. C

Solve the equation $\frac{3y + 14 - y}{2y + 1} = 2$ for the value of y.

	$\frac{3y + 14 - y}{2y + 1} = 2$
Combine the y-terms in the numerator of the left side:	$\frac{2y + 14}{2y + 1} = 2$
Multiply both sides by 2y + 1:	$2y + 14 = 2(2y + 1)$
Multiply out the right side:	$2y + 14 = 4y + 2$
Subtract 2y from both sides:	$14 = 2y + 2$
Subtract 2 from both sides:	$12 = 2y$
Divide both sides by 2:	$\frac{12}{2} = y$
	$6 = y$

40. A

There are 16 ounces in a pound, so in an ounce there is $\frac{1}{16}$ of a pound. The 39-ounce box weighs $39\left(\frac{1}{16}\right)$ pounds. This larger box costs 91¢, so the cost per pound of this 39-ounce box is $\frac{91}{39\left(\frac{1}{16}\right)}$, or $\frac{91}{39} \times 16$¢ per pound. The 18-ounce box weighs $18\left(\frac{1}{16}\right)$ pounds. The cost per pound of the smaller 18-ounce box is $\frac{48}{18\left(\frac{1}{16}\right)}$, or $\frac{48}{18} \times 16$¢ per pound. The ratio of the cost per pound of the larger box to the cost per pound of the smaller box is $\frac{\left(\frac{91}{39} \times 16\right)}{\left(\frac{48}{18} \times 16\right)}$. Now find the value of $\frac{\left(\frac{91}{39} \times 16\right)}{\left(\frac{48}{18} \times 16\right)}$.

$$\frac{\left(\frac{91}{39} \times 16\right)}{\left(\frac{48}{18} \times 16\right)}$$

Divide the numerator and the denominator of this fraction by 16: $= \frac{\left(\frac{91}{39}\right)}{\left(\frac{48}{18}\right)}$

To divide by a fraction, invert that fraction and multiply: $= \frac{91}{39} \times \frac{18}{48}$

Divide the numerator and denominator of $\frac{91}{39}$ by 13 and the numerator and denominator of $\frac{18}{48}$ by 6: $= \frac{7}{3} \times \frac{3}{8}$

Cancel a factor of 3 from the denominator of $\frac{7}{3}$ and the numerator of $\frac{3}{8}$: $= \frac{7}{8}$

The ratio is $\frac{7}{8}$. The decimal equivalent of $\frac{7}{8}$ is 0.875. The ratio is 0.875:1.

41. C

The phrase "is to" appearing in this question is related to the meaning of the word ratio. For example, the phrase "4 is to 17" means the ratio of 4 to 17. The sentence "3 is to 12 as 7 is to 28" says (correctly) that the ratio of 3 to 12 is equal to the ratio of 7 to 28.

Run through the answer choices until you find the correct one that works.

(A): The ratio of 16 to 8 is $\frac{16}{8}$, or 2. The ratio of $\frac{x}{6}$ to $\frac{x}{3}$ is $\frac{\left(\frac{x}{6}\right)}{\left(\frac{x}{3}\right)} = \frac{x}{6} \times \frac{3}{x} = \frac{1}{2}$. The ratios are not the same, so (A) is not correct.

(B): The ratio of 4 to 8 is $\frac{4}{8}$, or $\frac{1}{2}$. The ratio of $\frac{x}{6}$ to $\frac{x}{12}$ is $\frac{\left(\frac{x}{6}\right)}{\left(\frac{x}{12}\right)} = \frac{x}{6} \times \frac{12}{x} = \frac{12}{6} = 2$. The ratios are not the same, so (B) is not correct.

(C): The ratio of 12 to 8 is $\frac{12}{8}$, or $\frac{3}{2}$. The ratio of $\frac{x}{6}$ to $\frac{x}{9}$ is $\frac{\left(\frac{x}{6}\right)}{\left(\frac{x}{9}\right)} = \frac{x}{6} \times \frac{9}{x} = \frac{9}{6} = \frac{3}{2}$. The ratio of 12 to 8 is equal to the ratio of $\frac{x}{6}$ to $\frac{x}{9}$, and (C) is correct.

42. D

This is a good question to solve by picking a number. Always pick numbers that are easy to work with. In percent questions, it is often good to pick 100, and this is the case with this question. It does not matter if the numbers you pick are not what you would expect from everyday life. What matters is that the numbers you pick are easy to work with and consistent with everything the question says. Let the list price of the car be \$100. The dealer bought the car at 75% of the list price, so he bought the car for 75% of \$100, which is \$75. The dealer sold the car for 93% of \$100, which is \$93. His profit was \$93 – 75, or \$18. The percent profit is the percent that the profit is of the amount the dealer spent to buy the car, so the percent profit is the percent that 18 is of 75. Expressed as a fraction, we have $\frac{18}{75}$, and we just have to convert this fraction to a percent: $\frac{18}{75} = \frac{18}{75} \times 100\% = \frac{6}{25} \times 100\% = 6 \times 4\% = 24\%$.

43. D

This question can be solved by picking a number for the original volume of the container or letting a variable represent the original volume. Let's solve this question by letting the original volume be represented by the variable x. From 11:30 AM to 2:00 PM of the same day there are $2\frac{1}{2}$ hours. The number of half-hours in $2\frac{1}{2}$ hours is $2\frac{1}{2} \times 2$, or 5.

From 11:30 AM to 12 noon,
the volume doubles from x to 2x.

From 12 noon to 12:30 PM,
the volume doubles from 2x to 4x.

From 12:30 PM to 1:00 PM,
the volume doubles from 4x to 8x.

From 1:00 PM to 1:30 PM,
the volume doubles from 8x to 16x.

From 1:30 p.m. to 2:00 p.m.,
the volume doubles from 16x to 32x.

So the volume increased from
x at 11:30 AM to 32x at 2:00 PM.

In general, the percent increase is equal to

$$\frac{\text{Amount of increase}}{\text{Original amount}} \times 100\%.$$

Here, the percent increase is $\frac{32x - x}{x} \times 100\% = \frac{31x}{x} \times 100\% = \frac{31}{1} \times 100\% = 31 \times 100\% = 3{,}100\%$.

44. C

Call the number of teachers N. Because the ratio of teachers to students is 1:8, or 1 to 8, the number of students is 8N. The number of teachers increased by 10%. The fractional equivalent of 10% is 0.1, so this year the number of teachers is N + 0.1N = 1.1N. The number of students also increased by 10%, so the new number of students is 8N + 0.1(8N) = 8N + 0.8N = 8.8N. The ratio of the teachers to students this year is the ratio 1.1N to 8.8N, which in fractional form is $\frac{1.1N}{8.8N}$. Simplify this fraction. $\frac{1.1N}{8.8N} = \frac{1.1}{8.8} = \frac{11}{88} = \frac{1}{8}$. The ratio this year is $\frac{1}{8}$, which is a ratio of 1:8, or 1 to 8.

45. D

Rearrange $\sqrt{0.4761}$ using the law of radicals, which says that $\sqrt{\frac{a}{b}} = \sqrt{\frac{a}{\sqrt{b}}}$.

$$\sqrt{0.4761} = \sqrt{\frac{4{,}761}{10{,}000}} = \frac{\sqrt{4{,}761}}{\sqrt{10{,}000}} = \frac{\sqrt{4{,}761}}{100}$$

Now use a little guesswork to find what $\sqrt{4{,}761}$ is equal to. The number 4,761 under the radical sign is, for our purposes here, relatively close to 4,900, which is 70^2, so $\sqrt{4{,}900} = 70$ and $\sqrt{4{,}761}$ is close to and a little bit less than $\sqrt{4{,}900}$, which is 70. If we test 69 by squaring it to see if we get 4,761, we find that $69^2 = 69 \times 69 = 4{,}761$, so it works, and $\sqrt{4{,}761} = 69$. Getting back to our work with $\sqrt{0.4761}$, we then find that

$$\sqrt{0.4761} = \frac{\sqrt{4{,}761}}{100} = \frac{69}{100} = 0.69$$

46. A

This question can be solved by picking a value for one of the variables in the equations $\frac{8a}{9} = \frac{2b}{3}$ and $0.5b = \frac{4c}{5}$, finding the values of all variables, and then finding out how many a's will equal 24 c's. Because a and c are the variables of interest, let's pick a value for one of these variables that is easy to work with. Because c is in the equation $0.5b = \frac{4c}{5}$, let's let $c = 5$ so that the 5 in the denominator of the fraction on the right can cancel with the 5 in the numerator of that fraction when c is replaced with 5.

Plug 5 for c into the equation $0.5b = \frac{4c}{5}$ and find the value of b that results. $0.5b = \frac{4(5)}{5}$, $\frac{1}{2}b = 4$, and $b = 8$. Now substitute 8 for b into the equation $\frac{8a}{9} = \frac{2b}{3}$ and find the corresponding value of a. Therefore $\frac{8a}{9} = \frac{2b}{3}$, $\frac{8a}{9} = \frac{2(8)}{3}$, and dividing both sides of this last equation by 8 gives $\frac{a}{9} = \frac{2}{3}$, so $a = \frac{2}{3}$, $9 = 2 \times 3 = 6$, and thus $a = 6$ and $c = 5$. We want to know how many a's equal 24 c's. Well, 24 c's is 24(5), or 120. We want to figure out how many a's equal 120, where $a = 6$; i.e., we want to figure out what number multiplied by 6 equals 120. That number is 120 divided by 6, which is 20. So 20 a's equal 24 c's. (A), or 20, is correct.

47. B

Call the number of patients the dentist saw in August N. In September, he saw $\frac{1}{3}$ more patients than he did in August, so in September he saw $N + \frac{1}{3}N = 1\frac{1}{3}N$ patients. Because the increase from September to October will require multiplying $1\frac{1}{3}N$ by another fraction, it is more convenient to work with $\frac{4}{3}N$ rather than $1\frac{1}{3}N$, and so the number of patients he saw in September was $\frac{4}{3}N$. In October, he saw $\frac{1}{5}$ more patients than he did in September, so the number of patients he saw in October was

$$\left(\frac{4}{3}N\right) + \frac{1}{5}\left(\frac{4}{3}N\right) = \left(\frac{4}{3}N\right)\left(1 + \frac{1}{5}\right) = \frac{4}{3}N\left(\frac{6}{5}\right) = \frac{24}{15}N = \frac{8}{5}N.$$

The number of patients he saw in October was $\frac{8}{5}N$, and the question tells us that he saw 240 patients in October. Therefore, $\frac{8}{5}N = 240$, $8N = 240(5)$, and $N = \frac{240(5)}{8} = 30(5) = 150$. He saw 150 patients in August, and (B) is correct.

This answer can be checked in not a lot of time. Suppose that he saw 150 patients in August. In September he saw $\frac{1}{3}$ patients more than the 150 he saw in August, so in September he saw $150 + \frac{1}{3}(150) = 150 + 50 = 200$ patients. In October, he saw $\frac{1}{5}$ patients more than the 200 he saw in September, so in October he saw $200 + \frac{1}{5}(200) = 200 + 40 = 240$ patients. Now 240 is the right number of patients seen in October, so we know that 150 is the correct number of patients seen in August, and we have now checked that (B) is indeed correct.

48. C

Let's use the variable x in place of the question mark (and the parentheses that contain it). Then we want to find x where 90% of $40 = \frac{5}{6}$ of x. The fractional equivalent of 90% is $\frac{9}{10}$, and the word *of* means "times," so $\frac{9}{10}(40) = \frac{5}{6}x$. Solve this equation for x.

$$\frac{9}{10}(40) = \frac{5}{6}x$$

$$9(4) = \frac{5}{6}x$$

$$36 = \frac{5}{6}x$$

$$36(6) = 5x$$

$$216 = 5x$$

$$x = \frac{216}{5} = 43.2$$

49. D

Translate the information in the question stem into math. Let R be the number of toys that Rebecca has and let J be the number of toys that Jennifer has. The first sentence says that Rebecca has twice as many toys as Jennifer does. This means that $R = 2J$. The second sentence says that if Jennifer gives Rebecca four of her toys, Jennifer will have one-fourth the number of toys that Rebecca has. We're letting J be the number of toys that Jennifer has and we're letting R be the number of toys that Rebecca has. If Jennifer gives Rebecca four toys, then Jennifer will have four fewer toys, or $J - 4$ toys, whereas Rebecca will have four more toys, or $R + 4$ toys, so $J - 4 = \frac{1}{4}(R + 4)$. Now we have the two equations $R = 2J$ and $J - 4 = \frac{1}{4}(R + 4)$, which we can solve for the value of R. There are various ways these two equations can be solved. To solve for R directly, let's solve the equation $R = 2J$ for J in terms of R, and then plug the value of J, which is in terms of R, into the equation $J - 4 = \frac{1}{4}(R + 4)$. Dividing both sides of the equation $R = 2J$ by 2 gives $J = \frac{R}{2}$. Now plug $\frac{R}{2}$ for J into the equation $J - 4 = \frac{1}{4}(R + 4)$, and we get the equation $\frac{R}{2} - 4 = \frac{1}{4}(R + 4)$. Solve this equation for the value of R.

$$\frac{R}{2} - 4 = \frac{1}{4}(R + 4)$$

Multiply both sides by 4 to get rid of both denominators: $4\left(\frac{R}{2} - 4\right) = 4\left[\frac{1}{4}(R + 4)\right]$

Multiply out each side: $2R - 16 = R + 4$

Subtract R from both sides: $R - 16 = 4$

Add 20 to each side: $R = 20$

Therefore, Rebecca has 20 toys, and (D) is correct.

50. E

Substitute the values of a, b, and c into the expression $(b \times a) + \frac{1}{c}$. The question stem gives us the values of c and a. We'll have to do just a little work to find the value of b. Because $\frac{1}{b} = 4$, $1 = 4b$, and $b = \frac{1}{4}$. You could also have found the value of b if you realized that $\frac{1}{b} = 4$ says that the reciprocal of b is 4, so b must be $\frac{1}{4}$. Now substitute 10 for a, $\frac{1}{4}$ for b, and $\frac{2}{5}$ for c into the expression $(b \times a) + \frac{1}{c}$, and then

$$(b \times a) + \frac{1}{c} = \left(\frac{1}{4} \times 10\right) + \frac{1}{\left(\frac{2}{5}\right)} = \frac{5}{2} + \frac{5}{2} = \frac{10}{2} = 5.$$

Compute Your Score

Raw Score	Survey of Natural Sciences: Biology 1–40	General Chemistry 41–70	Organic Chemistry 71–100	Physics	Reading Comprehension	Quantitative Reasoning
50	–	–	–	–	–	400
49	–	–	–	–	400	–
48	–	–	–	–	–	400
47	–	–	–	–	390	–
46	–	–	–	–	390	–
45	–	–	–	–	–	400
44	–	–	–	–	380	–
43	–	–	–	–	380	400
42	–	–	–	–	–	–
41	–	–	–	–	370	–
40	400	–	–	400	360	390
39	400	–	–	–	350	–
38	400	–	–	400	–	370
37	400	–	–	–	350	–
36	400	–	–	400	340	–
35	390	–	–	–	–	360
34	380	–	–	380	340	–
33	380	–	–	–	330	350
32	360	–	–	360	–	–
31	360	–	–	–	320	–
30	350	400	400	350	310	340
29	340	390	400	–	300	–
28	340	380	400	330	–	330
27	330	370	400	–	290	–
26	320	360	390	320	280	–
25	320	350	380	–	–	310
24	310	340	370	310	270	–
23	310	340	360	–	260	300
22	300	330	350	300	–	–
21	290	320	350	–	250	–
20	290	320	340	280	240	290
19	280	310	330	–	230	–
18	270	310	330	270	–	280
17	270	300	320	–	220	–
16	260	300	320	260	220	–
15	260	290	310	–	–	260
14	260	280	300	240	210	–
13	250	280	300	–	210	230
12	240	270	290	220	–	–
11	230	260	280	–	210	–
10	220	260	270	200	210	220
9	210	250	260	–	200	–
8	210	240	250	200	–	200
7	200	230	240	–	200	–
6	200	220	230	200	200	–
5	200	210	220	–	–	200
4	200	200	210	200	200	–
3	200	200	200	–	200	200
2	200	200	200	200	–	–
1	200	200	200	–	200	–
0	200	200	200	200	200	200

Total Score

Raw Score (RS)	Scaled Score (SS)	Raw Score (RS)	Scaled Score (SS)	Raw Score (RS)	Scaled Score (SS)
240	400	150	320	60	200
238	400	148	320	58	200
236	400	146	310	56	200
234	400	144	310	54	200
232	400	142	310	52	200
230	400	140	310	50	200
228	400	138	300	48	200
226	400	136	300	46	200
224	400	134	300	44	200
222	400	132	300	42	200
220	400	130	290	40	200
218	400	128	290	38	200
216	400	126	290	36	200
214	400	124	290	34	200
212	400	122	290	32	200
210	400	120	280	30	200
208	390	118	280	28	200
206	390	116	280	26	200
204	380	114	270	24	200
202	380	112	270	22	200
200	380	110	270	20	200
198	380	108	270	18	200
196	380	106	260	16	200
194	370	104	260	14	200
192	370	102	260	12	200
190	370	100	260	10	200
188	360	98	260	8	200
186	360	96	250	6	200
184	360	94	250	4	200
182	360	92	250	2	200
180	350	90	240	0	200
178	350	88	240		
176	350	86	240		
174	350	84	230		
172	350	82	230		
170	350	80	220		
168	340	78	220		
166	340	76	220		
164	330	74	220		
162	330	72	210		
160	330	70	210		
158	330	68	200		
156	330	66	200		
154	320	64	200		
152	320	62	200		